D1689182

OXFORD MEDICAL PUBLICATIONS

Audiology and audiological medicine

Volume 2

Audiology and audiological medicine

Volume 2

Edited by

H. A. BEAGLEY

Consultant Otologist and Consultant in Charge of the Department of Electrophysiology, The Royal National Throat, Nose and Ear Hospital, London
Honorary Lecturer in the Institute of Laryngology and Otology, University of London
Honorary Lecturer, Imperial College, London

OXFORD
OXFORD UNIVERSITY PRESS
NEW YORK   TORONTO
1981

Oxford University Press, Walton Street, Oxford OX2 6DP
London   Glasgow   New York   Toronto
Delhi   Bombay   Calcutta   Madras   Karachi
Kuala Lumpur   Singapore   Hong Kong   Tokyo
Nairobi   Dar es Salaam   Cape Town
Melbourne   Wellington

and associate companies in
Beirut   Berlin   Ibadan   Mexico City

© The several contributors listed on pages xi–xv, 1981

All rights reserved. No part of this publication may be reproduced, stored in a retrieval system, or transmitted, in any form or by any means, electronic, mechanical, photocopying, recording, or otherwise, without the prior permission of Oxford University Press

This book is sold subject to the condition that it shall not, by way of trade or otherwise, be lent, re-sold, hired or otherwise circulated without the publisher's prior consent in any form of binding or cover other than that in which it is published and without a similar condition including this condition being imposed on the subsequent purchaser

British Library Cataloguing in Publication Data
Audiology and audiological medicine.
  – (Oxford medical publications).
  1. Hearing disorders
  2. Audiology
  I. Beagley, H A
  617.8'9   RF290   80–41814
  ISBN 0–19–261154–2

Set by Western Printing Services Ltd, Bristol
Printed in Great Britain by the Thetford Press, Norfolk.

Preface

This volume has been compiled with medical people interested in audiology primarily in view. Audiology is increasingly significant in medicine and surgery and indeed audiological medicine has recently been recognized as a medical specialty in the UK, as it is in many European countries.

The subject matter covers all clinical aspects of medical audiology. Considerable emphasis has also been placed on certain subjects where the scientific substrate is somewhat advanced with respect to routine clinical practice, but which will become steadily of greater importance. For this reason subjects such as ultrastructure of the inner ear and its innervation as well as the pathophysiology of the Eustachean tube have been treated in some detail. Other subjects treated extensively are forensic audiology and industrial audiology, noise control, and compensation, as well as psychological and psychiatric aspects of hearing loss and paedoaudiology.

Inevitably some basic subjects are dealt with in a more introductory manner. A case in point is the chapter on the psychophysics of hearing. This information is basic to many aspects of audiology and has been presented accordingly. But psychophysics is a major scientific study in its own right and those who would like to pursue this subject further are referred to the standard texts which deal with it. Similarly, no attention has been paid to the vestibular labyrinth and its disorders as this is generally considered to be a separate, if related, subject, albeit one of considerable importance.

While the uses, advantages, disadvantages, and implications of various audiological procedures have been treated in the same depth, little space has been allotted to describing, step by step, the mechanics of carrying out such tests and the book cannot be regarded as being simply a technical manual. Instead the philosophy and the rationale behind the procedures and their clinical implications are dealt with predominantly. On the other hand in the case of some of the newer procedures such as electrophysiological tests of hearing a certain amount of practical advice has been included which may prove helpful to some readers.

It is a matter of deep regret that Professor Ingelstedt died between the time that his manuscript was received and its publication in this book. Those who knew Professor Ingelstedt are aware of his significant contributions to the important matter of Eustachean tube function and his comprehensive treatment of this subject in Chapter 29 is a fitting memorial.

London HAB
March 1981

Contents

List of contributors   xi

VOLUME 1
SECTION 1   BASIC SCIENCES
1. Clinical anatomy of the auditory part of the human ear   3
   T. NICOL AND K. K. CHAO-CHARIA
2. Structure of the cochlear duct   50
   C. A. SMITH
3. Neuroanatomy of the cochlea   72
   H. SPOENDLIN
4. Physiology of the ear   103
   A. R. D. THORNTON
5. Psychophysics of hearing pertaining to clinical audiology   117
   L. L. ELLIOTT
6. Acoustics in audiology   133
   J. J. KNIGHT
7. Acoustics of normal and pathological ears   145
   J. J. ZWISLOCKI

SECTION 2   INSTRUMENTATION
8. Audiometers   161
   M. C. MARTIN
9. Instrumentation for electric response audiometry   186
   A. R. D. THORNTON
10. Hearing aids   200
    M. C. MARTIN
11. Acoustic impedance bridges   228
    J. J. KNIGHT

SECTION 3   PATHOLOGY OF DEAFNESS
12. Pathology of the ear   245
    L. MICHAELS AND M. WELLS
13. Genetically determined hearing defects   302
    G. R. FRASER

SECTION 4   ADULT AUDIOLOGY
14. Clinical tests of auditory function in the adult and the school-child   319
    R. HINCHCLIFFE
15. Clinical audiometry   365
    S. D. G. STEPHENS
16. Speech audiometry   391
    J. D. HOOD
17. Diagnosis of acoustic neuroma   415
    W. P. R. GIBSON

viii *Contents*

18. The role of drugs in audiological medicine — 441
    R. HINCHCLIFFE
19. Surgical management of deafness in adults: the external and middle ear — 482
    J. B. BOOTH
20. Surgical management of deafness in adults: the inner ear — 506
    A. W. MORRISON
21. Auditory rehabilitation — 516
    S. D. G. STEPHENS
22. Cochlear implants: pathophysiological considerations — 541
    J. TONNDORF
23. Drug ototoxicity — 573
    G. J. MATZ AND S. A. LERNER

VOLUME 2

SECTION 5 PAEDO-AUDIOLOGY
24. Syndromes associated with hearing loss — 595
    L. FISCH
25. Diagnosis of hearing loss in infants and young children — 640
    M. V. BICKERTON AND H. A. BEAGLEY
26. Education of the hearing-handicapped child — 663
    H. KERNOHAN, G. LUCAS, AND V. MUTER
27. Non-organic hearing loss in children — 685
    H. A. BEAGLEY
28. Surgical treatment of conductive deafness in children — 694
    N. SHAH

SECTION 6 ACOUSTIC IMPEDANCE AND TUBAL FUNCTION
29. Clinical use of acoustic impedance testing in audiological diagnosis — 707
    J. JERGER AND D. HAYES
30. Physiology and pathophysiology of the middle ear—Eustachian tube system — 723
    S. INGELSTEDT

SECTION 7 ELECTROPHYSIOLOGICAL TESTS OF HEARING
31. Bio-electric potentials available for electric response audiometry: indications and contra-indications — 755
    H. A. BEAGLEY AND L. FISCH
32. Auditory myogenic responses — 769
    E. DOUEK
33. Electrophysiological tests of hearing — 781
    H. A. BEAGLEY
34. Sedation and anaesthesia in audiological medicine — 809
    J. N. T. HUTTON
35. Radiology in audiological diagnosis — 816
    P. D. PHELPS

SECTION 8 FORENSIC AND PSYCHOLOGICAL ASPECTS OF AUDIOLOGY

36. Hearing conservation programmes — 829
    M. E. BRYAN AND W. TEMPEST
37. Industrial hearing loss: compensation in the United Kingdom — 846
    W. TEMPEST AND M. E. BRYAN
38. Compensation for industrial hearing loss: the practice in the United States — 861
    A. GLORIG
39. Compensation for industrial hearing loss: the practice in Canada — 880
    P. W. ALBERTI
40. Compensation for industrial hearing loss: the practice in Australia — 896
    J. MACRAE AND R. A. PIESSE
41. Non-organic hearing loss in adults — 910
    P. W. ALBERTI
42. Forensic audiology — 932
    R. HINCHCLIFFE
43. Some psychosocial aspects of deafness — 961
    J. C. DENMARK
44. Tinnitus — 974
    P. D. JACKSON

Index — 995

Contributors

P. W. ALBERTI
Department of Otolaryngology,
University of Toronto,
Toronto, Canada

H. A. BEAGLEY
The Royal National Throat, Nose and Ear Hospital,
London

M. V. BICKERTON
Royal National Throat, Nose and Ear Hospital,
London

J. B. BOOTH
The London Hospital,
Whitechapel,
London

M. E. BRYAN
Audiology Group,
University of Salford,
Salford

K. K. CHAO-CHARIA
Institute of Laryngology and Otology,
University of London

J. C. DENMARK
Whittingham Hospital,
Whittingham,
Preston

E. DOUEK
Hearing Research Group,
Guy's Hospital,
London

L. L. ELLIOTT
Northwestern University,
Evanston,
Illinois, U.S.A.

L. FISCH
Institute of Laryngology and Otology,
London

G. R. FRASER
Lister Hill National Center for Biomedical Communications,
National Library of Medicine,
Bethesda, U.S.A.

W. P. R. GIBSON
Royal National Throat, Nose and Ear Hospital
and Hospital for Nervous Diseases (Queen Square),
London

A. GLORIG
Otologic Medical Group Inc.,
Los Angeles, U.S.A.

D. HAYES
Baylor College of Medicine,
Houston, U.S.A.

R. HINCHCLIFFE
Institute of Laryngology and Otology,
University of London

J. D. HOOD
Medical Research Council Hearing and Balance Unit,
National Hospital for nervous diseases,
London

J. N. T. HUTTON
Department of Anaesthetics,
Royal National Throat, Nose and Ear Hospital,
London

S. INGELSTEDT ✠
ENT Department,
Malmö General Hospital,
Sweden

P. D. JACKSON
Institute of Laryngology and Otology,
University of London

J. JERGER
Baylor College of Medicine,
Houston, U.S.A.

H. KERNOHAN
Wall Hall College of Further Education,
Radlett, Hertfordshire

J. J. KNIGHT
Institute of Laryngology and Otology,
University of London

S. A. LERNER
Department of Medicine,
University of Chicago,
U.S.A.

G. LUCAS
Nuffield Hearing and Speech Centre,
Royal National Throat, Nose and Ear Hospital,
London

J. A. MACRAE
National Acoustic Laboratories,
Australian Department of Health,
Sydney, Australia

M. C. MARTIN
Scientific and Technical Department,
The Royal National Institute for the Deaf,
London

G. J. MATZ
Department of Surgery,
University of Chicago,
U.S.A.

L. MICHAELS
Department of Pathology,
Institute of Laryngology and Otology,
University of London

A. W. MORRISON
The London Hospital,
Whitechapel, London

V. A. MUTER
Nuffield Hearing and Speech Centre,
Royal National Throat, Nose and Ear Hospital,
London

T. NICOL
Department of Clinical Anatomy,
Institute of Laryngology and Otology,
University of London

P. D. PHELPS
Department of Radiology,
The Royal National Throat, Nose and Ear Hospital
London

R. A. PIESSE
National Acoustic Laboratory,
Australian Department of Health,
Sydney, Australia

N. SHAH
The Royal National Throat, Nose and Ear Hospital,
London

C. A. SMITH
Department of Otolaryngology,
University of Oregon School of Medicine,
Oregon, U.S.A.

H. H. SPOENDLIN
Universitätsklink fur Hals-, Nasen- und Ohrenkrankheiten,
Innsbruck, Austria

S. D. G. STEPHENS
Adult Auditory Rehabilitation Centre,
The Royal National Throat, Nose and Ear Hospital,
London

W. TEMPEST
Audiology Group,
University of Salford, Salford

A. R. D. THORNTON
Medical Research Council Institute of Hearing Research,
Royal South Hants Hospital,
Southampton

J. TONNDORF
Columbia University,
New York, U.S.A.

M. WELLS
Department of Pathology,
Institute of Laryngology and Otology,
University of London

J. J. ZWISLOCKI
Institute for Sensory Research,
Syracuse University,
New York, U.S.A.

Section 5
Paedo-audiology

24 Syndromes associated with hearing loss

L. FISCH

THE IMPORTANCE OF SYNDROMES

The knowledge and recognition of syndromes with hearing impairment as part of the clinical picture is important to all workers in audiological medicine. It helps not only with early detection of hearing loss but also with its diagnosis and prognosis. All children who belong to one of the syndromes should have their hearing tested fully as soon as possible. Children with an already diagnosed hearing impairment who show some signs or symptoms of one of the syndromes, should be investigated fully. A detailed knowledge of these syndromes helps with better understanding of the nature of the hearing loss. The discovery of the connections between the defective hearing system and other disorders can lead to a better understanding of causation of deafness.

CLASSIFICATION

A strictly logical classification is not possible as yet because of many gaps in our knowledge concerning these syndromes. However, as our understanding of the fundamental causes of these disorders increases a more logical structure is emerging. This is reflected in the terminology. For a long time the colloquial term 'mongolism' was the one used for a well-known condition in children because of certain superficial appearances. Later it was named as Down's syndrome, but as a chromosome disorder the more precise or appropriate term is 'trisomy 21'. Similarly 'gargoylism' advanced to Hurler's and Hunter's syndrome and now, as a more detailed knowledge is available concerning the basic disorder, the terms 'mucopolysaccharidosis I' or 'II' etc. indicate more appropriately that a relatively large number of genetically different disorders exists in this group of particular abnormalities of metabolism of the high molecular carbohydrate compounds of the intracellular matrix.

In this chapter the syndromes are grouped as much as possible according to the fundamental disorder of the tissues or systems involved in the abnormality. First of all it is useful to group all the syndromes into non-genetic and genetic ones. The most important non-genetic conditions are the rubella syndrome and athetoid cerebral palsy. The following is a list of genetic syndromes:

Ectodermal dysplasia (anhidrotic type)
Disorders of keratinization
    Twisted hair (pili torti)

- Onychodystrophy
- Keratosis palmaris and plantaris
- Dystrophy of nails

Collagen defects in genetic disorders of connective tissue
- Osteogenesis imperfecta
- Marfan's syndrome

Bone abnormalities
- Osteitis deformans (Paget's disease)
- Leontiasis ossea
- Osteopetrosis (Alberg–Schönberg disease)
- Apert's syndrome
- Crouzon's disease
- Split hand and foot syndrome
- Kniest disease
- Achondroplasia

Mucopolysaccharidosis
- Hurler's syndrome
- Hunter's syndrome
- Marotaux–Lamy syndrome

Branchial arch abnormalities
- Treacher Collins syndrome
- Pierre Robin syndrome

Klippel–Feil syndrome

Moebius syndrome

Myopathies of genetic origin
- Kearn's syndrome
- Myopathy with lactic acidosis
- Muscular dystrophy

Retinal degeneration and ocular anomalies
- Usher's syndrome (retinitis pigmentosa)
- Laurence–Moon–Biedl syndrome
- Cockayne's syndrome
- Refsum's syndrome
- Leber's disease
- Cogan's syndrome
- Vogt–Kayangi syndrome

Kidney abnormalities
- Alport's syndrome
- Renal tubular acidosis
- Urticaria and amyloidosis
- Hyperprolinaemia
- Congenital kidney abnormalities

Thyroid dysfunction
- Pendred's syndrome
- Congenital hypothyroidism

Pigmentation abnormalities
    Waardenburg's syndrome (the 'white forelock syndrome')
    Early greying syndrome
Hirschprung's disease
Neuropathies
    Hereditary sensory radicular neuropathy
    Friedrich's ataxia
    Ataxic neuropathy
Chromosome disorders
    Down's syndrome
    Turner's syndrome (?)
Heart disorder
    Jervell–Lange-Nielsen syndrome
Blood disorder
    Fanconi syndrome

DISORDERS OF ECTODERMAL DERIVATIVES

Remembering the ectodermal origin of the otocyst and, in turn, of the cochlea, it is not surprising to find that hearing defects are present in syndromes in which the basic disorder is an abnormality of ectodermal derivatives. These disorders include ectodermal dysplasias and abnormalities of keratinization.

Ectodermal dysplasia

Cases of hereditary ectodermal dysplasia tend to fall into two groups: the hidrotic and anhidrotic forms according to involvement of sweat glands. They share common abnormalities of the teeth, nails, and hair, one or all of which may be expressed in a single individual, but they are determined by different genetic mechanisms. The hidrotic form with normal or elevated sweat electrolytes usually results from the action of an autosomal dominant gene, whereas the anhidrotic form (decreased number of sweat glands) appears to be determined by the action of a sex-linked recessive gene.

It is the hidrotic type which is associated with sensorineural hearing loss combined with a variety of congenital anomalies such as polydactylism and syndactylism (of fingers or toes); small dystrophic nails; primary and secondary dentition are delayed; many teeth are missing or misshapen; fingernails and toenails are often small and dystrophic.

The concentrations of electrolytes in the sweat glands (sodium and chloride concentrations) are elevated. These concentrations increase with age. The sensorineural hearing loss is a high-frequency one.

A number of inconstant features, which at times are associated with the major signs of the syndrome, include obliteration of the superior labial gingival sulcus, orthopaedic deformities of the lower extremities, mental retardation, ocular anomalies, genital anomalies, and hepatosplenomegaly.

In the anhidrotic type the following abnormalities can be noted: abnormal or sparse teeth; sparse or brittle hair; saddle nose and congenital ozeonas. In this condition there is a greatly decreased number of sweat glands in the skin and consequently no perspiration. Hearing impairment was reported, but it is not a consistent part of the syndrome. The condition is largely restricted to males.

FURTHER READING
ROBINSON, G. C., MILLER, J. R., and BENSINSON, J. R. (1962). Familial ectodermal dysplasia and sensori-neural deafness and other anomalies. *Pediatrics, Springfield* **30**, 797.

Dermatoglyphics

Dermatoglyphic analysis (the study of finger prints, palm lines, and ridges) can contribute to the diagnosis of some of the syndromes. For example, there is a typical appearance of palm print in Down's syndrome. Since the skin is involved in ectodermal dysplasia (and many other conditions) one might expect to find characteristic dermatoglyphic changes (Priest 1967). Dermatoglyphic analyses of anhydrotic ectodermal dysplasia reveals ridge disruption in all areas of the palms and soles. There is also a tendency for the patterns to be vestigial, particularly in the third and fourth interdigital and plantar hallucal areas. The C and D digital triradi tend to be absent, vestigial, or displaced, and the C and D palmar lines are impossible to trace or stop without going anywhere. It is of interest to note that the carrier's mothers have some but not all of these patterns.

Thus dermatoglyphics may prove to be another clinical measure for diagnosis of patients with anhydrotic ectodermal dysplasia and of the carriers or less affected females.

Onychodystrophy

Congenital dystrophy or absence of the nails are anomalies which occur in a variety of forms. A few or all of the nails may be involved. The abnormality may be the only malformation present, or it may be associated with developmental defects of the teeth and the pilosebaceous apparatus as part of a more widespread congenital ectodermal defect.

In children affected by this condition the nails of all fingers and toes may show dystrophic changes which exist from birth. The nails do not grow. The sensorineural hearing loss is very severe and congenital.

FURTHER READING
FEINMESSER, M. and ZELIG, S. (1961). Congenital deafness associated with onychodystrophy. *Archs Otolar.* **74**, 507.

Pili torti

In the pili torti syndrome there is a peculiar abnormality of the hair. The hair shaft shows a more or less tightly twisted configuration through its longitudinal axis. Individual hairs can be flattened or have an irregular cross section. The twists can be incomplete and vary in direction. The hair is untidy, dry, brittle, and easily broken, the result, in the most extreme cases, being that the scalp hair is only a few centimetres long and women may find it necessary to wear a wig. The eyebrows and eyelashes can also be deformed.

The condition is related to a congenital pilar defect which occurs more frequently in women than in men. Even at birth the hair can be abnormal, but changes in most cases reveal themselves in the first or second year of life. In less pronounced cases an improvement at puberty has been postulated by some authors.

The characteristic absence of hair growth, which may involve all or part of the scalp is usually recognized during the second year of life. Pili torti is usually transmitted by an autosomal recessive gene but in some cases a dominant mode of inheritance occurred.

The hearing loss is sensorineural. The familial occurrence of this syndrome suggests that there may be clinical variants and only one of these is associated with hearing loss.

FURTHER READING

BJORDSTAD, B. (1965). Pili torti and sensorineural loss of hearing. *Proc. 17th Meet. Northern Dermatological Soc.* Copenhagen.
—— and ROAR, Th. (1965). Pili torti and sensory-neural loss of hearing. *Proc. Finno-Scand. Ass. Derm.* 3–12.
ROBINSON, G. C. and JOHNSTONE, M. M. (1967). Pili torti and sensory neural hearing loss. *J. Pediat.* **70**, 621–3.

Knuckle pads, leukonychia, and deafness syndrome

In this syndrome keratodermic skin changes appear on the palms and soles, combined with leukonychia (white nails) and a mixed type of hearing loss. Knuckle pads are fibrous thickenings (wart-like growths) over the knuckles. Leukonychia is due to incomplete or otherwise imperfect keratinization of the nail plate. These anomalies are inherited together as an autosomal dominant condition. The chief phenotypic expression, the sensorineural hearing loss, is a simple dominant trait. Other components seem to show incomplete penetrance.

FURTHER READING

BART, R. S. and PUMPHREY, R. E. (1967). Knuckle pads, leukonychia and deafness. *New Engl. J. Med.* **26**, 202–7.

Dermatological abnormalities and hearing defects

Hearing loss can be associated with a variety of dermatological abnormalities in different syndromes. Apart from the conditions in which skin abnormalities are obvious, as it is the case in disorders of keratinization ('twisted hair', onychodystrophy, keratosis palmaris, dystrophy of nails), cutaneous anomalies may also appear in Refsum's disease and Cockayne's syndrome (see in group of syndromes with retinitis pigmentosa) and Hunter's syndrome (mucopolysaccharidosis II).

Disorders of pigmentation in the skin are present in the Waardenburg's syndrome and associated 'pigmentation–hearing' disorders.

ABNORMALITIES OF CONNECTIVE AND BONY TISSUES

Collagen defects in genetic disorders of connective tissue

The basic defect in certain heritable disorders of connective tissue is an abnormality in the structure of collagen (a defect in the collagen molecules themselves). Two disorders in this category can be associated with hearing impairment: osteogenesis imperfecta and Marfan's syndrome.

OSTEOGENESIS IMPERFECTA

Osteogenesis imperfecta is marked by a fragility of the bone (brittle bones) associated with a blue sclerosa (McKusick 1966) and hearing loss of conductive type similar to otosclerosis owing to fixation of the stapes (Alberti and Parkannen 1963) or stapes anomalies (Hall and Røhrt 1968). The blue colour of the sclerosa varies. In some cases it is minimal. Bony deformities occur from old fractures.

MARFAN'S SYNDROME

Individuals with this syndrome are thin, tall, with skeletal and ocular defects. The fingers are long and spidery. Scoliosis, hammer toe, pigeon breast, and dolichocephaly are other anomalies present in the condition. The hearing loss can be conductive, sensorineural, or mixed, according to the extent of anomalies reaching the structures connected with hearing.

It has been reported that the collagen synthesized by fibroblasts from patients with Marfan's syndrome is abnormally soluble, but no other evidence for the site of molecular defect has been found in this disorder, or in osteogenesis imperfecta, despite intensive research efforts in several laboratories. Obviously not all of the connective tissue disorders can have a defect in collagen molecules themselves and basic lesions will no doubt be found in other components of the extracellular matrix and at sites in metabolic pathways where the reason for the effect on the structural integrity of connective tissues is not so directly apparent.

FURTHER READING

BENSON, P. F. (1974). Collagen defects in genetic disorders of connective tissue. *Devl Med. child Neurol.* **16**, 531–8.

KELEMEN, G. (1965). Marfan's syndrome and the hearing organ. *Acta oto-lar.* **59**, 23–32.

PRIEST, R. E., MOINUDDIN, J. F., and PRIEST, J. H. (1973). Collagen of Marfan's syndrome is abnormally soluble. *Nature, Lond.* **245**, 264.

Bone and skeletal abnormalities associated with hearing loss

Abnormality of bone or connective tissues can cause a conductive or sensorineural hearing loss by distorting the normal anatomy or architecture of the external, middle, or internal ear or of the internal auditory meatus. The same applies to skeletal abnormalities secondary to a fundamentally metabolic disorder. A good example of such abnormalities is produced by the severe skeletal disorders in the mucopolysaccharidoses.

Several distinctive disorders of bone tissue are especially associated with hearing impairment: osteitis deformans (Paget's disease); leontiasis ossea; and osteopetrosis with syndactyly (Alberg-Schönberg disease). A variety of skeletal abnormalities should be included in this group of conditions: achondroplasia; Kniest disease with spondylometaphyseal dysplasia; Apert's syndrome; Crouzon's disease, and 'split hand and foot' syndrome.

OSTEITIS DEFORMANS (PAGET'S DISEASE)

The disease arises from an increase in the number and activity of osteoclasts, with a compensatory increase in bone formation. This leads to an increase in bone formation and to a gross disorder of the normal lamellar structure of the collagen of the ground substance. The best recognized clinical picture is one of a gross enlargement of the skull and marked bowing of the femur and tibia. Expansion of bones around foramina at the base of the skull can lead to neurological disorders. Hearing loss occurs frequently and may be conductive, sensorineural, or mixed.

FURTHER READING

PAGET, T. (1878). *Rev. Med. Chirurg. Soc., Lond.* **61**, 41.
BARRY, H. C. (1969). *Paget's disease of bones.* E. and S. Livingstone, Edinburgh.

LEONTIASIS OSSEA

This is a rare condition in which hypertrophy of the face and head is prominent. First the head shows enlargement and later the facial bones enlarge also. Pressure within the skull may cause headaches; hearing loss and optic atrophy occur from pressure or distortion of the anatomical structures of the relevant sensory system.

OSTEOPETROSIS WITH SYNDACTYLY (ALBERG-SCHÖNBERG DISEASE)

Osteopetrosis is characterized by a generalized increase in density of the bones, noted in X-rays, corresponding to an increased specific gravity of the bone tissue in which the proportions of calcium, phosphate and collagen are within normal limits.

It has been suggested that the primary fault is deficiency of osteoclastic activity (Weinmann and Sicher 1955), which would explain also the deficient bone remodelling that is usually present to some degree.

Apart from a conductive hearing loss a sensorineural one may develop as a result of pressure of thickened bone on relevant structures. Bilateral lower motor neurone facial palsy may appear. A markedly thickened right malleus was seen on otoscopy with associated conductive hearing loss. Because of narrowing of the external auditory meati, in some cases otoscopic examination may be difficult or impossible.

The disorder begins *in utero* in some cases, but in others it has been observed to develop during childhood. Osteopetrosis is congenital and may be sporadic or familial. Usually it is inherited as a recessive characteristic, sometimes as a dominant one.

A rare disease which has some features in common with Alberg-Schönberg's disease and also thought to be due to developmental errors is 'Craniometaphysial dysplasia' (Jackson, Albright, Drewry, Hanelin, and Rubin 1954). In this increased bone density is restricted to the skull and face, combined with abnormal metaphysial moulding as found in familial metaphysial dysplasia (Pyle's disease). Thickening of the face and calvarium is greater than is usual in osteopetrosis and thickening confined to the diaphysis of the large limb bones, often associated with increased density of parts of the skull.

FURTHER READING

ALBERG-SCHÖNBERG, H. (1904). Rontgenbilder einer seltener Knochenerkrankung. *Munch. Med. Woschr.* **51**, 365.

—— (1907). Eine bisher nicht beschriebene Allgemeinerkrankung des Skelettes im Rontgenbild. *Fortschr. Geb. RöntgStrahl.* **11**, 261

ACHONDROPLASIA

In this type of dwarfism, with normal-sized trunk, large head and shortened extremities, the conductive hearing loss is the consequence usually of secretory otitis media. The nasal bridge is depressed. Sensorineural losses have been reported (Nelson 1964; Yarington and Sprinkle 1967) most probably due to deformities of the bony structures involving the auditory system.

KNIEST DISEASE

The main disorders here consist of spondylometaphyseal dysplasia, severe myopia, and cleft palate (not always present). In all cases conductive hearing loss is present, but sensorineural loss may also develop.

FURTHER READING

PFEIFFER, R. A., JÜNEMANN, G., TOLSTER, J., and BONER, H. (1973). Epihyseal dysplasia of the femoral head, severe myopia and perceptive hearing loss in three brothers. *Clin. Genet.* **4**, 141.

SPRANGER, J. and NIEDEMAN, H. R. (1966). Dysplasia spondyloepiphysasia congenital. *Lancet* **ii**, 642.

APERT'S SYNDROME

The appearance of the child with this syndrome is characteristic: craniofacial deformities include maxillary hypoplasia, shallow orbits causing proptosis, and acrocephaly (tower skull) (Fig. 24.1). Fused digits (syndactyly) give an appearance of a 'lobster claw' hand (Fig. 24.2). Talipes is also present.

Deformities of the skull are secondary to bi-coronal craniosynthesis. The metopic suture may remain open. Cleft palate is present. Proptosis occurs at varying degrees according to the degree of shallowness of orbits.

The hearing loss, of varying degrees, is conductive. Fixation of the stapes is observed in some cases (Gorlin and Pindborg 1964).

CROUZON'S DISEASE

This is a condition similar to Apert's syndrome, as far as the craniofacial deformities are concerned (Crouzon 1912). Atresia of the external auditory canals is present, with conductive loss; but, as in all conditions associated with severe skeletal abnormalities, sensorineural loss can develop.

SPLIT HAND AND FOOT SYNDROME

A variety of deformities of the hand are noted in this condition. The phalanges of the middle finger may be lacking in one hand, while the third and fourth fingers present syndactyly in the other one.

In the feet, the phalanges of the middle toe may be missing, while on the other side the phalanges of the second toe are absent with the metatarsal lying under the metacarpal of the big toe and fused with it. One hand can be normal while the phalanges of the middle finger are absent on the other side.

A great variety of expressivity is often encountered. Minor signs can be present in members of the family. For example, in one family of a child affected by the syndrome, a stiff thumb was found in the maternal grandfather, in two sisters, and in a son of one of them.

The sensorineural hearing loss is of a high-frequency type.

Genetically, the condition is dominant.

FURTHER READING

WILDERVANCK, I. S. (1963). Perceptive deafness associated with split-hand and foot, a new syndrome? *Acta genet., Basel* **13**, 161–9.

DIGITAL ABNORMALITIES

Digital abnormalities are recognized in many of the developmental bone diseases. In some, such as Ollier's disease, chondro-osteodystrophy, achondroplasia, and arachnodactyly, they are clearly due to involvement of the digits in the generalized bone disorder. However, in acrocephalosyndactyly, myositis ossificans progressiva, pseudohypoparathyroidism, Laurence–Moon–Biedl syndrome and several other rare diseases, the digital abnormalities appear as if due to a distinct but associated gene. Syndactylism and hypoplastic distal phalanges in osteopetrosis seem to be another example of the latter group.

If a child is presented for examination of hearing and a digital abnormality is noted, an investigation should be carried out concerning the possibility of one of these syndromes being present.

FURTHER READING

STRASBURGER, A. K., HAWKINS, M. R., ELDRIDGE, R., HARGRAVE, R. L., and MCKUSICK, V. A. (1965). Symphalangism: genetic and clinical aspects. *Bull. Johns Hopkins Hosp.* **117**, 108–27.

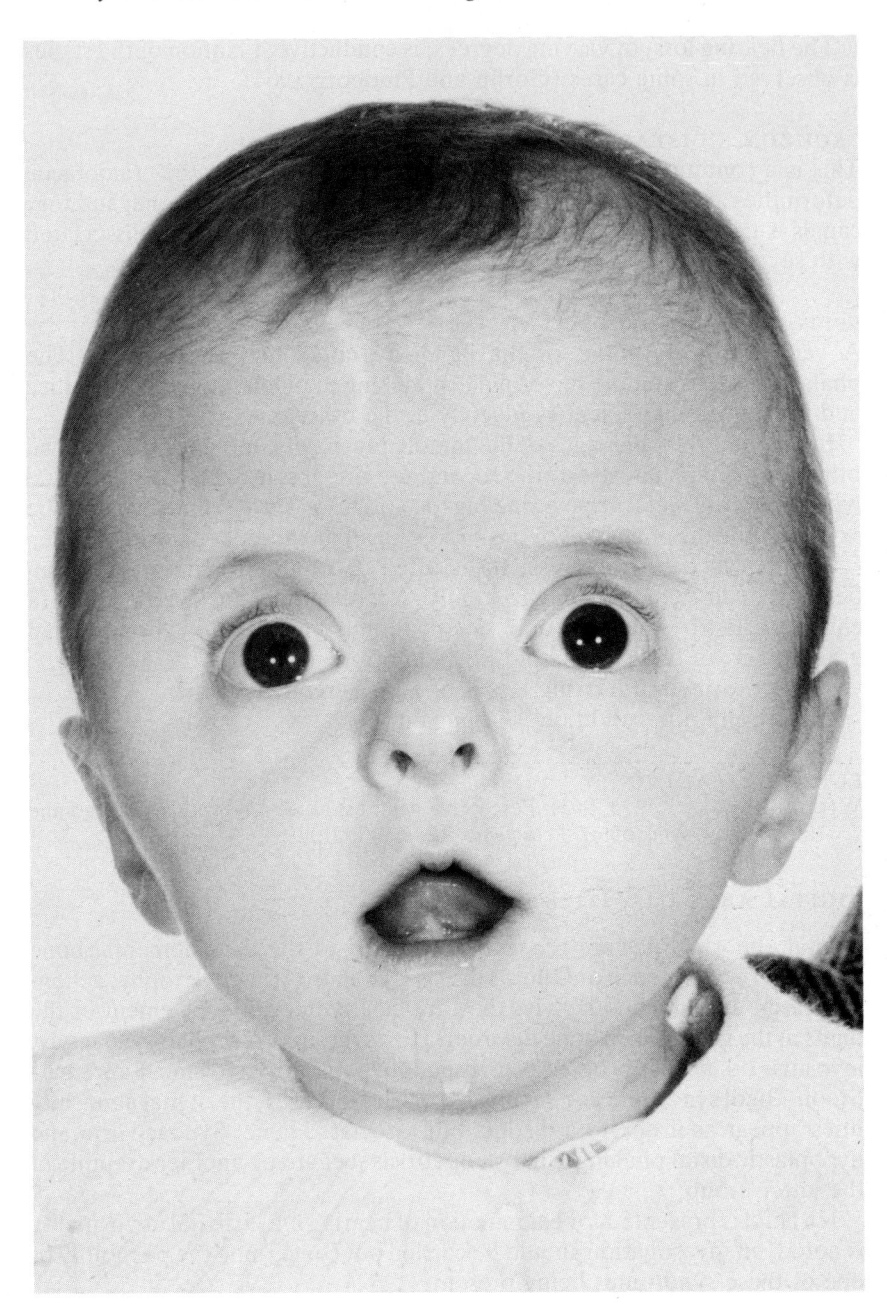

Fig. 24.1(a). Apert's syndrome (face) showing the severe cranial and facial deformities associated with this syndrome. (By kind permission of Mr I. W. Broomhead, Hospital for Sick Children, London.)

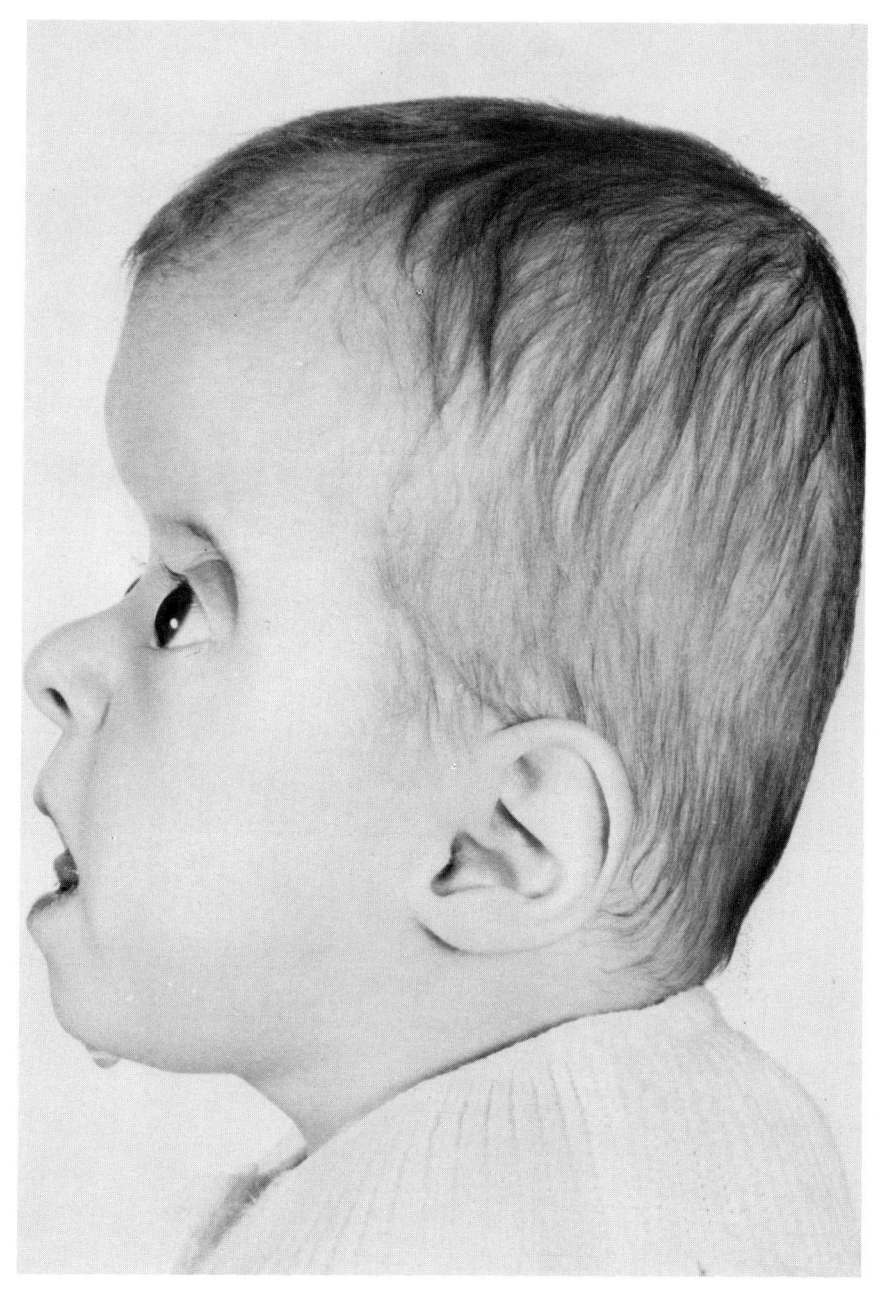

Fig. 24.1(b).

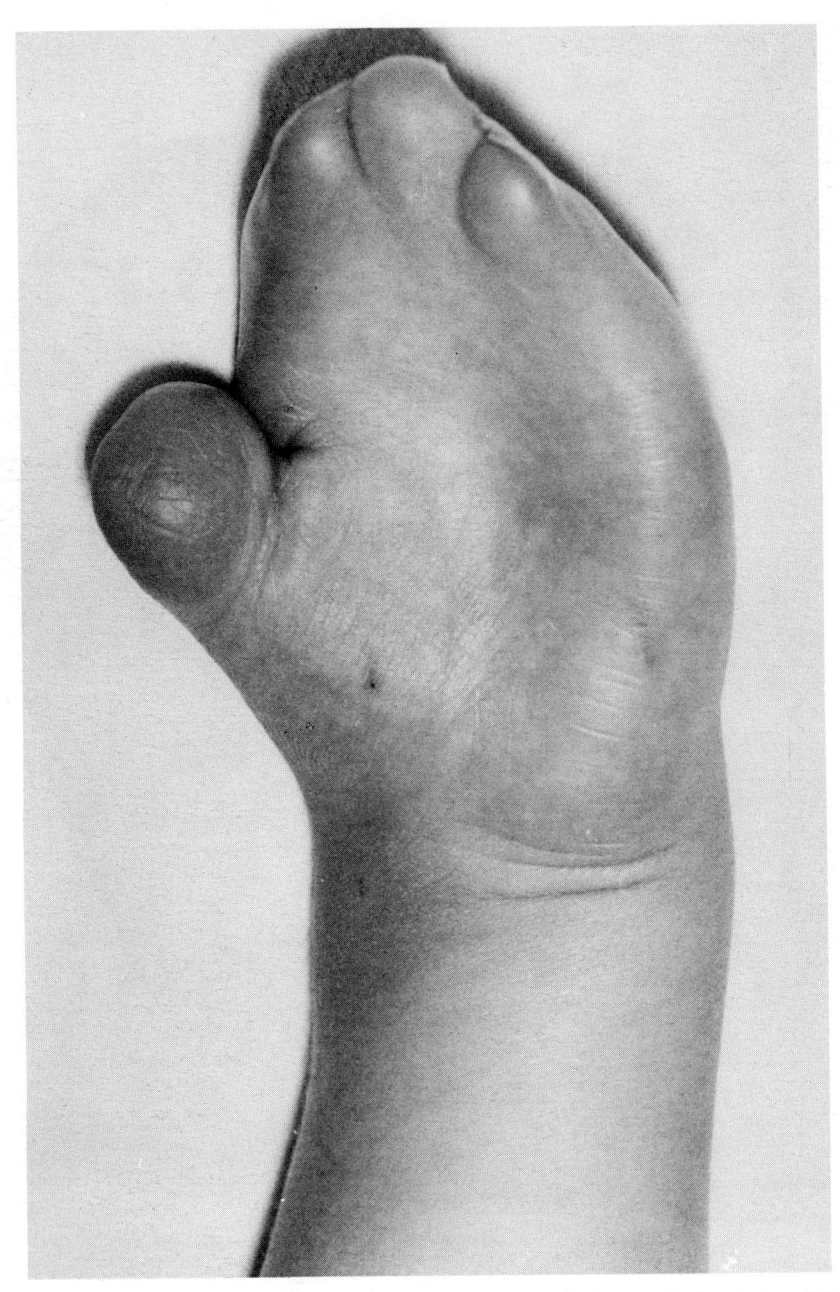

Fig. 24.2 (a). Apert's syndrome (hands) showing the 'lobster claw' type of deformity in a child affected by this syndrome. (By kind permission of Mr I. W. Broomhead, Hospital for Sick Children, London.)

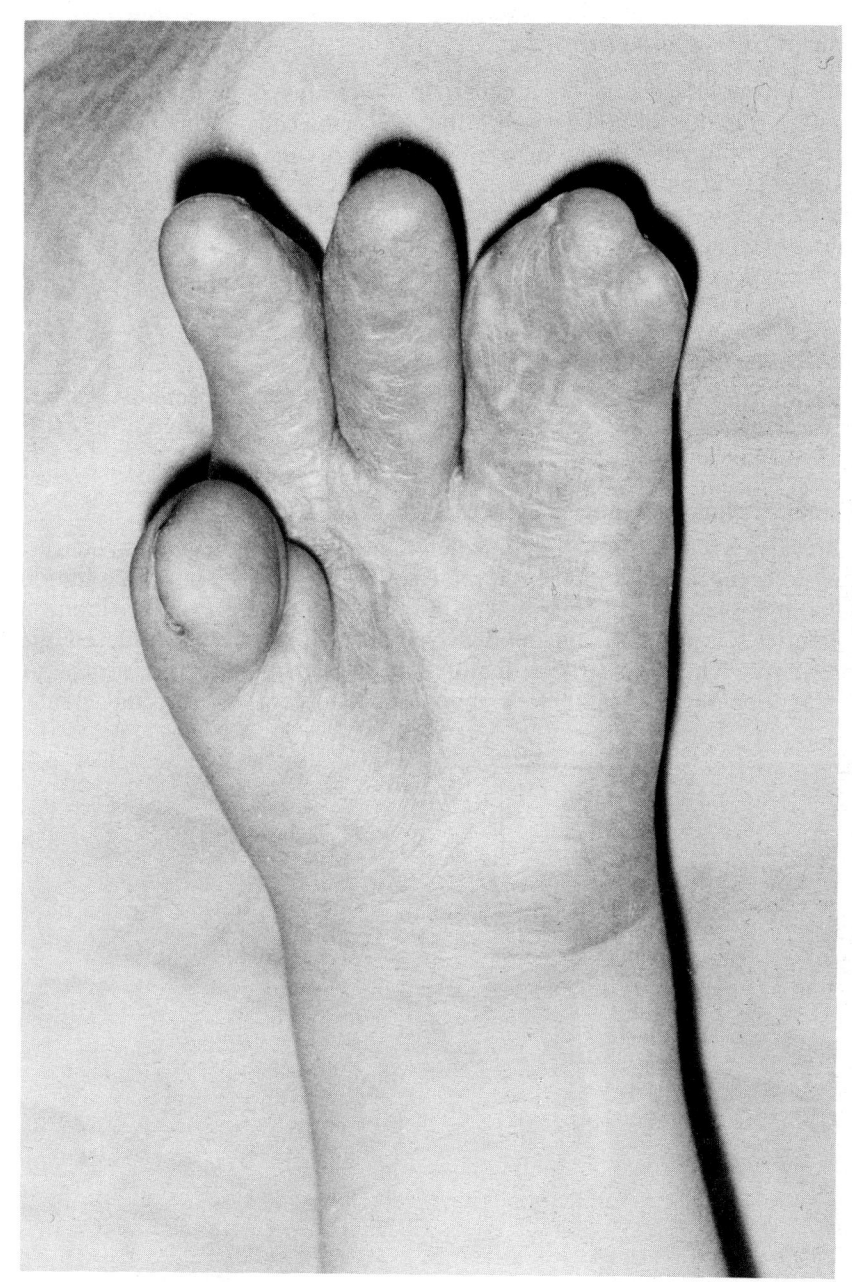

Fig. 24.2 (b).

MUCOPOLYSACCHARIDOSES

The mucopolysaccharidoses are a group of heritable diseases characterized by abnormalities of metabolism of the high molecular carbohydrate compounds of the intracellular matrix. What was originally considered to be a number of variants of 'Gargoylism' is now recognized as a group of separate heritable diseases with phenotypical similarities. They are due to a variety of mutant gene products involved in the metabolism of mucopolysaccharides.

The two principal clinical manifestations of this disorder are Hurler's and Hunter's syndromes.

Hurler's syndrome (mucopolysaccharidosis I)

This has the following clinical characteristics: skeletal deformities; marked corneal opacity and somatic changes; and severe mental retardation. It is inherited in an autosomal recessive fashion.

Hunter's syndrome (mucopolysaccharidosis II) (Fig. 24.3)

This has characteristic marked skeletal deformities and somatic changes, but no corneal clouding; mental retardation is only moderate. In addition hearing loss is present. It is inherited in an X-linked recessive fashion.

Hurler's syndrome, mucopolysaccharidosis I, may be considered the prototype. The most striking features are moderate dwarfism, grotesque facial appearance, protuberant abdomen, joint contractures, and mental

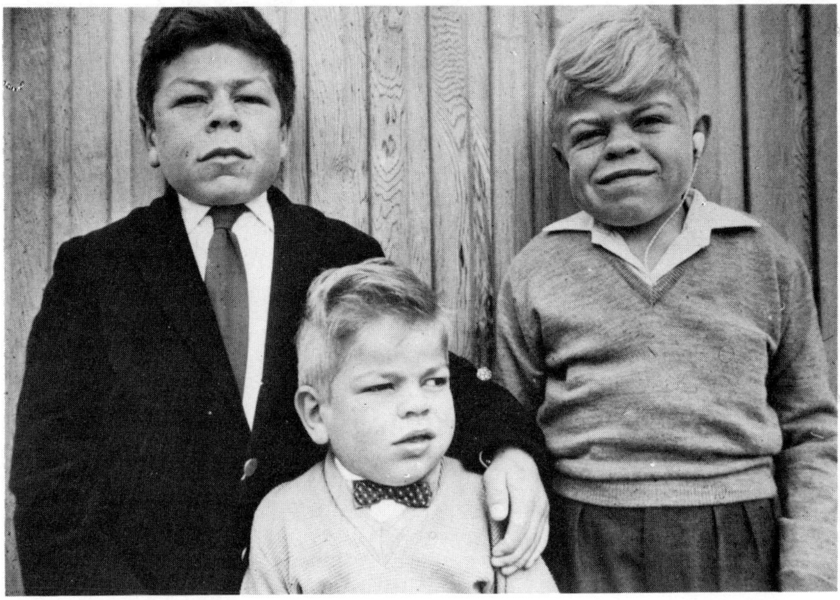

Fig. 24.3. Hunter's syndrome. The facial characteristics of children affected by this syndrome gave rise to the former name of 'gargoylism'.

retardation. The large head frequently shows a prominent ridge along the sagittal suture. Hypertelorism is evident even in young infants who do not yet show the full-blown syndrome.

The bridge of the nose is depressed under a prominent forehead frequently covered by an abnormal amount of dark, coarse hair. Contractures of the hips, knees, ankles, elbows, and fingers are common. The liver and spleen are markedly enlarged. Umbilical and inguinal hernias are frequent. The skin is usually thick. Heart damage, which results from deformity of the valves as well as the coronary arteries, leads to congestive failure, a common cause of death. Corneal clouding is a prominent feature of Hurler's syndrome, but rarely occurs in Hunter's syndrome. In contrast, hearing loss is more prominent in Hunter's syndrome.

Available evidence suggests that most of these diseases are characterized by defects in degradation, particularly of dermatan sulphate and heparin sulphate, with consequent storage of incompletely degraded products in the lysosomes.

Eleven variants of the mucopolysaccharidoses and related disorders have been recognized, all genetically autosomal recessive, but one—Hunter's syndrome—is X-linked and this is the one which is particularly associated with pronounced sensorineural hearing loss; however, as the recognition and diagnoses of the various types is improving, it transpires that several other types are also associated with hearing impairment. Fisch (1980) reported that all the children affected by one of the types of mucopolysaccharidoses which he had examined had hearing impairment. In many cases the hearing loss is conductive, of considerable degree, and very troublesome. This is often superimposed on a moderate high-frequency sensorineural loss which can remain undiagnosed for a long time.

Marotaux–Lamy syndrome (mucopolysaccharidosis type 6)

In this type of mucopolysaccharidosis mental ability can be normal. The affected children are of short stature; there is bilateral clouding over the cornea; bony changes can be detected by X-ray; there is an increased creatinin ratio in the urine and inclusion bodies are found in peripheral blood leukocytes. The enzyme arylsulphatase-B activity in leukocytes is virtually absent.

Because of the small depressed nose and Eustachian malfunction there is often secretory otitis media causing a considerable degree of conductive hearing loss. This is resistant to treatment and repeated myringotomies prove useless. A very moderate sensorineural high-frequency loss is masked by the conductive one which can be much more pronounced.

The main disability is hearing and vision impairment. Provided these are compensated for, in the case of hearing-loss by amplification, a child with this type of mucopolysaccharidoses can make very good progress educationally.

Hearing loss in mucopolysaccharidoses of all types

Some of the disorders in this group of abnormality are rare, but in many children the condition goes unrecognized. With better diagnostic facilities an increasing number of children are identified. Reports have been received about hearing impairment in a number of types. For example, Fisch (1980) reports of a child examined at an audiology centre because of suspected hearing loss eventually being diagnosed by a paediatrician as suffering from 'aspartylglycosaminuria' (or A-glycosaminuria). According to Rossiter (personal communication) this was only the second family diagnosed in Great Britain. Progressive mental retardation, increasing gargoyle-like features, umbilical herniae, deepening voice, severe infections during early childhood, especially ear, nose, and throat ones, and skeletal abnormalities are signs of this distressing condition.

One should accept that all types of mucopolysaccharidoses are associated with hearing impairment; because of osteoporosis (as part of the skeletal abnormalities) and ENT infections, conductive losses are inevitable and probably in all cases there is also a high-frequency sensorineural loss present. For this reason as soon as one of these conditions is diagnosed in a child, a full audiological investigation should be carried out as a routine.

FURTHER READING

DORFMAN, A. (1972). The molecular basis of the mucopolysaccharidosis. *Triangle* **11**, 43.

HUNTER, C. (1917). A rare disease in two brothers. *Proc. R. Soc. Med.* **10**, 104–16.

HURLER, G. (1919). Ueber einen Typ Multipler Abartungen vorviesend am Skelett-system. *Z. Kinderheilk.* **24**, 220–34.

LAMY, M., MAROTEAUX, P., and BADER, J. P. (1957). Etude génétique du gargoilisme. *Fr. génét. Hum.* **6**, 156.

MAROTEAUX, P., LAMY, M., and BERNEUX, J. (1957). *Presse méd.* **65**, 1205.

BRANCHIAL ARCH ABNORMALITIES

Treacher–Collins syndrome

This syndrome is discussed in this chapter in greater detail because certain aspects concerning its nature, assessment, and treatment are applicable to many other syndromes. The commonest feature of the syndrome is a hypoplasia of the malar bones and maxillae so that the nose tends to dominate the face, but the malformation of the zygomatic region consists not only of a hypoplasia of the malar bones but also of defects in the zygomatic arches. This results from a non-fusion of the temporal process of the malar bone with the zygomatic process of the temporal bone. The hypoplasia of the malar bone gives an oblique position to the whole orbit and thus contributes to the 'antimongoloid' palpebral fissures. The lower orbital margin falls away laterally, thereby causing obliquity of the palpebral fissure. The characteristic facial appearance of individuals with this syndrome is therefore chiefly due to the formation of the palpebral fissures which slope downwards (Fig. 24.4). Often, there is a notching of the eyelid. The 'notch', which can be large or small, is in the lower lid at the transition between the medial two-thirds and the lateral third. Lashes on the medial two-thirds are either absent or poorly developed. Both sight and the functioning of the extra-ocular musculature are normal.

Once known this syndrome is readily recognized. Malformations of the middle ear are common and it is not unusual to find absence of the middle-ear

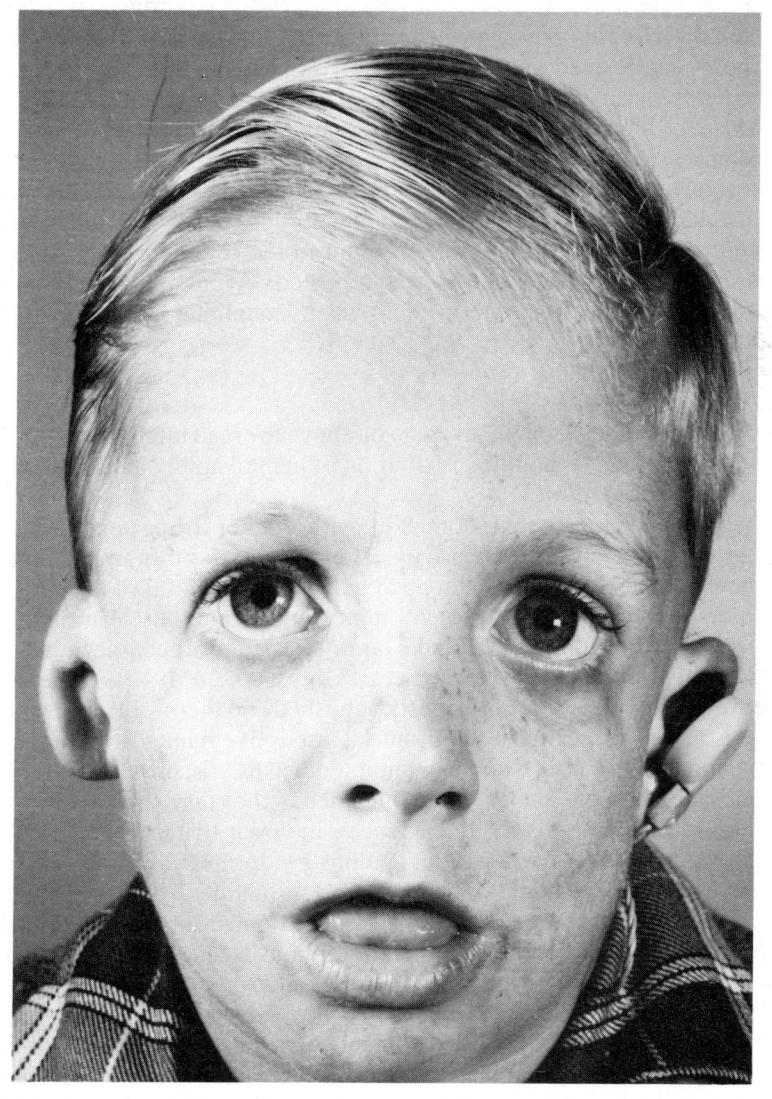

Fig. 24.4. Treacher–Collins syndrome. A typical facial appearance of a child affected by this syndrome.

cleft or gross malformations of the ossicles with fusion of the malleus and incus. The middle ear, incus, and stapes can be absent, but the middle-ear cavity and internal ear can be normal. The drum and middle ear is often diminished. The drum may be replaced by a bony plate. The malleus and the incus are often fused into one single bone. The long process of the incus can be hypoplastic and continues in a deformed and hypoplastic stapes, fixed in a narrow oval window. The edge of the footplate and the margin of the oval window are not so distinct as normally, but the appearance is different from that of otosclerosis.

More severe cases may show microtia and meatal atresia. The pinnas are commonly malformed and a great variety of abnormalities have been described. Malocclusion and malformation of the teeth can also exist. The palate can be high and arched. Further anomalies can be present: hypoplasia of the nasal sinuses; blind fistulas between the angles of the mouth and the ears; atypical hair growth in the form of tongue-shaped processes of the hairline extended towards the cheeks; and absence of the parotid gland. 50 per cent of the recorded cases are present in the complete form. In some cases associated hydronephrosis was reported. A possibility of a kidney abnormality should be borne in mind when examining children with this syndrome.

MENTALITY

Many authors remark on the average or above average intelligence of these individuals. It seems that the distribution of mental ability is the same as in the normal population.

The mode of inheritance is dominant, with a rather strong penetrance and a great variability in the expressivity. There seems to be an increase in the incidence of this syndrome with each generation. Several of the 'normal' members of the families present minor malformations. Chromosome studies by Livingstone (1959) and Maran (1964) have been negative.

Treacher–Collins described two cases in 1900. In 1949 Franceschetti reviewed most of the cases previously published and therefore in Europe his name is associated with the syndrome. Descriptive names have also been given and of these 'dysostosis mandibulofacialis', is probably the most appropriate. Other names have included, 'the first arch syndrome', 'Bilateral facial agenesia', and 'bird face'. In Great Britain and the United States it is known as the Treacher–Collins syndrome.

The mechanism of causation of the abnormalities gave rise to much speculation and consequently abnormal development of the first branchial arch was the object of considerable attention. McKenzie (1958) suggested that a defect of the stapedial artery causes maldevelopment in the region of the first visceral arch, whose vessels the stapedial artery normally supports during the critical phase of development. Vascular supply during the first two months of embryonal development in this region is critical. Its hazardous existence depends on the relay of blood via three successive vessels: the first aortic arch, the stapedial artery, and the external carotoid artery, each of which in turn takes over the dominant supply. Early vascular changes due to an abnormality in the arteries could be responsible for malnutrition and the maldevelopment in the derivatives of the first arch. This portion of the first visceral arch suffers then from a temporary deficiency in its blood supply by occlusion or failure of the maxillary artery at an early age. The stapedial artery is a short-lived vessel in the human embryo. It passes through the stapes, supplying the structures derived from the posterior end of the second visceral arch and affixing itself to the stem of the supra-orbital artery. A defect of the stapedial artery causes maldevelopment not only in its own field of supply but also in the region of the first visceral arch whose vessels the stapedial artery normally supports during the critical phase between the disappearance of the first aortic arch and the full development of the external carotid artery, just after the formation of the primitive face.

When examining children affected by the Treacher–Collins syndrome, it is important not to jump to conclusions on the basis of superficial or subjective appearances. These children often look unattractive, are very hard of hearing, and have serious communication difficulties; when they are older serious emotional disturbances also develop because of their appearance. One can easily at this stage form a very pessimistic view concerning the prognosis. But good otolaryngological and audiological care can give very good results. Furthermore, one should strongly resist the temptation to explore surgically the middle ear. Major cosmetic surgery should be postponed for as long as possible. The right time for this should be selected by a joint consultation of everybody concerned, that is the audiological physician, the paediatrician, the remedial teacher, and the plastic surgeon.

FURTHER READING

AXELSSON, A., BROLIN, I., ENGSTROM, H., and LIDEN, G. (1963). Dysostosis mandibulo-facialis. *J. Lar. Otol.* **79**, 575–92.
HALL-JONES, J. (19??). The Treacher–Collins Syndrome. *N. Z. med. J.* **64**, 25–9.
HERBERTS, G. (1961). Otological observations on the 'Treacher–Collins Syndrome'. *Acta oto-lar.* **54**, 457–65.
HOLBOROW, C. A. (1961). Deafness and the Treacher–Collins Syndrome. *J. Lar. Otol.* **77**, 978–84.
MCKENZIE, J. and CRAIG, J. (1955). Mandibulo-facial dysostosis Treacher–Collins Syndrome). *Archs Dis. Child.* **30**, 391–5.
WILDERVANCK, L. S. (1960) Dysostotis mandibulo-facialis (Franceschetti-Zwahlen) in four generations. *Acta genet. med. Gemell.* **9**, 447–51.
WILLE-JORGENSEN, A. (1962). Dysostosis mandibulo-facialis (Franceschetti). Report of two atypical cases. *Acta ophthal.* **40**, 348–57.

Pierre Robin syndrome

The anomalies in this branchial arch abnormality consists of micrognathia, glossoptosis, cleft palate, and multiple middle- and inner-ear abnormalities. Basically these are architectural malformations rather than neural or end-organ developmental anomalies. A palatal cleft is also present in over 50 per cent of cases. Multiple anomalies in the ear include: abnormal narrowing of the crus commune–utricle junction, superiorly located crus commune and posterior semicircular canal, underdeveloped modiolus, absence of the bony septum between the middle and apical coil, abnormally small internal auditory meatus, abnormal direction of internal auditory canal, large cartilaginous mass around the superior semicircular canal and in the tympanic end of the fissula ante-fenestrum; small facial nerve, large facial bony canal dehiscence, and anomalies of the stapes.

Clinically, the newborn infant with this syndrome experiences episodes of cyanosis with difficulty in breathing and swallowing. The respiratory distress is characteristically relieved by placing the infant in the prone position, thereby allowing the tongue to fall forward. These infants are often described in the literature as having a 'bird-like' face. The palatal defects vary from only a high arched palate without a cleft to a complete cleft of the hard and soft palate. The combination of improved surgical and mechanical forms of therapy with good nursing care has resulted in a good prognosis for the majority of cases.

The hearing loss is a mixed one, varying in degrees according to the extent of the architectural malformations of structures of the hearing system.

FURTHER READING
IGARASHI, M, FILIPPONE, M. V., and ALFORD, B. (1976). Temporal bone findings in Pierre Robin syndrome. *Laryngoscope, St. Louis* 1679–87.

Klippel–Feil syndrome

The principal anomaly of this syndrome consists of fused cervical vertebrae. This gives an appearance of the head sitting on shoulders or of a very short webbed neck (Fig. 24.5). This abnormality is associated with abducens palsy and restricted bulbi of one or both eyes, that is an inward retraction of the bulb of the eye when looking with the affected eye in the direction of the nose. Spina bifida occulta may be present and apart from the cervical vertebrae sometimes also the upper thoracic ones are fused. There is a severe, almost total congenital sensorineural hearing loss. Some of the above mentioned abnormalities may be lacking as is the case in many syndromes. Males are rarely affected by this condition. For example, in a survey of 51 cases only 4 of them were males (Wilderwanck, Hoeksema and Penning 1965).

Deafness is the consequence of extension of the abnormality with the petrous bone. The bony capsule of the labyrinth is maldeveloped. Vestibular disorder is almost invariably present. Normal vestibular function is rarely found in those children with this syndrome who are deaf.

The mode of heredity is not quite clear. Polyfactorial inheritance is most likely. Among the relatives of many individuals affected by this condition one can find 'short necks', spina bifida operta, hydrocephalus, or birth of children with anencephaly. All these anomalies belong to the so called 'status dysraphicus' anomaly caused by incomplete closure of the neural plate.

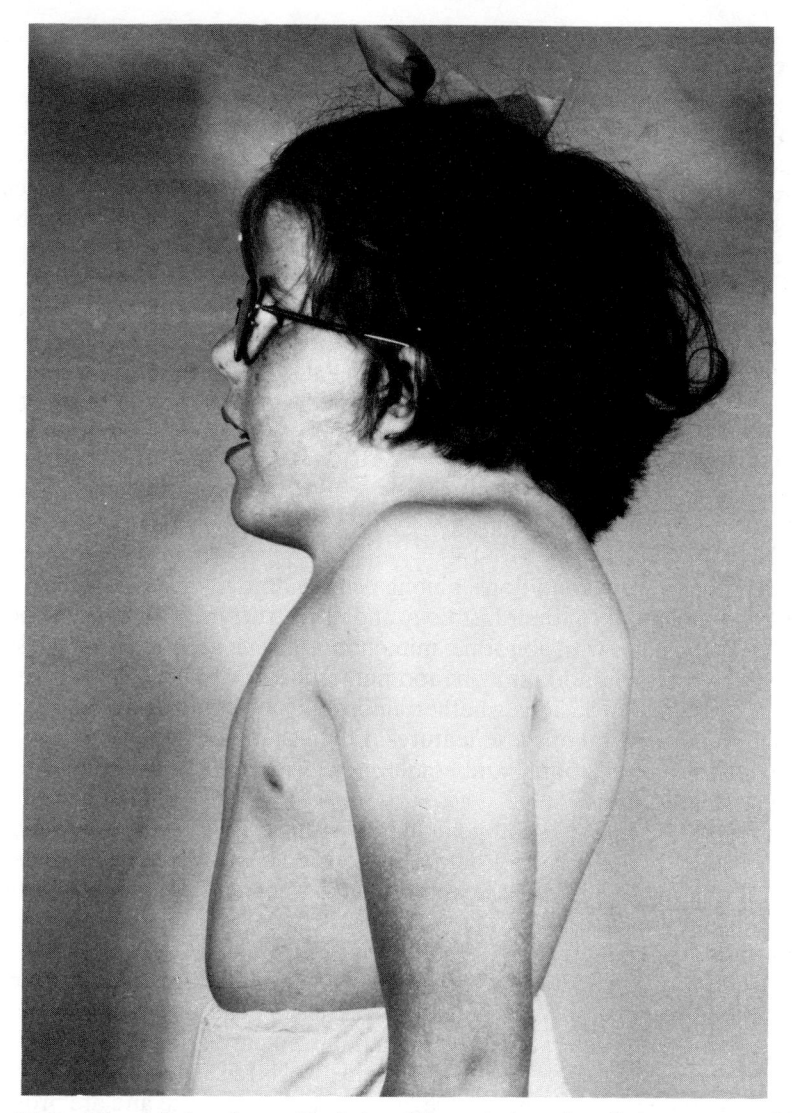

Fig. 24.5. Klippel–Feil syndrome. The fusion of the cervical vertebrae limits movement of the head which is set deeply between the shoulders.

FURTHER READING

McLay, K. and Maran, A. G. D. (1969). Deafness and the Klippel–Feil syndrome. *J. Lar. otol.* **83**, 175–84.

Wildervanck, L. S. (1960). Een cervico-oculo-acusticus syndroom. *Ned. Tijdschr. Geneesk.* **104**, 260–5.

—— Hoeksema, P. E., and Penning, L. (1965) Radiological examination of the inner ear of deaf-mutes. *Acta oto-lar.* **61**, 445–53.

Moebius syndrome

The principal feature of this syndrome is produced by an agenesis or hypoplasia of brainstem nuclei (the sixth and seventh nerve nuclei are involved). Because of lateral and medial rectus paralysis the eyes can not be abducted (paresis of lateral gaze). Facial diplegia; auricular malformation; micrognathia; and absence of hands, feet, fingers, or toes may occur. In some cases there is a paralysis of the tongue.

The Moebius syndrome may also present as a facial weakness in the newborn, usually as a facial diplegia. Congenital absence of pectoral muscles and talipes equinovarus were found in some cases.

Hearing loss is reported in about 15 per cent of cases. Inner-ear abnormalities can be confirmed in some cases by radiography. Also an absence of the stapes and oval and round windows has been reported (Livingstone and Delohunty 1968).

MYOPATHIES OF GENETIC ORIGIN

Newly discovered conditions among 'congenital myopathies' were described on the basis of their histology and ultrastructure. Numerous reports of muscle biopsies with abnormal mitochondria have appeared in the last 15 years. The mitochondria may be too numerous, irregular in shape or size, contain unusual inclusions whether amorphous or paracrystalline in form, or may show several of these features. Often there is also accumulation of lipid in the muscle fibres and sometimes an excess of glycogen without defects in glycolysis.

Here we are interested in genetic myopathies with abnormal mitochondria because two of the syndromes in this group are associated with sensorineural hearing loss, Kearns' syndrome and myopathy with lactic acidosis.

Kearns' syndrome

In its full form this syndrome comprises mitochondrial myopathy, external ophthalmoplegia, ptosis, pigmentary retinal degeneration, sensorineural hearing loss, cerabellar ataxia, growth failure, heart block, and sometimes dementia and spasticity. The CSF protein level is raised (Kearns and Sayre, 1958). The symptoms begin between 3 and 12 years of age and are progressive. Death may result from heart block or from a spongiform encephalopathy.

Mitochondrial change may also be seen in the cerebellum in ataxic patients (Schneck, Adachi, Briet, Wollintz, and Volk 1973). Partial forms of the syndrome are frequent, especially the combination of progressive external ophthalmoplegia and mitochondrial myopathy with or without retinal changes. The sensorineural hearing loss, initially a high-frequency one, is progressive, becoming quite severe.

The full syndrome has been recorded only in sporadic cases and so the genetic position is obscure.

Myopathy and lactic acidosis

The combination of muscular weakness, excessive fatigue, short stature, and episodic vomiting may be associated with lactic acidosis (Tarlow, Lake, and Lloyd 1973). In a similar syndrome, in which sensorineural hearing loss exists, fatigue, progressive growth failure, mild myopathy, episodic vomiting, and lassitude, cardiomyopathy, and mild retinal pigmentation are associated with lactic and pyrexic acidosis and hyperalaminaemia (Hackett, Bray, Ziter, Nyhan, and Creer 1973).

Muscular dystrophy

Congenital sensorineural hearing loss was reported in muscular dystrophy of recessive inheritance, associated with retinal detachment later and progressive muscle wasting. The same applies to severe infantile muscular dystrophy.

RETINAL DEGENERATION AND OCULAR DISORDERS

Usher's syndrome (retinitis pigmentosa)

The two main features of the syndrome are retinal degeneration and progressive sensorineural hearing loss. Vestibular ataxia, cataract, mental defect, and psychosis are found in many cases. The majority of patients show ataxia in the form of a swinging gait and the degree is related to the degree of hearing loss. The incidence of psychosis, mainly schizophrenic-like illness, is over 20 per cent. This may be attributed to the stress of hearing loss and the inexorably progressive loss of vision in early adult life.

The rod and cone layer of the retina is involved primarily. It is interesting to note the basic disorder causing the degeneration as it may be relevant to the causation of damage in the cochlea: the retina depends greatly on carbohydrate metabolism. There is some evidence to show a decline in the anaerobic glycolysis in the retina before changes are apparent histologically.

Children with this syndrome are difficult to educate and manage. Behavioural problems increase with age; the hearing loss is progressive and, generally, the prognosis is very bad.

The mode of inheritance is recessive.

FURTHER READING
USHER, C. H. (1914). On the inheritance of retinitis pigmentosa with notes of cases. *R. Lond. ophthal. Hosp. Rep.* **19**, 130–236.

Syndromes with retinal degeneration distinct from retinitis pigmentosa of Usher's syndrome

It seems that in a significant number of children with severe congenital deafness the hearing impairment is associated with pigmentary degeneration in the retina. Some of the syndromes associated with retinal degeneration are distinct from retinitis pigmentosa and thus form a group which may be confused with Usher's syndrome. These include the association of dwarfism, retinal degeneration, and deafness in Cockayne's syndrome; the deafness sometimes found in the Laurence–Moon–Biedl syndrome; and Hallgren's and Refsum's syndromes.

Hearing loss and retinal degeneration may appear either separately or jointly during the course of certain lipidoses, such as Niemann–Pick disease (Oppikofer 1935) and juvenile amaurotic idiocy or cerebromacular degeneration (Wibau 1931; Steinberg *et al.* 1937; Loebell 1938). In the Laurence–Moon–Biedl syndrome retinal degeneration is associated with the main disorders of obesity, hypogenitalism, myopia, polydactily, and low mental ability. Hearing loss (sensorineural) is not always present but was observed in a proportion of cases (Burn 1950).

Alstrom, Hallgren, Nilsson and Asunder (1959) reported a condition in which there was an association of diabetes mellitus, sensorineural hearing loss, obesity, and pigmentary degeneration of the retina. They considered the syndrome to be a distinct genetic and clinical entity. They drew attention to the similarity of the Laurence–Moon–Biedl syndrome to the one they described. It seems that this condition is a homozygous manifestation of a recessive gene mutation at a different locus to that responsible for the Laurence–Moon–Biedl syndrome. The hearing loss develops in late childhood or adolescence.

COCKAYNE'S SYNDROME

This is characterized by dwarfism, lipodistrophy of the face, light sensitivity, skeletal abnormalities, mental deterioration, and cerebellar ataxia in association with retinitis pigmentosa. Progressive sensorineural hearing loss is part of the syndrome. The mode of inheritance is recessive.

FURTHER READING

COCKAYNE, E. A. (1936). Dwarfism with retinal atrophy and deafness. *Archs Dis. Child.* **11**, 1.

WALLEY, P. J. and FINK, C. N. (1963). Cockayne's syndrome with chromosomal analysis. *Am. J. Dis. Child.* **105**, 204–8.

HALLGREN'S SYNDROME

In this syndrome, retinitis pigmentosa is associated with nystagmus, vestibular cerebellar ataxia, mental retardation, and severe congenital sensorineural hearing loss.

REFSUM'S SYNDROME

In this syndrome the retinal pigmentation is irregular (hemeralopia and concentric constriction of the visual field). Refsum called the disorder 'heredopathia atactica polyneuritiformis'. The salient features are, apart from the atypical retinitis, chronic polyneuritis with progressive paresis of distal parts of limbs and decreased or absent reflexes, ataxia (cerebellar), and increased cerebrospinal fluid protein with normal cell count.

Sensorineural hearing loss is present in many cases. Abnormal electrocardiographic changes, pupillary abnormalities, and skin changes resembling ichthyosis are also noted.

Although this is a relatively rare condition, it is of interest in the context of syndromes associated with hearing loss because it is one of the few 'inborn metabolisms' associated with hearing impairment. The understanding of the mechanism causing the hearing defect may lead to better understanding of causation of deafness in general.

The chief biochemical abnormality in Refsum's disease is the presence of comparatively large quantities of phytanic acid in the blood. The enzyme for the reaction which normally breaks down phytanic acid is missing in patients with the disease. Deficiency of this enzyme may adversely affect nervous metabolism and the phytanic acid accumulation is a secondary effect which does not cause the symptoms (Steinberg et al. 1967). This and many other syndromes, as already mentioned elsewhere, need further study which should lead to an understanding of the association of hearing defect with other disorders.

FURTHER READING

HALLPIKE, C. S. (1967). Observations on the structural basis of two rare varieties of hereditary deafness, etc. Ciba Foundation Symposium (ed. A. V. S. De Reuch). Little Brown, Boston.

REFSUM, S. (1946) Heredopathia Atactic Polyneuritiformis. *Acta psychiat. scand.* (Suppl.) 38, 1–303.

—— SOLOMONSER, L., and SHOTVEDT, M. (1949) Heredopathia Atactic Polyneuritiformis in children. *J. Pediatr.* 35, 335.

Ocular disorders other than retinal degeneration

Many conditions with various ocular disorders associated with hearing defect are known.

LEBER'S DISEASE

Here the main disorders are tapetoretinal degeneration or retinal aplasia, leading to severe visual handicap from birth and hearing loss. It is probably inherited in an X-linked manner and is known to be associated with widespread neurological disease (Wilson 1963; Bruyn and Went 1962).

COGAN'S SYNDROME

Here the symptoms consist of redness of the eyes, lacrimation, blepharospasm, and blurred sight as a result of interstitial keratitis. It is associated with vertigo, nausea, tinnitus, and usually profound deafness. Interstitial keratitis consists of deep patchy corneal infiltrates which tend to fluctuate in distribution and intensity.

As the hearing loss appears, the symptoms of nausea, vomiting, and vertigo disappear. A progressive sensorineural hearing loss becomes severe and permanent. Total visual loss is rare. The vestibulo-auditory dysfunction may occur concomitantly with, precede, or follow the visual symptoms, usually within three months.

Cogan's syndrome appears to be found primarily in young adults of either sex, usually in the second to third decades, although it has been seen as early as ten years of age and as late as 60 years of age. The aetiology of this syndrome remains unknown although it is thought to represent probably a manifestation of a systematic disease, most likely of collagen.

FURTHER READING
ALBRITE, J. P. and RESNICK, D. M. (1961) *Archs Otolar.* **74**, 501–6.
COGAN, D. G. (1945). Syndrome of non-syphilitic interstitial keratitis and vestibulo-auditory symptoms. *Archs Ophthal.* **33**, 144–9.

VOGT–KAYANGI SYNDROME
In this syndrome severe bilateral uveitis (inflammation of the pigmentary layer of the eye) is accompanied by vitiligo, alopecia, poliosis and hearing loss. Retinal detachment and deafness may occasionally be present. It usually occurs in adults. The conspicuous feature is the severe prolonged bilateral uveitis. Several weeks to months following onset and as the uveitis gradually subsides, changes in skin and hair occur. The vitiligo is usually symmetric and appears especially on face, neck, and trunk. Alopecia areata may appear in patches or in some instances there is total loss of hair. Poliosis or premature greying of hair, eyebrows, and eyelashes occurs. Tinnitus and partial to complete deafness are usually bilateral.

The course of this disorder is chronic and may continue for many months. Hair and skin changes usually disappear. Ear symptoms frequently resolve but in some cases may progress to partial or total deafness. Impairment of vision may improve gradually but seldom returns to normal. Partial or complete blindness secondary to glaucoma may result. No satisfactory treatment is known.

FURTHER READING
LEWIS, G. M. and ESPLIN, B. M. (1949). Vogt–Kayangi syndrome. *Archs Derm. Syph.* **59**, 526–30.

KIDNEY ABNORMALITIES

Alport's syndrome
Patients with Alport's syndrome are usually asymptomatic for years. The most common and earliest finding is symptomless haematuria and albuminuria in early childhood. When specifically sought, these have been found in the first week or so of life. In the majority of affected males the disorder proceeds insidiously to chronic nephritis from which they die, usually before reaching the age of 30, and sometimes much earlier. Sensorineural hearing

loss of high-frequency type develops gradually and progresses to a severe degree.

Females are seldom severely affected and most seem to have a normal expectation of life despite recurrent or continuous albuminuria. Some have a minor high-frequency loss for frequencies above 4000 Hz. Hearing loss in this syndrome seldom precedes nephritis. Some of the patients develop vestibular symptoms and electronystagmography shows a symmetrical paresis to thermic stimulation.

Several observers have also commented on the occurrence of various congenital ocular defects in their patients. Particular mention has been made of cataracts and of sphereophakia. It is estimated that about 15 per cent of cases have these ocular lesions.

The following description of a clinical example shows the progression of the syndrome.

A 5-year-old boy was sent for examination because of a 5 week history of an episode of blood-stained urine. This was painless and not associated with a previous sore throat although there was illness at the time, but he had no urinary symptoms. For a week before admission he had a further episode of blood-stained urine which cleared up within 2 or 3 days.

A general examination showed no abnormality and he looked a fit boy, but the aortagram on the left side showed a small renal artery which appeared to supply the upper pole of the kidney. Biopsy of the upper pole of the left kidney contained an average of 70 glomerulae which showed some increase in cellularity with wide open capillaries in which red cells were seen.

He was regularly examined at the audiology department. He had a minor high-frequency loss which gradually deteriorated along with deterioration of his kidney condition. When seen again at the age of 12, his hearing loss was severe. He was transferred to a unit for partially hearing children. His difficulties gradually increased.

Alport's syndrome is considered to be probably the most common dominantly inherited condition associated with sensorineural hearing loss. However, there are some doubts about the transmission of the syndrome as a whole.

The renal lesion is transmitted as a partially sex-linked dominant trait and most other workers seem to agree with this view. There is less agreement on the mode of inheritance of the deafness. According to Hamburger, Crosmier, Lissae, and Waffha (1956) it is by a particularly sex-linked recessive gene, but Perkoff (1967) suggests that it is linked with the renal lesion in some as yet unknown way.

The cause of Alport's syndrome is not known. Temporal bone studies show destruction of cochlear and vestibular neuroepithelium. It is assumed, according to one view, that there is a genetic defect in an enzyme system common to parts of the renal, auditory, and vestibular and ocular tissues. This is purely speculative. According to another view (Beaney 1964) subjects with diminished renal function excrete some drugs which may have an ototoxic effect at a slower rate than normally and the concentration may therefore stay high for a longer time. The hair cells may be exposed to the effect of the drug longer than usual. Obviously, the connection between renal and auditory abnormality requires further detailed studies.

FURTHER READING

ALPORT, A. C. (1927). Hereditary familial congenital haemorrhagic nephritis. *Br. med. J.* **i**, 504.

FRASER, J. S. (1965). Association of congenital deafness with goitre (Pendred's syndrome). *Ann. hum. Genet.* **28**, 201–49.

Renal tubular acidosis

One of the signs of this syndrome is nephrocalcosis. Renal calculi can be readily seen in abdominal radiographs. The main complication consists of renal calculi, but renal function gradually improves. The hearing loss associated with this syndrome is a sensorineural high-frequency one.

Individuals with this condition are characteristically of small stature and in children the condition is discovered occasionally during investigation of lack of growth. Most cases occur sporadically. Reported familial cases appear to behave as of autosomal dominant inheritance.

FURTHER READING

NONCE, W. E. and SWEENEY, A. (1971). Evidence for autosomal recessive inheritance of the syndrome of renal tubular acidosis with deafness. *Birth Defects, Orig. Artic. Ser.* **7**, 70.

Urticaria, amyloidosis, and deafness

This is also a dominantly inherited condition (as Alport's syndrome and renal tubular acidosis) but the kidney disease and hearing loss is associated with a specific metabolic abnormality. It consists of frequently recurrent transient attacks of an urticaria-like rash with severe constitutional upset; progressive sensorineural hearing loss; premature loss of libido and relative infertility; hyperglobulinaemia; nephropathy; amyloidosis, and minor physical anomalies.

The main characteristics of this complex are inherited in a dominant fashion and show anticipation in successive generations but no sex-linkage and when transmitted are tightly linked together.

FURTHER READING

MUCKLE, T. J. and WELLS, M. (1962). Urticaria, deafness and amyloidosis: a new heredo-familial syndrome. *Q. Jl Med.* **31**, 235–48.

Hyperprolinaemia

Scriver, Schafer, and Efron (1961) described a condition of familial nephritis with deafness and epilepsy, associated with hyperprolinaemia and the excretion of excessive amounts of glycine, L-proline, and L-hydroxy-proline in the urine. Additional abnormalities are photomyoclonus, diabetes mellitus, and cerebellar dysfunction.

Seizures, mental retardation, and sensorineural hearing loss are present in some persons with this abnormality. Menkes (1974) reported that in hyperprolinaemia photosensitive epilepsy is part of the syndrome. Genetically the condition is autosomal recessive.

Epilepsy and hearing loss syndromes

Epilepsy has been reported in a few syndromes associated with hearing loss. Apart from hyperprolinaemia it was reported in Unvericht's syndrome, in which myoclonic epilepsy is associated with hearing impairment (Latham and Munro 1938; May and White 1968). Herman, Aguilar, and Sachs (1964) reported a syndrome with epilepsy, hearing loss, nephropathy, and diabetes mellitus.

Congenital kidney abnormalities associated with hearing impairment

The association of congenital kidney abnormality with abnormalities of ear and hearing has been reported by many observers. Although a more systematic study is still necessary, there is little doubt that an association of congenital kidney abnormalities and aural disorders does occur in a significant number of cases.

In many such cases one kidney is smaller than the other (in three-quarter of the cases the right kidney is the smaller one). A small kidney occurs in 0.97 per cent of the population. These are cases of hypoplasia with normal architecture and function of the kidney. In children with deformities of the external ear, especially combined with maldevelopment of the facial bones (as in Treacher Collins syndrome) it is recommended to investigate the urinary tract.

In extreme cases one kidney may be missing altogether. This is so in the Hallerman–Streif syndrome. Fisch (1980) reported a child with this syndrome who had a progressive sensorineural hearing loss, initially a high-frequency one. The child was also of low mental ability and had in addition a moderately deformed auricle. The child's sister also had a progressive sensorineural hearing loss.

Children with kidney abnormalities should be considered to be at risk in having or possibly developing a hearing impairment and therefore they should be tested as a routine.

THYROID DYSFUNCTION

Pendred's syndrome

Pendred's syndrome is characterized by an invariable association with an inborn error of thyroxine synthesis at the level of organic incorporation of trapped iodine in the thyroid gland. This abnormality is associated with sensorineural hearing loss of a severe degree and goitre.

The hearing loss is congenital, but the goitre develops during childhood. In a very few recorded cases the goitre was congenital or appeared in infancy. More commonly it appears in middle childhood and is not prominent, especially in males, till an even later stage. The hearing loss is, however, congenital.

Diagnosis of Pendred's syndrome presents no difficulty, especially when facilities exist to test the response of thyroid to perchlorate. An impaired capacity of the thyroid to convert inorganic iodine to organic compounds is shown by discharge of radio-iodine when perchlorate or thiocyanate is administered. Potassium perchlorate, given one hour after a dose of radioactive iodide, discharges a variable amount from the thyroid gland, showing that trapped iodide has not been incorporated into organic form. In Pendred's syndrome the perchlorate test is positive.

Although the majority of children with Pendred's syndrome are mentally normal, mental subnormality is not incompatible with the diagnosis and may be associated with the hypothyroidism that affects a minority of cases during critical periods of early childhood. Confusion between goitrous cretinism and Pendred's syndrome is liable to occur in such individuals, but it is important not to confuse these very different conditions.

The inheritance of this syndrome is recessive.

FURTHER READING
PENDRED, V. (1896). Deaf–mutism and goitre. *Lancet* **ii**, 532.
TROTTER, W. R. (1960). The association of deafness with thyroid dysfunctions. *Br. med. Bull.* **16**, 92.

Congenital hypothyroidism

Hypothyroidism is a clinical condition associated with a decrease in the circulating level of thyroid hormone. Thyroid hormone has a widespread action on the body and increases cellular metabolism. Cellular metabolism slows down in hypothyroidism and in its congenital form it has a devastating effect on growth and development. The failure to detect it early after birth can lead to permanent brain retardation. When signs such as mental retardation are noted, brain damage has occurred.

Hearing loss is often reported in this condition. The cause is, however, very different as compared with Pendred's syndrome. Temporal-bone pathology showed hyperostosis of the bone of the promontory, large cochlear aquaducts, and fibrous tissue obliterating the round window niche (Paparella, 1969). Superimposed conductive losses are frequent. In many affected infants unusual deformity of the external ears was observed (Walsh 1979).

In the context of syndromes with hearing impairment, the importance of congenital hypothyroidism is underestimated. Partial hearing losses can go unrecognized in these children because full threshold audiometry is possible only later than is the case in mentally and physically normal children. The symptoms of hypothyroidism are numerous and clinically it is difficult to diagnose early. The early detection of partial hearing loss, as part of the condition, can be even more difficult.

Fortunately, it is now possible to detect congenital hypothyroidism by a screen test based on the radioimmunoassay of thyroxin. It can be done on a tiny sample of dried blood. Those babies who have a thyroxin level below the third centile can be detected. Further detailed investigation can then be carried out to confirm the diagnosis of hypothyroidism. When confirmed, thyroxin-replacement therapy is instituted, although the replacement dosage of thyroid hormone is still a matter for consideration.

Screening for congenital hypothyroidism is now established in many countries. The incidence of congenital hypothyroidism varies from country to country (1 in 3500 to 1 in 5180). In Great Britain a screening programme in Peterborough revealed an incidence of 1 in 3600 (Walsh 1979). If this is reflected throughout the country, 150 children are born each year who are at risk. This is then a considerable reservoir of children with partial hearing loss which can often go undetected or remain so for a long time during childhood. This is, hopefully, one of the groups of children whose hearing loss will be preventable by effective screening and treatment.

FURTHER READING
DE VOS, J. A. (1963). Deafness in hypothyroidism. *J. Lar. Otol.* **77**, 390–414.

Genetic and endemic goitre

The clinical symptoms of genetic goitre are similar to endemic goitre, so that areas with a high incidence of the disease are unlikely to distinguish the smaller proportion of goitres caused by inherited defects. According to certain views, deafness accompanies endemic goitre when the goitre is associated with poor nutritional status. Endemic goitre seems to be accompanied by a high incidence of deafness in poorer countries, but not in countries where nutritionally conditions are better (Greenwald 1959).

Thyroid dysfunction and hearing loss

Much speculation has taken place to clarify the relationship between thyroid dysfunction and hearing impairment. Experimental work is beginning to throw some light on this relationship in Pendred's syndrome. Experiments were carried out with thyroidectomized guinea pigs. They were maintained in a hypothyroid state for varying periods of time. Histochemical studies were then carried out. Results indicated that hyaluronidase-sensitive mucous substances were increased in the scalae of the inner ear. As a consequence of increased deposition of acid mucopolysaccharides and the relationship of potassium to sodium in endolymph and perilymph was found to be markedly altered. Marked swelling of the chambers of the inner ear was noted, and this was believed to represent hydropic induction by acid mucopolysaccharide, with consequent alteration of electrolyte relationships ('electrochemical theory'). Acid mucopolysaccharide was also found in significant quantities in the region of the acoustic nerve, producing a compression phenomenon of the nerve. This was most marked in the region of Rosenthal's canal of the lamina spiralis ossea. This finding supports a 'mechanical theory' for hearing disturbance.

A further possibility, arising from the close relation between the thyroid gland and vitamin A on one hand and between the hearing system and vitamin A on the other, should be considered. A vitamin-A-deficient diet disturbs the embryonic development of the thyroid gland, as pointed out by Van Dyke (1945). It is possible that the separation of the endolymphatic space and the space in the tunnel of Corti depends on a proper balance of vitamin A metabolism. When the separation is disturbed or breaks down, the mixing of the potassium-rich endolymph with the potassium-poor 'Cortilymph' can lead to damage of unmyelinated nerve fibres. It is also important to note that the vitamin A content of the inner ear is ten times higher than that of any other tissue except the liver.

PIGMENTATION ANOMALIES
Waardenburg's syndrome
The principal features of this syndrome are as follows: A pigmentation defect which can appear as, (i) 'a white forelock', (a white streak of hair in front, usually just over the central point of the forehead); (ii) lack of pigmentation in one or both eyes (if in both eyes, they are translucently blue; if in one, the condition is named as heterochromia iridium; (iii) patches of depigmented areas in the skin (these can be clearly visible, but often a depigmented area can be detected only under ultraviolet light).

The next characteristic sign in this syndrome is a peculiar deformity of the eyelids; the inner corner of the eyelids is shortened because the upper eyelid turns vertically downwards and thus increasing the distance between the inner edges of the two eyes. This gives a superficial impression of a wide nasal bridge or even a sideway displacement of the eyes. In fact the distance between the centre of the pupils of the two eyes is perfectly normal. The facial appearance in this syndrome when all these signs are present is quite characteristic (Fig. 24.6).

A sensory neural hearing loss is part of the syndrome. This can be a profound bilateral deafness or a unilateral one or a partial hearing loss which is somewhat unusual being a predominantly low-frequency sensory neural impairment. A combination of the two patterns of hearing loss in the same person is possible: a profound, almost total deafness in one ear and a partial low-frequency loss in the other one. Mental ability is not affected. Also, physically these people are normal.

As is the case in many syndromes, the genetical penetrance of each sign varies and only in the minority of affected individuals are all the classical signs present at the same time. All possible combinations may occur in an affected person: profound hearing loss, heterochromia of the iris, white forelock, but without an eyelid deformity; or a white forelock, eyelid abnormality, profound hearing loss, but normal eye colour etc. This condition is inherited in a dominant autosomal (that is non-sex chromosomal)

Pigmentation anomalies 627

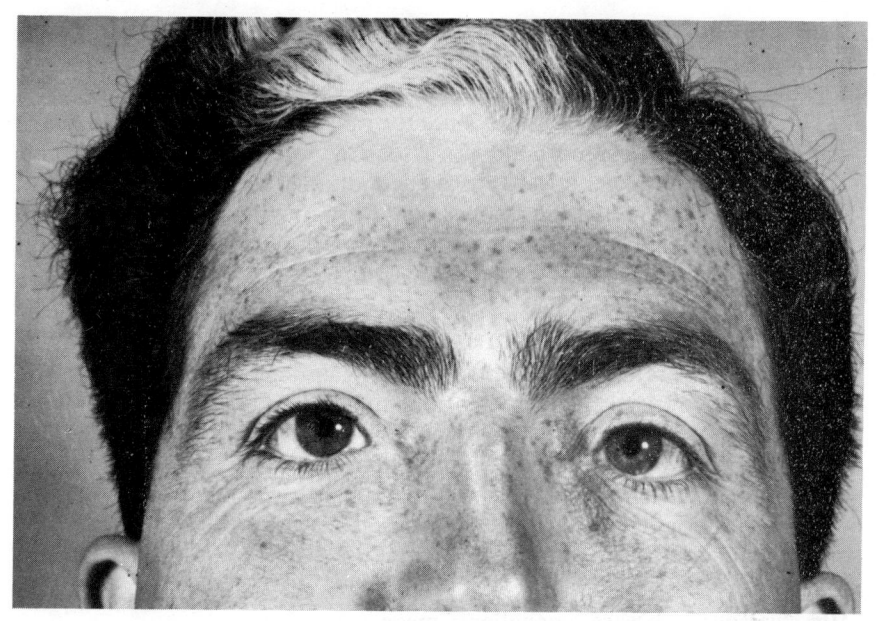

Fig. 24.6. Waardenburg's syndrome. A white forelock, an eyelid abnormality (at the inner canthus), and heterochromia of the irides produce the immediately recognizable signs of this syndrome.

manner. In a parent (father or mother) the full syndrome may be present or only some of the signs. The syndrome can be traced back often to several generations and consistently transmitted in one form or another.

The asymmetrical nature of many of these abnormalities is an indication that they are remote effects of the gene. As it is the case in Hirschsprung's disease, the fact that ganglion cells are affected indicates that the deleterious affect of the gene acted on the cells in the neural crest before differentiation of these cells into more complex tissues or organs occurred.

The age long mystery of the connection between deafness and pigmentation disorder (the mystery of the 'blue-eyed deaf cat') was resolved following the suggestion by Fisch (1959) that the source of the common genesis of both disorders rests in a genetical fault in the neural crest at the initial stages of foetal development. It has been confirmed by meticulous investigations that the inner ear and the organ of Corti originate from the cells of the neural crest. Also, almost all body pigments have the same origin.

Normally, cutaneous melanocytes migrate in foetal life from the neural crest to the basal layer of the epidermis, where they are found in the ratio of one melanocyte to ten basal cells. In this site they synthesize melanosomes which are then transferred via the dentritic processes of the melanocytes to the surrounding keratinocytes.

The enzymes dopa-oxidase and tyrosinase are essential for melanin synthesis. In albinism melanocytes are present in normal numbers in the epidermis, but they are non-functioning. Albinism is not associated with hearing disorder. In Waardenburg's syndrome, the melanocytes in the depigmented areas are present, but contain abnormal melanosomes.

The Waardenburg's syndrome is not the only clearly defined condition in which pigmentation abnormality is associated with hearing impairment. There is a variety of genetically distinct conditions. For example, in one of these 'pigmentation hearing disorders', severe deafness is associated only with lack of pigment development in the iris of both eyes, but no other abnormalities are present.

THE EARLY GREYING SYNDROME

This is again genetically distinct from the Waardenburg's syndrome. The main feature consists of early greying of hair in one of the parents and one or more of the children may be born with a severe sensory neural congenital deafness or occasionally only with unilateral hearing loss. The bilateral hearing loss can appear often as a predominantly high-frequency type.

The early greying can be traced back to several generations. There are no other abnormalities. Physically and mentally these children are not affected.

Hirschsprung's disease (aganglionic megacolon)

Hirschsprung's disease is a disorder of intestinal motility caused by an absence of parasympathetic ganglion cells from the submucosal and myenteric plexuses of the gut. The numerous reports of an association of this syndrome with congenital deafness indicate that this should be now classified as one of the conditions in the context of this group of syndromes.

The connection between the inner-ear disorder and the one in the intestine is of special interest. McKusick (1973) focused the attention on the fact that the cells of the myenteric plexus are believed to originate from the neural crest. Fisch (1959) advanced the theory of the connection between deafness and pigmentation disorders based on the embryological origin of both of the organ of Corti and body pigments (see p. 627). Similarly a genetic defect which causes a defect in migration of neuroblasts before the twelfth week of gestation causes the disorder in Hirschsprung's aganglionic megacolon and in the inner ear.

Beilschowsky and Schofield (1962) discovered that a considerable number of piebald mice suffered from megacolon associated with marked reduction of the myenteric ganglion and this indicated that the gene affected the neural crest before its differentiation into melanoblasts and ganglionic primordia. Of additional interest is the observation that there are several conditions known or suspected to be associated with an increased risk of Hirschsprung's disease, including Down's syndrome and neuroblastoma. Similarly, Hirschsprung's aganglionic megacolon is probably caused by a defect in migration of neuroblasts before the twelfth week of gestation.

FURTHER READING
SINNNER, R. and IRVINE, D. (1973). Hirschsprung's disease and congenital deafness. *J. med. Genet.* **4**, 337.

NEUROPATHIES

Sensory radicular neuropathy

Sensorineural hearing loss was originally described in this condition by Hicks (1922) when he drew attention to a family in which several members had 'perforated ulcers of the feet and were deaf'. There is loss of sensation in the feet with absence of ankle reflexes and down-going plantar reflexes, with prolonged sensory conduction latencies of the ulnar and median nerves.

The hearing loss is a high-frequency type and progressive. Tinnitus is also present in some cases. Apart from the sensorineural hearing loss there are also vestibular changes. Absent vestibular responses were noted. Ataxia has been observed in some patients (Denny-Brown 1951), especially at night.

The atrophy of the cochlear and vestibular ganglia parallel the atrophic process in the spinal ganglia. It is interesting to note that hearing loss and vestibular disturbances are the only cranial nerve findings.

FURTHER READING
FITZPATRICK, D. B., HOOPER, R. E. and SEIFE, B. (1976). Hereditary deafness and sensory radicular neuropathy. *Archs Otolar.* **102**, 552–7.

Friedrich's ataxia

Friedrich's ataxia is the classical progressive non-neoplastic ataxia of childhood. The condition develops insidiously, usually during the first decade, and the child may be first diagnosed as a 'clumsy' child. Subsequently, there is a spontaneous gaze nystagmus, absent knee jerk, extensor plantar responses, and impaired position and vibration sense. High-frequency sensorineural hearing loss develops.

The inheritance is autosomal recessive.

Ataxic neuropathy

This syndrome has been studied in detail in Nigeria by Hinchcliffe, Osuktokun, and Adenga (1972). They investigated an endemic ataxic neuromyelopathic syndrome. The fully developed syndrome, termed 'Nigerian nutritional ataxic neuropathy', comprises myelopathy with predominant involvement of the posterior columns of the spinal cord, bilateral optic atrophy, sensorineural hearing loss, and symmetrical peripheral polyneuropathy. The condition is more prevalent in areas with a high cassava consumption. Cassava contains high concentrations of a cyanogenic glycoside, linamarin. The presumption is, therefore, that the disorder is primarily due to chronic cyanide intoxication consequent on high cassava consumption.

FURTHER READING
HADDOCK, D. R. W., EBRAHIM, M. B., and KAPUR, B. B. (1962). Ataxic neurological syndrome found in Tanganyika. *Br. med. J.* **ii**, 1442-3.

Ataxia in childhood

Since even the healthy infant has poor balance and imprecise movements, ataxia cannot usually be demonstrated until the end of the first year of life. Since muscular hypotonia is not uncommonly seen in ataxic patients in general, this sign may be the first indication of congenital ataxia.

Several syndromes associated with hearing impairment include ataxia as one of the major symptoms: Friedrich's ataxia; ataxic neurological syndromes; retinitis pigmentosa (Usher's syndrome); Hallgren's syndrome (Hallgren 1959); cerebellar ataxia and sensorineural hearing loss; and Refsum's syndrome.

Ataxia will, of course, also be part of the picture of an acute labyrinthine failure, which may occur at any age. This condition is characterized by sudden loss of hearing and of vestibular function, so that there is also nausea, vomiting, and acute vertigo. The condition may occur without any apparent precipitating factor, or it may be a complication of a suppurative otitis media. Fortunately, the condition is invariably unilateral.

An acute ataxia, the acute cerebellar syndrome of childhood (Blau and Sheehan 1958), occurs about 7-10 days after a viral infection. It is characterized by ataxia, spontaneous nystagmus, and intention tremor. Spontaneous recovery occurs within a few weeks. One should not forget that ataxia can also be associated with medulloblastoma and cerebellar astrocytoma.

CHROMOSOME DISORDERS

A limited number of investigations have been carried out to find out whether chromosome abnormalities exist in some groups of children with hearing impairment. The only syndrome associated with hearing impairment and undoubtedly caused by a chromosome disorder is Down's syndrome (trisomy 21). In Turner's syndrome a hearing loss has been found occasionally, but it is still doubtful whether these cases are sufficiently numerous to include it in this group.

DOWN'S SYNDROME

This is a well known disorder, previously named 'mongolism'. The chromosome abnormality is more precisely defined as 'trisomy 21'. The outstanding sign is mental retardation. Physically these children are easily recognized because of the characteristic brachicephaly, epicanthus, small depressed nose, broad flat head with typical dermatoglyphical signs (Fig. 24.7).

Conductive hearing loss and serous otitis media is almost always present, in varying degrees. However, in many children there is also a moderate sensorineural, principally high-frequency loss.

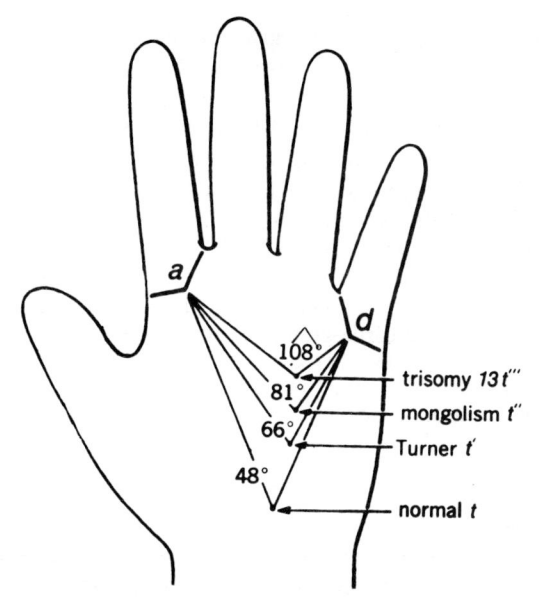

Fig. 24.7. Dermatoglyphics. The study of palm lines shows abnormalities in certain chromosome disorders.

TURNER'S SYNDROME

In this chromosomal disorder (trisomy 18) one of the physical signs consists of 'webbing' of the neck. Often this extends as far as the external ear and can narrow down the meatal orifice, especially when the auricle is flattened over the mastoid bone. One should note this possibility when the hearing of children with Turner's syndrome is tested by audiometry. The pressure of the large earphone can easily cause an occlusion of the meatal orifice and the resulting audiogram can simulate a moderate hearing loss. These children are also mentally retarded and not easy to test in clinics without adequate audiological facilities for children. As already mentioned, it has not been reliably ascertained whether hearing loss is part of the clinical picture of this syndrome.

FURTHER READING
SZPUNAR, J. and RYBAK, M. (1968). Middle ear disease in Turner's syndrome. *Archs Otolar.* **87**, 34–40.

JERVELL AND LANGE-NIELSEN SYNDROME

This relatively rare syndrome was first described by Jervell and Lange-Nielsen in 1957 in four of six sibs of a family. Fainting attacks occurred in three of the deaf children who died at the ages of four, five, and nine years respectively. The attacks of unconsciousness, probably Adams–Stokes types, caused by ventricular fibrilation, are usually provoked by mental stress or exercise. The electrocardiogram shows striking abnormalities and is characterized mainly by a gross prolongation of the QT interval, with abnormal T waves and is diagnostic of this condition. The hearing loss is severe. Cerebral dysrhythmia is said to occur in some cases.

Genetically, the deafness and cardiac lesion are pleiotropic effects of an abnormal gene in homozygous form, but the chain of causation involving the combination of the defects is unknown.

FURTHER READING
FRASER, G. R., FROGGETT, P., and JAMES, T. N. (1964). Congenital deafness associated with electro-cardiographic abnormalities, fainting attacks and sudden death. *Q. Jl Med.* **33**, 361–85.
FRIEDMAN, I., FRASER, G. R., and FROGGETT, P. (1966). Pathology of the ear in the cardio-auditory syndrome. *J. Lar. otol.* **80**, 451–70.
See also Chapters 12 and 13.

FANCONI SYNDROME

The main signs of this syndrome are congenital hypoplastic anaemia associated with multiple developmental defects. The pathogenesis of congenital hypoplastic anaemia is not clear. In many cases the disorder occurs sporadically in a child who is otherwise completely well, in the absence of other aetiological agents. These cases are assumed to result from a chance defect in the chromosomal mechanism for development of the bone marrow. In a child with sensorineural hearing loss (a high-frequency type), examined by the author, there was underdevelopment of the bones, so that the skeletal age was two to four years less than the chronological age. There was hypogenesis of the left thumb and agenesis of the right thumb and two carpal bones of the right hand. There was maldevelopment of the bones of the right foot.

FURTHER READING
ESTREN, S., SUESS, J. F. and DAMESHEK, W. (1947). Congenital hypoplastic anemia associated with multiple developmental defects (Fanconi syndrome). *J. Hemat.* **2**, 85–93.
SILVER, H. K., BLOIR, N. C., and KEMPE, C. H. (1952). Fanconi syndrome. *Am. J. Dis. Child.* **83**, 14.

NON-GENETIC SYNDROMES
ATHETOID CEREBRAL PALSY
Hyperbilirubinaemia is the cause of athetoid cerebral palsy, which is often associated with sensorineural hearing loss. Thirty per cent of all athetoid cerebral palsied children have a hearing impairment which can cause serious communication difficulties. The cause is the destruction of nerve cells in the cochlear nuclei by bilirubin which penetrated into the brain (kernicterus).

A level of bilirubin in the blood of a child with haemolytic disease which is considered as 'safe' from the point of view of causing cerebral palsy, may still cause damage in the cochlear nuclei. All children who have had neonatal jaundice should be considered to be at risk in respect of a high-frequency loss and their hearing should be tested until it can be proved to be normal. The audiogram has a characteristic pattern: this is a high-frequency loss but with the maximum degree of impairment in the 2000 Hz area as illustrated in Fig. 24.8. This is a good example of the relation between the type of congenital hearing loss (as readily revealed by the audiometric patterns) and its aetiology (Fisch 1955).

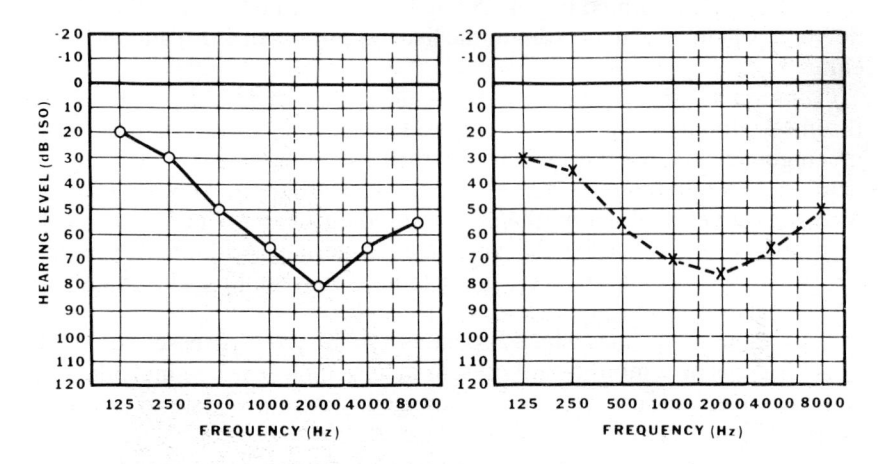

Fig. 24.8. Audiogram of a patient with hyperbilirubinaemia.

Cerebral palsied children may not be able to make normal use of the various accessory devices associated with sensory perception. These are almost invariably connected with muscular activity (e.g. trying to localize a source of a stimulus by turning the head). They have consequently difficulty in learning effectively from experience about happenings in the environment. These difficulties are often complicated by distractibility and perceptual problems. When in addition there is also a hearing impairment, the consequences can be serious. Unless the impairment is discovered in good time and steps are taken to alleviate its effects, a child will be badly affected by these additional disabilities.

All children with cerebral palsy of any type should have their hearing tested as soon as possible. If a hearing impairment is not discovered, even a very moderate one, the child may not learn to communicate and naturally this will affect his future in a decisive way. A very severely physically handicapped person with knowledge of language and ability to communicate it, may be better off than a moderately handicapped one without adequate language and with an inability to communicate.

RUBELLA SYNDROME

The rubella syndrome is a multisystem disease caused by infection during the first trimester of pregnancy. Foetal damage by rubella virus may result either from disruption of chromosomes or endothelial cell damage and thrombosis in small foetal blood vessels. Chromosomal damage induces infected cells to divide more slowly and the organs of rubella-infected children are therefore smaller and tend to have a subnormal number of cells (general miniaturization of the foetus). If this occurs during or before the critical period of organogenesis, multiple congenital defects may occur. Endothelial cell damage and thrombosis lead to tissue necrosis which may further affect malformed organs. Such defects may be found in the central nervous system, the myocardium, the liver, the organ of Corti and the inner ear.

Common transient features of the rubella syndrome are: low birth weight, thrombocytopenic purpura, hepatosplenomegaly, bone lesions, and meningoencephalitis. Permanent characteristic features are as follows: hearing loss, pulmonary stenosis, mental retardation, behavioural disorders, cataract and microphthalmos, retinopathy, patent ductus arteriosus, cryptorchidism, microcephaly, and inguinal hernia. Additional disorders observed are: myopia, diabetes, myocardial abnormalities, glaucoma, and dermatoglyphic abnormalities.

As in most syndromes which appear as a multisystem disease, not all the possible signs or symptoms are present in any single affected individual. In some cases only a few systems are damaged while other systems escape or are only slightly affected. In the rubella syndrome the multiplicity or degree of damage depends on many circumstances, some of them not fully understood. However, it is certain that various systems are most vulnerable during a critical stage of development, when the metabolic needs are very great during a high rate of cellular division.

The organ of Corti develops very rapidly during foetal life and its growth is completed by the twelfth week of pregnancy. Because of the high rate of cell division it is especially vulnerable to damage by virus infection at the critical stage. The maximum of damage probably occurs when the virus reaches the organ of Corti at the time of highest rate of cellular division.

The sensorineural hearing loss is characteristic for this syndrome. Almost invariably hearing is impaired to about the same degree for all the frequencies tested by pure-tone audiometry, thus producing more or less a flat audiogram. There are, of course, variations in this pattern and often it is a trough-sloped graph, with maximum impairment in the middle range of frequencies (see Fig. 24.9). Another very characteristic feature is the asymmetry of the hearing loss. Often the differences between the two ears are considerable, one severely and one very moderately or slightly affected. Unilateral hearing loss, as an extreme case of this asymmetry, is not a rare occurrence, as discovered by Jackson and Fisch in 1958 in a carefully controlled study. Reports concerning progression of the hearing loss as a characteristic part of the condition could not be confirmed. Undoubtedly in a certain percentage of cases a deterioration can be observed, but our own observations confirmed that in *all* types of congenital hearing loss in

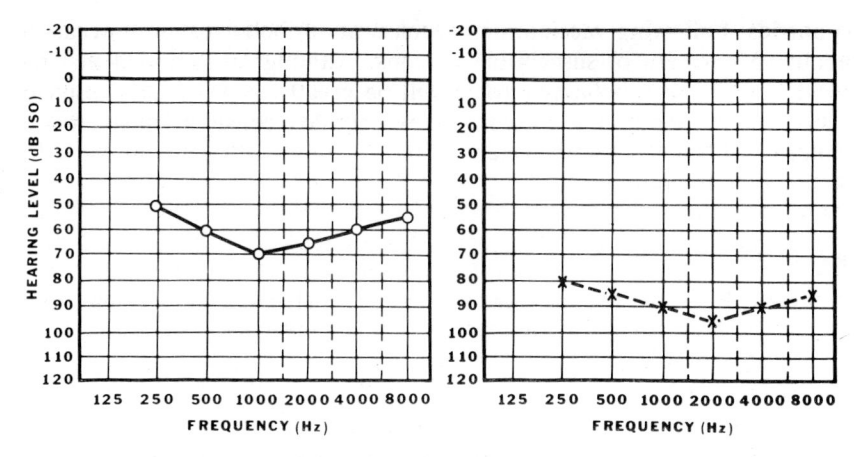

Fig. 24.9. Audiogram of a patient with a hearing loss due to maternal rubella.

children, including those who belong to any of the syndromes described in this chapter, a deterioration or progression of the impairment can be observed in a certain percentage of cases for a variety of reasons.

From the diagnostic point of view (when investigating a possible cause of hearing loss in a child), much depends on the accuracy of the history given by the pregnant woman and on the form of questioning of the doctor taking the history. It should be particularly stressed that 'history taking' by a questionnaire, to be completed by the patient, is often a most unreliable method.

In practice, it is often difficult for the doctor to decide when exposure to infection took place. If it is a recent contact (within the past 14 days) it is safer to collect blood on two occasions, separated by about a week, for testing to indicate any significant change in antibody titre. If there is no change the patient is already immune. A past history of rubella means little unless it was confirmed virologically. Full details of the patient's exposure to rubella must be known in order to make a serological assessment.

Following exposure to a rubella-like illness, infection can be contracted only if three conditions are satisfied simultaneously: (i) the patient must be susceptible; (ii) she must be exposed to a genuine case of rubella; and (iii) she must contract the infection as a result of close and prolonged contact with an infected person (rubella is less easy to catch than, for example measles or varicella) during the vulnerable stage of pregnancy (first trimester).

Many patients claim to have had rubella on more than one occasion. Virologically confirmed clinical re-infection is a very rare occurrence. Naturally acquired disease is followed by a very high rate of immunity. No woman has ever had more than a single congenitally infected infant (apart from rare cases of identical twins being infected).

Fortunately, this is yet another category of hearing impairment which is preventable. A vaccination programme of some sort operates now in many countries. Following vaccination a persistent antibody response occurs in about 95 per cent of susceptible persons. Although it is hoped that the incidence of the rubella syndrome will be greatly reduced as a result of vaccination programmes, one can still expect that a considerable number of children with hearing impairment as part of this syndrome will occur for some years to come.

REFERENCES

ALBERTI, P. W. R. M. and PARKANNEN, J. V. (1963). Stapedial otosclerosis: recent histochemical & histopathological observations. *Laryngoscope, St. Louis* **73**, 1184–200.

ALSTROM, C. H., HALLGREN, B., NILSSON, L. B. and ASUNDER, H. (1959). Retinal degeneration combined with obesity, diabetes mellitus & neurogenous deafness. *Acta psychiat. neurol. scand.* **34**, Suppl. 129.

BEANY, G. P. E. (1964). Otolaryngological problems arising during the management of severe renal failure. *J. Lar. Otol.* **78**, 507–15.

BEILSCHOWSKY, M. and SCHOFIELD, G. C. (1962). Studies on megacolon in piebald mice. *Aust. J. exp. Biol. Med. Sci.* **40**, 395–404.

BERRY, G. A. (1889). Note on a congenital defect (colomba of the lower lid). *Ophthal. Hosp. Rep., Lond.* **12**, 255–7.

BLAU, M. E. and SHEEHAN, J. C. (1958). Acute cerebellar syndrome of childhood. *Neurology, Minneap.* **8**, 538.

BRUYN, G. W. and WENT, L. N. (1964). A sex-linked heredo-degenerative neurological disorder associated with Leber's optic atrophy. Part 1. Clinical Studies. *J. neurol. Sci.* **1**, 59.

BURN, R. A. (1950). Deafness and Laurence–Moon–Biedl syndrome. *Br. J. Ophthal.* **34**, 64–88.

CHOLE, R. A. and QUICK, C. A. (1978). Estimate of vitamin A in the guinea pig cochlea. *Ann. Otol.* **87**, 380–2.

CROUZON, O. (1912). Disostose cranio-facial héréditaire. *Bull. Soc. méd. Hosp., Paris* **35**, 545–55.

DARWIN, C. (1859). *On the origin of species.* Murray, London.

DENNY-BROWN, D. (1951). Hereditary sensory radicular neuropathy. *J. Neurol. Neurosurg. Psychiat.* **14**, 237–52.

DEOL, M. S. (1970). The relationship between abnormalities of pigmentation and of the inner ear. *Proc. R. Soc.* **175**, 201–17.

FISCH, L. (1955). The aetiology of congenital deafness and audiometric patterns. *J. Lar. Otol.* **69**, 479–93.

—— (1959). Deafness as part of a hereditary syndrome. *J. Lar. Otol.* **73**, 355–382.

FRANCESCHETTI, A. and KLEIN, D. (1949). Mandibulo-facial dysotosis; a new hereditary syndrome. *Acta Ophthal.* **27**, 143–224.

—— FRANCOIS, J., BABEL, J., and DE ROUCK, A., et al. (1963). Les Hérédo-dégénerescences chorio-retiniennes (dégén. tapeto-retiniennes), 2 Vols. Masson, Paris.

GARDENER-MEDWIN, D. (1977). Children with genetic muscular disorders. *Br. J. hosp. Med.* **17**, 314–49.

GORLIN, R. J. and PINDBORG, J. J. (1964). *Syndromes of the head and neck*, pp. 138–45. McGraw-Hill, New York.

GREENWALD, I. (1960). Endemic goitre: heredity, deficiency, intoxication or infection. In *Clinical endocrinology*, Vol. 1 (ed. E. B. Astwood) pp. 123–32. Grune and Stratton, New York.

HACKETT, T. N. JR., BRAY, P. F., ZITER, F. A., NYHAN, W. L., and CREER, K. M. (1973). A metabolic myopathy associated with chronic lactic acidemia, growth failure and nerve deafness. *J. Pediat.* **83**, 426–31.

HALL, J. G. and RØHRT, T. (1968). The stapes in osteogenesis imperfecta. *Acta oto-lar.* **65**, 345–8.

HALLGREN, B. (1959). Retinitis pigmentosa combined with congenital deafness, vestibulo-cerebellar ataxia and mental abnormality in a proportion of cases. *Acta psychiat. scand.* Suppl. 138.

HAMBURGER, J., CROSMIER, J., LISSAE, J., and NAFFHA, J. (1956). Sur un syndrome familial de nephrophathie avec surdité: *J. Urol. Méd. chir.* **62**, 113–24.

HERMAN, C., AGUILAR, M. J. and SACHS, O. (1964). Hereditary photomyoclonus associated with diabetes mellitus, deafness, nephropathy and cerebral dysfunction. *Neurology, Minneap.* **14**, 212–21.

HICKS, E. P. (1922). Hereditary perforating ulcer of the foot. *Lancet* **i**, 319–21.

HINCHCLIFFE, R., OSUKTOKUN, B. O., and ADENGA, A. O. G. (1972). Hearing levels in Nigerian ataxic neuropathy. *Audiology* **11**, 218–30.

JACKSON, A. D. M. and FISCH, L. (1958). Deafness following maternal rubella: Results of a prospective investigation. *Lancet* **ii**, 1241–4.

JACKSON, W. P. V., ALBRIGHT, F., DREWRY, G., HANELIN, J., and RUBIN, M. I. (1954). Metaphyseal dysplasia, epiphyseal dysplasia, diaphyseal dysplasia, and related conditions; familial metaphyseal dysplasia and craniometaphyseal dysplasia; their relation to leontiasis ossea and osteopetrosis; disorders of "bone remodeling". *Archs intern. Med.* **94**, 871–85.

JERVELL, A. and LANGE-NIELSEN, F. (1957). Congenital deaf-mutism, functional heart disease with prolongation of the QT interval and sudden death. *Am. Heart J.* **54**, 59–68.

KEARNS, T. P. and SAYRE, G. P. (1958). Retinitis pigmentosa, external ophthalmoplegia and complete heart block: unusual syndrome with histologic study in one of two cases. *Archs Ophthal.* **60**, 280–9.

LATHAM, A. D. and MUNRO, T. A. (1938). Familial myoclonus epilepsy associated with deaf-mutism in a family showing other psychobiological abnormalities. *Ann. Eugen.* **8**, 166–75.

LIVINGSTONE, G. L. (1959). The establishment of sound conduction in congenital deformities of the external ear. *J. Lar. Otol.* **73**, 231–41.

—— and DELOHUNTY, J. E. (1968). Malformations of the ear associated with congenital ophthalmic and other conditions. *J. Lar. Otol.* **82**, 495–504.

MCKENZIE, J. (1958). The first arch syndrome. *Archs Dis. Child.* **33**, 477–86.

MCKUSICK, V. A. (1966). *Heritable disorders of connective tissue*, 3rd edn. Mosby, St. Louis.

—— (1973). Congenital deafness and Hirschsprung's disease. *New Engl. J. Med.* **288**, 691.

MARAN, A. G. D. (1964). The Treacher Collins syndrome. *J. Lar. Otol.* **78**, 135–51.

MAY, D. L. and WHITE, H. H. (1968). Familial myoclonus, cerebellar ataxia and deafness: specific genetically determined disease. *Archs Neurol., Chicago* **19**, 331–8.

MENKES, J. H. (1974). Introduction: the treatment of paroxysmal disorders. *Pediatrics, Springfield* **53**, 529–30.

MUNRO, M. (1956). Sensory radicular neuropathy in a deaf child. *Br. med. J.* **i**, 541–4.
NELSON, W. E. (1964). *Text book of pediatrics*, 8th edn. Saunders, Philadelphia.
OPHEIM, O. (1968). Loss of hearing following the syndrome of van der Hoeve–de Kleyn. *Acta oto-lar.* **65**, 337–44.
OPPIKOFER, E. (1935). Histologische Ohrveränderungen bei Niemann-Pickscher Krankheit. *Z. Hals. Nasen u. Ohrenheilk.* **39**, 77–84.
PAPERELLA, M. M. (1969). *Sensorineural deafness in children.* Medical Audiology Workship, Veil, Colorado.
PERKHOFF, G. T. (1967). The hereditary renal diseases. *New Engl. J. Med.* **277**, 79–85; 129–38.
PRIEST, J. H. (1967). Dermatoglyphics in ectodermal dysplasia. *Lancet* **ii**, 1093.
SCHAFER, I. A., SCRIVER, C. R., and EFRON, M. L. (1962). Familial hyperprolinemia, cerebral dysfunction and renal anomalies occurring in a family with hereditary nephropathy and deafness. *New Engl. J. Med.* **267**, 51–60.
SCHNECK, L., ADACHI, M., BRIET, P., WOLLINTZ, A., and VOLK, B. W. (1973). Ophthalmoplegia with morphological and chemical studies of cerebellar and muscle tissue. *J. neurol. Sci.* **19**, 37–44.
SCRIVER, C. R., SCHAFER, I. A., and EFRON, M. L. (1961). New renal tubular amino-acid transport system and a new hereditary disorder of amino-acid metabolism. *Nature, Lond.* **192**, 672–3.
SHAPIRA, Y., CEDERBAUM, S. D., CONCILLA, P. A., NIELSSEN, D., and LIPPE, B. M. (1975). Familial poliodystrophy, mitochondrial myopathy and lactate acidaemia. *Neurology, Minneap.* **25**, 614.
STEINBERG, D., HERNDON, J. H. JR, UHLENDORF, B. W. *et al.* (1967). Refsum's disease: nature of the enzyme defect. *Science, N.Y.* **156**, 1740–2.
TARLOW, M. J., LAKE, B. D., and LLOYD, J. K. (1973). Chronic lactic acidosis in association with myopathy. *Archs Dis. Child.* **48**, 489–92.
TREACHER COLLINS, E. (1900). IX Congenital abnormalities: cases 8 & 9 with symmetrical congenital notches in the outer part of each lower lid and defective development of the malar bones. *Trans. ophthal. Soc. U.K.* **20**, 190–2.
VAN DYKE, J. H. (1942). The development of ultimobranchial cysts in the thyroid gland of rats on a vitamin A deficient diet. *Anat. Rec.* **82**, 451.
—— (1943). The behaviour of ultimobranchial tissue in the post-natal thyroid gland of sheep. *Anat. Rec.* **85**, 342.
—— (1944). Behaviour of ultimobranchial tissue in the post-natal thyroid gland: the origin of cystadenoma in the rat. *Anat. Rec.* **88**, 369–91.
—— (1945). The behaviour of ultimobranchial tissue in the post-natal thyroid gland; epithelial cysts, their relation to thyroid parenchyma and to new growths in thyroid gland of young sheep. *Am. J. Anat.* **76**, 201–51.
WAARDENBURG, P. J. (1951). A new syndrome combining developmental anomalies of the eyelids, eyebrows and nose root with pigmentary defects of the iris and head hair and with congenital deafness. *Am. J. hum. Genet.* **3**, 195–253.
WALSH, M. P. (1979). Screening for neonatal hypothyroidism. *Br. J. hosp. Med.*, 28–36.
WEINMANN, J. P. and SICHER, H. (1955). *Bone and bones, fundamentals of bone biology*, 2nd edn.
WIBAU, F. (1931). XXXI Studien über Retinitis Pigmentosa. *Klin. Mbl. Augenheilk.* **87**, 298–307.
WILSON, J. (1963). Leber's hereditary optic atrophy; some clinical and aetiological considerations. *Brain* **86**, 347–62.

WILDERWANCK, L. S., HOEKSEME, P. E., and PENNING, L. (1965). Radiological examination of the inner ear of deaf-mutes presenting the cervico-oculo-acusticus syndrome. *Acta oto-lar.* **61**, 445–53.

YARINGTON, C. T. and SPRINKLE, P. (1967). Hearing problems in certain forms of osteodystrophy. The chondrodystrophies. *Eye Ear Nose Throat Mon.* **46**, 1136–8.

25 Diagnosis of hearing loss in infants and young children

M. V. BICKERTON and H. A. BEAGLEY

HISTORICAL INTRODUCTION

In 1911 the Chief Medical Officer of the Board of Education in his annual report wrote 'Among the requirements of a satisfactory scheme of medical inspection is that of applying a hearing test to every child who is old enough to respond' (Board of Education 1911). This was the first occasion on which a routine hearing check had been recommended by a Statutory Authority, and the hearing of live speech was to be used for testing. It was not until 1930 that the gramophone audiometer was introduced by the school health service of Birmingham, London, and the London Borough of Tottenham (Board of Education 1931). In the 1940s pure-tone audiometry began to replace gramophone audiometry and it was at about this time that Professor Sir Alexander and Lady Ewing at Manchester University and Miss Edith Whetnall at The Royal National Throat, Nose, and Ear Hospital in London were urging the need for the diagnosis of hearing handicaps before the age of two years. This led to clinics being established for the diagnosis of the hearing-impaired children, with facilities for auditory training and parent guidance.

PRESENT-DAY ARRANGEMENTS

There is now a scheme for the screening of both pre-school and school-age children throughout the United Kingdom. Those who are suspected of having a hearing loss are referred to the many audiology centres attached both to hospitals and to health centres throughout the country for diagnosis of deafness and its treatment, where practicable, and for the management of any remaining hearing loss which is not amenable to medical or surgical treatment. The methods and principles of diagnosis and management of hearing impaired children will be illustrated by reference to the Nuffield Hearing and Speech Centre in London where both authors have clinical responsibilities and to the Hertfordshire Area Health Authority where one of us (MVB) has overall clinical responsibility.

The Hertfordshire Area Health Authority covers an urban and semi-rural area north of London, where in 1976 there was a population of 217 900 children under the age of 15 years. The Nuffield Hearing and Speech Centre is a department of The Royal National Throat, Nose, and Ear Hospital, London, and is essentially a reference centre devoted almost entirely to children suspected of hearing and speech defects. The total number of new cases attending the Centre in 1978 was 1130, while 4677 old cases were reviewed.

HEARING TESTING ENVIRONMENT

It is essential that audiology testing rooms should have a low ambient noise level and therefore, many centres now have purpose-built sound-treated rooms both for clinical examination and for audiometry. In order to give sufficient space for testing, the clinic room should measure not less than 6 × 5 metres (20 feet by 16 feet). Rooms used only for audiometry can be smaller, but there must be space for a parent to accompany the child. Very small rooms or booths become claustrophobic for the staff and particularly for the children. Ideally the sound treated rooms should be sited away from outside noise such as car parks and busy roads and away from sources of noise within the building, i.e. waiting rooms, play rooms, typewriters, passenger and goods lifts, etc. Noisy surroundings can lead to much wastage of time, and even more important, to unreliable test results. Audiology clinic rooms and test rooms should be provided in the plans for any new hospital or health centre. It would also be advantageous if all new schools had acoustically treated rooms away from the general noise of the school so that screening hearing tests can be performed in a low ambient noise level; such, unfortunately, is rarely the case today.

SCREENING TESTS OF HEARING

Although the progress of the child's hearing and speech is noted at each of the four routine developmental checks made by medical officers on children under 18 months of age, it is recommended by The Department of Health and Social Security (DHSS) that all babies, whether on the 'At Risk' register or not, should have a screening hearing test when the baby can sit unsupported, i.e. between the ages of 7–9 months. In Hertfordshire these routine tests are usually performed by health visitors; these specially trained nurses have an attachment to a group of general practitioners. It is one of their responsibilities to test the hearing of all the babies in the practice. The methods used are distraction tests based on the methods described by Ewing (1957) or the Stycar tests of hearing as described by Mary Sheriden (1968). These will be discussed later. Although every endeavour is made to test all babies, it must not be assumed that each baby has had the test for inevitably some are missed, e.g. through non-attendance or because of moving from one district to another, or as a result of immigration. In a survey in 1976 (Frost, Knight, and Sharp, unpublished) when 1092 babies were tested at the age of approximately 8 months by 20 health visitors in Hertfordshire 980 (89.7 per cent) passed on the first attempt, a further 97 (8.9 per cent) passed a few weeks later on the second or third attempts, and the 15 (1.4 per cent) who failed were referred for further investigation. Health visitors with the help of an assistant usually carried out these tests in a health centre as testing

642 Diagnosis of hearing loss in infants and young children

in home conditions had been found to be unsatisfactory. Similarly, testing single-handed is not a reliable procedure and is discouraged in Hertfordshire.

In order to determine the effectiveness of the method used in Hertfordshire a survey was undertaken of the 51 congenitally deaf children of under 5 years of age using hearing aids and of those referred initially to the Hertfordshire audiology service (42), it was found that 76 per cent of them had been diagnosed under the age of 13 months and 93 per cent by the age of 18 months (Fig. 25.1). The other nine children in the area using hearing aids had been referred initially to other diagnostic centres.

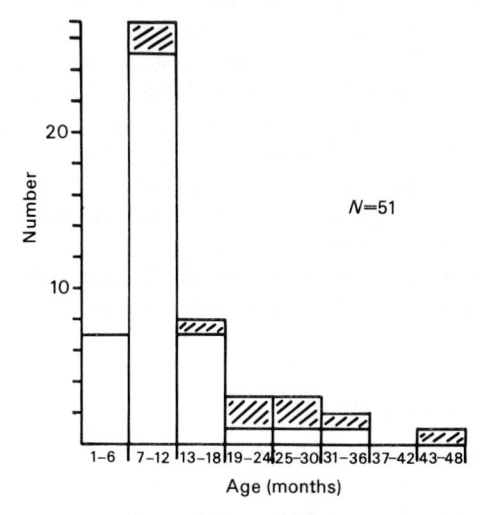

Fig. 25.1. This histogram shows the ages when the diagnosis of a hearing loss was made on all the children under the age of five years, using hearing aids and living in Hertfordshire in March, 1979 (51 in all). Those represented by the unshaded cells (42) were diagnosed initially by the Hertfordshire Audiology Service whereas the remaining nine (hatched) were referred initially to other centres outside Hertfordshire.

Infants of between 2 and 5 years of age have annual general developmental examinations; in infant welfare clinics these include an assessment of hearing and speech using age-appropriate spoken voice tests and language progress assessments. Where there is any doubt regarding the hearing or speech development an audiology referral for the under four year olds, or audiometric testing for the 4–5-year-old children can be arranged. In addition, all children having speech therapy, except those being treated for a stutter, are given a hearing test, usually a pure-tone audiogram (PTA). Children with other handicaps such as mental retardation, blindness or cerebral palsy are usually referred to an audiology centre for hearing assessment to determine whether or not there is a dual or multiple handicap. A psychological assessment is also obtained whenever this is considered appropriate.

During a child's first four terms at school there is a further routine screening test based on pure-tone audiometry (Fig. 25.2) and in the Hertfordshire Area Health Authority (AHA) this is repeated once in subsequent school years. In order to save time the children are divided into groups of about ten and are taken into a quiet room where the test is demonstrated to the whole group, then each child is tested individually, care being taken that each child fully understands the test before commencing. The child is asked to move a brick on a form-board, or any other play technique, whenever he hears a sound. The following six frequencies are used: 250, 500 1000, 2000, 4000, and 8000 Hz, all at 25 dB ISO. The time intervals between the sounds are varied and when necessary the sound is alternated between the two ears. A child who fails to hear *any two* of the six frequencies presented is referred for a complete pure-tone audiogram. This technique allows for large numbers of children to be tested quickly. With the co-operation of the teaching staff and helpers it may be possible to test as many as 50 children in a three-hour session. In 1976, 22 302 children were tested in 428 schools; the failure rate was 1655 or 7 per cent. Seasonal conditions can influence the failure rate, e.g. upper respiratory tract infections in February and March and allergic conditions in May and June. The lowest failure rate is usually in September. Care should be taken to ensure that audiometers are kept in good working order and are calibrated periodically (see Chapter 8).

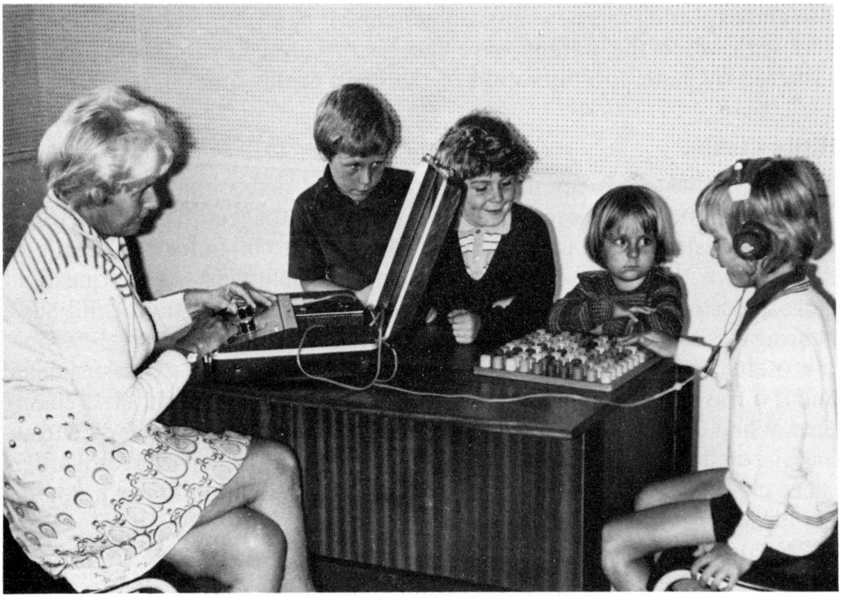

Fig. 25.2. School screening audiometry. The children behind the desk are watching one of their fellows being tested; this speeds up the explanatory process and increases the numbers of tests per hour. (Courtesy, the Editor *Nursing Mirror*.)

Children who fail this screening test are tested at a later date by means of a complete audiogram, preferably by both air and bone conduction. It is found that a child who has a hearing threshold of 30 dB or more in both ears usually has difficulty hearing both in the classroom and at home, and as long as this is not due to a transient condition, such as a common cold, further investigation and treatment is recommended. The school doctor and the general practitioner are informed of the results. With the case history and the result of the audiogram the child can be referred as required for otological or audiological opinions.

Besides these routine checks, a school child can be referred at any time for audiometry by school doctors, general practitioners, educational psychologists, teachers, or speech therapists should there be *any doubt* regarding his hearing. If the audiogram is outside normal limits further investigation can be instigated.

CLINICAL ASSESSMENT AT AN AUDIOLOGY CENTRE

It is of the utmost importance that a child coming for audiological assessment should find a happy and relaxed atmosphere at the assessment centre; toys and books in the waiting areas are of particular help to the child who is fearful of hospitals. It is recommended that white coats are not worn by the staff as this frequently arouses memories of injections. When a child comes into the room for assessment he should be given the opportunity of settling into and exploring this new environment and if he wishes he is given a toy to play with while the parents give the history. Much information can be gathered by general observation of the child at this time.

History taking

A detailed history is often the only means of determining the cause of deafness, as most diagnoses have to be made in retrospect. It is helpful to use a questionnaire for the initial history taking and to fill in further details on discussion with the parents. (See Appendix for Nuffield Centre questionnaire.) It is important to enquire if the parents think that their child has a hearing loss as it is found that parents who do suspect a loss are rarely wrong. It is useful to know the age of the child when the deafness was first suspected and if it was noticed initially by the parents or at a routine school screening test. When discovered on routine testing the child may have been hearing-impaired for a long period, even from birth and it may be difficult in these circumstances to convince the parents that their child has a hearing handicap.

The present history in a case of conductive hearing loss may reveal generalized upper respiratory tract infections, acute or chronic otitis media, tonsillitis, sinusitis, nasal obstructions, or discharge or the presence of allergies, any of which may affect the hearing. It must be remembered that any sensorineural loss can have a conductive overlay thereby adding to the disability, and as the conductive element is generally amenable to medical or surgical treatment this should be arranged.

Family history

The causes of hereditary deafness are described in Chapters 12, 13, and 24 and these are borne in mind when taking the family history. A very detailed enquiry is made when there are any cases with a family history of deafness. Parental consanguinity obviously increases the risk of hereditary deafness. Occasionally parents do not suspect a hearing loss in themselves and therefore it is sometimes helpful to test their hearing and also that of other members of the family, preferably by doing an audiogram; a characteristic pattern of hearing loss may then be seen, albeit of greater or lesser severity. Furthermore, deaf parents frequently fail to notice a hearing loss in their children particularly when the child has a little more hearing than they themselves, for in these instances the child will respond to sounds that the parents cannot hear and therefore the lesser degree of hearing loss is not appreciated. In the eight-year period (1970–7) when 2074 cases of sensorineural hearing losses were reviewed at the Nuffield Centre genetic causes accounted for 11.7 per cent.

Prenatal history

Details of the prenatal history, with particular note made of any infections or illnesses or of any drugs taken during the pregnancy, may reveal a possible cause of deafness. Rubella of pregnancy, particularly when occurring in the first trimester, has long been known to cause congenital abnormalities in the baby. A sensorineural hearing loss, commonly bilateral was diagnosed in 59 per cent of confirmed cases of congenital rubella in The National Congenital Rubella Surveillance 1971–5 (Sheppard, Smithells, Peckham, Dudgeon, and Marshall 1977).

This survey of 354 confirmed or suspected rubella cases showed that only 160 (45 per cent) mothers gave a history of rubella with a rash in pregnancy. A further 55 (16 per cent) mothers said that they had been in contact with rubella but had not suffered a subsequent clinical illness and 46 (13 per cent) had an undiagnosed rash. A rising titre in the absence of clinical signs was demonstrated in four women (1 per cent) and the remaining 89 (25 per cent) mothers were unaware of any contact with rubella, or had been well throughout their pregnancies. Therefore, from these figures it is obvious that a lack of history of rubella does not preclude the possibility of a rubella deafness. Between 1970 and 1977, according to the year in question, maternal rubella accounted for between 9.4 per cent and 15 per cent of the cases of sensorineural hearing loss referred to the Nuffield Centre. Peckham, Martin, Marshall, and Dudgeon (1979) give an extensive analysis of hearing and other defects in sero-positive children at the Nuffield Centre over the period 1972–5.

Congenital cytomegalovirus causes certain abnormalities of the central nervous system and is suspected of causing deafness in some cases. This infection is frequently asymptomatic and undiagnosed until the virus is discovered during routine investigation of the child's urine. Other virus infections during pregnancy, such as measles, influenza, chicken pox, mumps, or herpes simplex are also thought to be a possible cause of damage to the hearing of the developing foetus.

Drugs taken during pregnancy can damage the hearing of the foetus. Thalidomide given to pregnant women some years ago produced bizarre teratogenic effects, occasionally resulting in deafness from congenital abnormalities of the ears. McKinna (1966) reported two cases of congenital deafness in infants whose mothers had taken large doses of quinine prenatally. Conway and Birt (1965) warn that streptomycin taken in pregnancy can cause eighth nerve damage. Moreover, this antibiotic can cross the placental barrier (Robinson and Cambon 1964) (see Chapter 23).

Perinatal history

Difficulties in the perinatal period such as prematurity, asphyxia, kernicterus, and brain damage owing to birth trauma may cause a hearing loss. Babies who have a birth weight of less than 2.25 kg have an increased risk of damage during labour, as the tissues at this time are very susceptible to hypoxia and scattered haemorrhages can occur in the cochlear nuclei and auditory pathways.

Haemolytic disease of the newborn due to Rhesus incompatibility is now only rarely a cause of deafness because the babies who develop blood bilirubin levels of greater than 20 mg per cent are given exchange transfusions, and damage to the cochlear nuclei and auditory pathways is thereby generally prevented. The hearing loss sustained in the perinatal period from both hypoxia or jaundice is usually a high-tone loss. These cases may not be presented for diagnosis in early infancy, because the child is able to hear the vowels of speech which consist predominantly of lower frequencies, and he can learn to recognize the consonants by lip-reading. In these cases the presenting symptom may be a speech defect.

Past history

An inquiry should be made of any illnesses, head injuries or surgical operations the child may have had, and where possible note made of any treatment given. Meningitis can occasionally be a cause of a severe or total hearing loss. As the child will have been very ill the deafness may not have been noticed initially and speech deterioration may not present itself for a few weeks or even months after recovery from the illness. Since early rehabilitation of these children is vital to maintain speech patterns, it is recommended that every child who has had meningitis should, as soon as possible after the illness, have a hearing test.

A sensorineural hearing loss can be due to mumps; it is usually partial and unilateral and is generally followed by recovery, though total irreversible deafness can occur. In Finland 298 servicemen with mumps parotitis were investigated by Vuori, Lahikainen, and Peltoren in 1962 and there were 13 cases of deafness (4 per cent) one of which progressed to complete loss of hearing in one ear.

Head injuries resulting in trauma to the middle ear, cochlea, or auditory nerve and pathways may cause a unilateral or rarely a bilateral hearing loss.

An increasing number of drugs have been found to be ototoxic. As nearly all ototoxic drugs are eliminated through the kidneys, their ototoxicity is greater in cases of renal impairment with a rapid rise of the blood level of the drug. The following are some of the more common drugs known or suspected of being ototoxic: streptomycin, dihydrostreptomycin, neomycin, kanamycin, gentamycin, viomycin, framycetin, vancomycin, and polymyxin B. Neomycin and framycetin are too toxic for systemic use as they invariably cause deafness if used this way (Noone 1978). Ototoxic effects have also been suspected from the use of antibiotic ear drops and it can certainly occur when potentially ototoxic drugs, and especially neomycin, are used in the topical treatment of extensive skin infections, or burns. Similarly, the instillation of such drugs into large abscess cavities (e.g. empyema cavities) can lead to toxic blood levels owing to absorption from the extensive granulating surface of the infected cavity so treated.

The General Appearance of the Child

The child can be observed while he is playing in the clinic, for there may be evidence of a syndrome associated with hearing loss such as those described in Chapter 24 a case of Waardenburg's, Treacher–Collins', Klippel–Feil, or Hurler's syndrome for example may be very readily recognized. Careful watch can be made for any additional handicap, which may need treatment, or which may affect the future management of the child.

A detailed examination of the ears, nose, and throat is desirable in every child seen in the audiology clinic, but occasionally if the child is likely to be upset by such an examination, it may be preferable to leave this examination until the hearing has been tested. Ophthalmoscopy may be possible and helpful in some cases. The child's speech should be listened to so that the quality, intonation, and any defects of pronounciation, as well as the child's understanding of speech, can be noted and where necessary a referral for further investigation arranged.

HEARING TESTS

The baby can be tested by means of 'distraction' tests of hearing and the toddler may perform 'conditioned' tests of hearing, i.e. tests based on operant conditioning. The easiest time to use the distraction tests is at the age of about 7–9 months, when the baby will sit still on the mother's lap and will turn repeatedly to the testing sounds. When a mental age of 3 years is obtained the child should be able to give a reliable conditioned response, i.e. by giving a learned response when a sound is heard. Under the age of 6 months and between the ages of 18 months to 3 years variations of these standard tests are used to suit the abilities of the infant.

Distraction tests for the 6–18-month-old babies

The distraction tests as originally devised by the Ewings in Manchester, and those later described in great detail by Mary Sheridan in her Stycar tests of hearing are valuable tests for the 6–9-month-old babies both for the routine screening as well as the audiology clinic situation. Although the many people doing the test use their own variations of the basic scheme, the test sounds in common use are: (i) conversational voice; (ii) whispered voice; (iii) whispered 's' sound; (iv) high-tone rattle; (v) the rustle of thin cellophane paper (approx. 5 cm square); and (vi) the tinkle of a spoon on the rim of a china cup. All these sounds are of interest to a baby and it is when a baby is able to sit unaided and has normal hearing that he will usually respond by turning to whichever side these sounds are presented.

The conversational voice although it is of higher intensity than the required 30 dB has been included as many clinicians consider that once the mother has seen her baby respond, she relaxes and hence the baby settles, and the remaining tests can be performed; however, some clinicians, instead of using live voice *before* the other test sounds as described above, prefer to use it *after* the other sounds have been presented. All the other sounds are produced at an intensity of about 30 dB SPL which is comfortably above the threshold level of the normal baby's hearing.

Testing is performed with the baby sitting on the mother's lap facing an observer. The tester stands diagonally behind the baby, in order to be out of his field of vision, first on one side and then on the other, producing the test sounds for up to 10 seconds and if necessary repeating after a pause at a distance of 1 to $1\frac{1}{2}$ m from the baby (Fig. 25.3) and on the level of the baby's head. The tester should get into position very quietly and, after a pause, and with a minimum of movement, should produce the required sound. When the baby turns the tester should acknowledge the response. The observer who is seated in front of the mother and child uses a single toy or gentle movements of the hands to attract the baby's attention to the front prior to the test sounds. It is helpful as a variation for the observer occasionally to hide the toy or to stop hand movements prior to the testing sound, so that the baby is at maximum distractability at the crucial moment. Excessive efforts of the assistant to fix the child's attention can result in failure of the child to respond to the quiet test sounds. Should the baby get a toy in his hand, or especially if sucking an object, he may not be distracted by the test sound. A retarded child usually needs to hear the sound for a prolonged period before he responds (Figs. 25.4 and 25.5(a)–(d)).

Should a baby fail to respond to these quiet sounds, a louder sound should be used to obtain a response, e.g. a louder voice, or bringing the test sounds nearer the ear. The baby may respond to the portable free-field audiometer on any or all of the five frequencies at a distance of 1 metre from the ear at increasing intensities up to an 80 dB level. The more severely deaf child may need a loud shout, a loud xylophone tone or the bang of a drum before giving a response; the latter is probably a response to vibration.

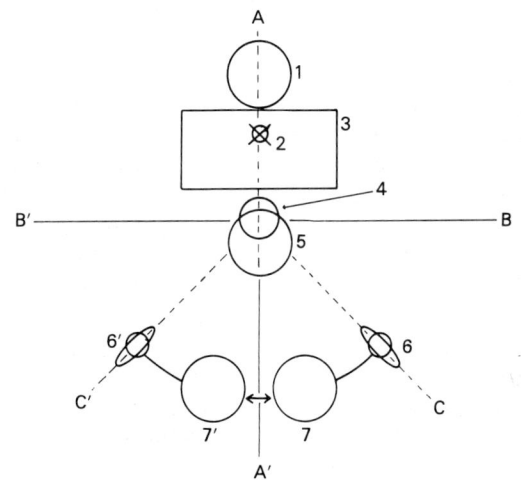

Fig. 25.3. This diagram shows the relative position of the mother (5), child (4), tester (7, 7') and the assistant (1) during distraction testing. Other features are the table (3)—which is optional—the toy (2) that the assistant uses to keep the child's eyes looking forwards as the sounds are presented at one or other side of the child (6, 6') by the tester. The lines AA' and BB' respectively are the child's visual axis and his inter-aural axis when looking straight ahead. The dotted lines drawn from the centre of the child's head to C and C', each at 45° to the axis AA', enclose the area in which the tester operates. Neither the tester's hand nor the noise maker should pass in front of these as there is then the danger that the child may detect them visually and give a false-positive response (see text).

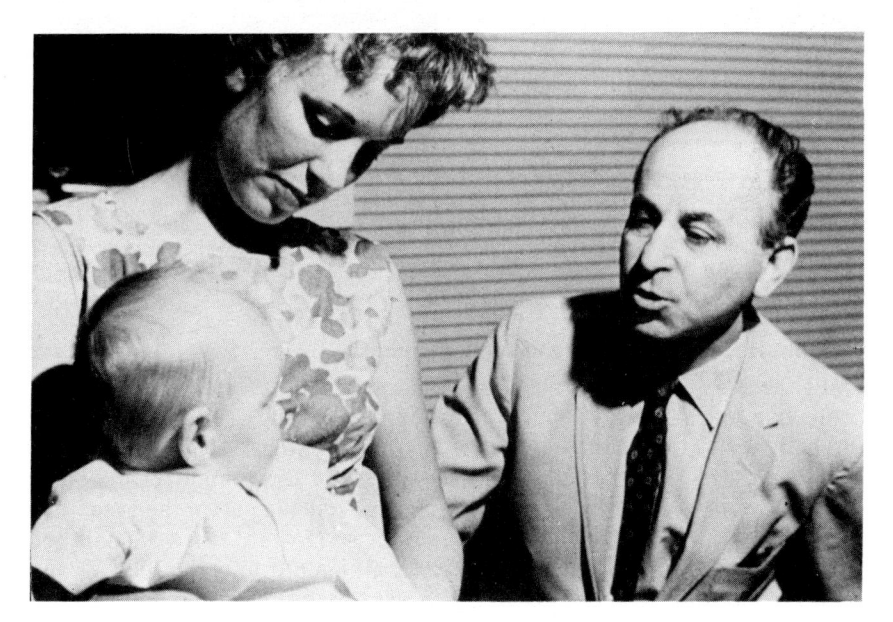

Fig. 25.4. A child turning to an 's–s–s' sound.

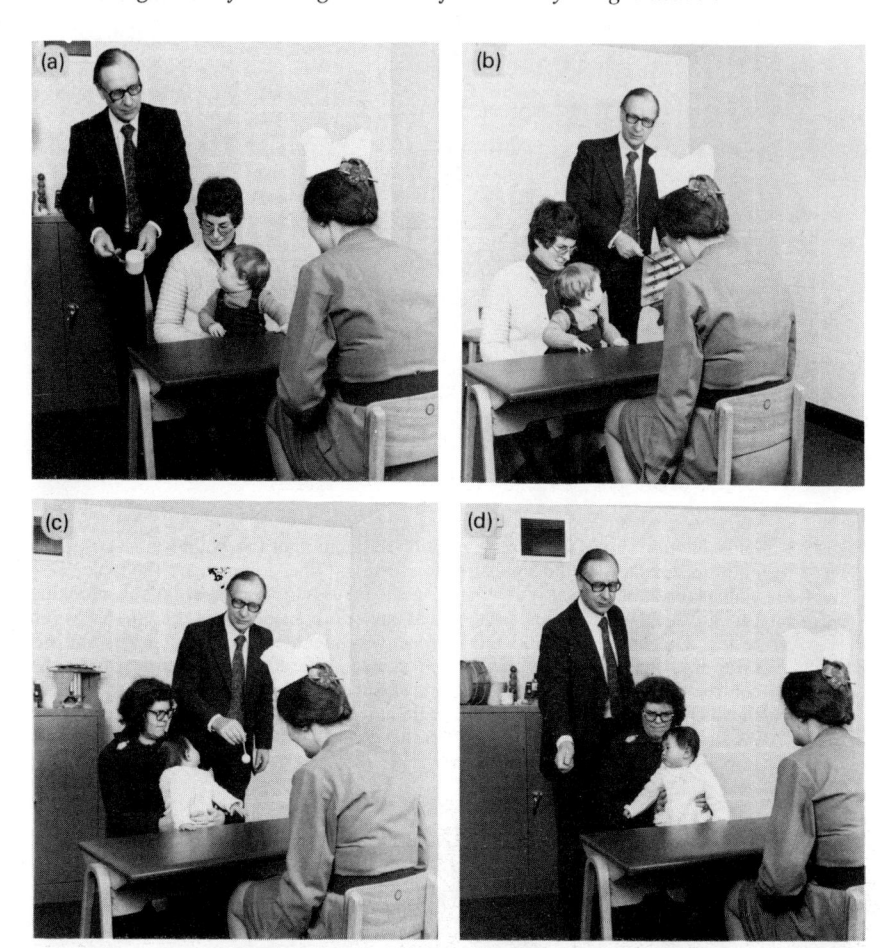

Fig. 25.5. A child responding (a) to the tinkling of a cup and spoon; (b) to a *very light* tap on a xylophone; (c) to a high-frequency rattle; and (d) to the crinkling of a piece of cellophane. In each case the child turned promptly and unambiguously to the source of the sound, suggesting normal auditory acuity. (Note that the xylophone is generally reserved for children who have failed to respond to quieter sounds.)

Hearing tests for the babies of under 6 months

Until the baby is 8 weeks old, he will respond to sound by a primitive protective reflex known as the Moro reflex. On hearing a sudden loud sound the baby will show a startle response by a jerky extension of the spine and limbs followed by a quick bowing movement of the arms over the chest usually accompanied by a cry and widening or screwing up of the eyes. At 6 weeks of age movements may momentarily be 'frozen' when a small bell held at a distance of 8–12 cm from the ear is rung gently for a few seconds and then repeated after a short pause; the eyes may then move towards the sound.

Babies of 4–6 months, before they are able to sit up unaided, often fail to respond to the previously described distraction or turning tests, but they may respond if the test is slightly varied as follows: the baby is held lying in the mother's lap (see Fig. 25.6) and the tester instead of standing behind the child, sits in front on a low stool close to the baby and with outstretched arms holding a sound producer in each hand slightly behind and on each side of the baby's head. For example, a piece of cellophane can be held in one hand and a high-tone rattle in the other, while a third sound can be produced by the voice. By this method the baby seems to find it easier to follow the arms of the tester and turn to sounds as they are repeated a number of times. For example, should the baby be looking at the rattle in the tester's left hand, a sound is made with the paper on the right and the hearing baby can be seen to turn; voice is then used to draw the baby's gaze back to the front. Care must be taken that the baby does not see the movement of the hand as the sound is being produced. Even if the baby responds in this way it is *strongly recommended* that he be retested with the more reliable distraction tests between the ages of 6–12 months or when he has reached the stage of being able to sit up unsupported.

Intensity of test sounds

When learning to do distraction tests of hearing on children it is very useful

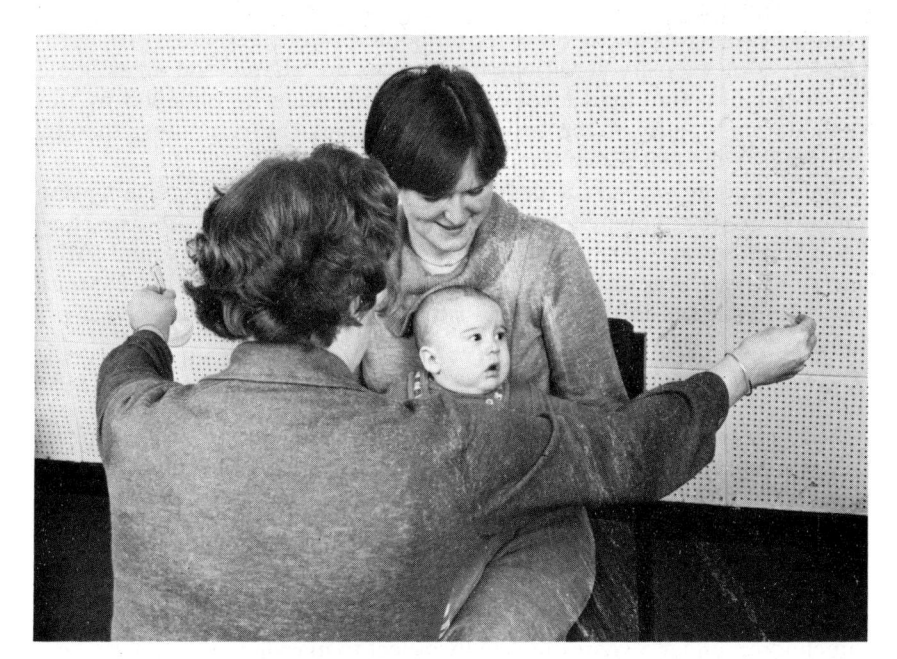

Fig. 25.6. A child of four months, too young to sit unsupported, is tested from the front by the tester who can use a noise maker in either hand (piece of cellophane, R, and a high frequency rattle, L) as well as voice. See text for a clear explanation of the uses and limitations of this test.

to measure the intensity of the test sounds with a sound level meter. It is very important not to use sounds louder than intended; this is unfortunately a frequent failing. Most testers, however, when they have learnt to estimate the intensity of sounds discard the sound level meter because they find it impossible to observe the child closely and at the same time watch the sound level meter, nor it is not possible to *repeat* the sound at progressively lower intensity levels without causing the baby to become habituated and unresponsive. So much can be learnt from keeping a close watch on the child's expression that we do not recommend the use of the sound level meter during the test procedure.

Tests with the portable free-field audiometer for children of 10 months–3 years

The portable free-field audiometer is an extremely useful instrument in the clinic room when working with young children. Pure tones of 250, 500, 1000, 2000, and 4000 Hz can be produced with intensities increasing in 5 dB steps from 0 dB–80 dB SPL at a distance of 1 metre. (See Chapter 8 for a description of the calibration technique for this type of audiometer.)

One method can be used with a baby of about 10 months to 2 years, who is placed on the mother's lap facing a table. The tester, who is seated on the other side of the table, positions the audiometer to one side of the baby and holds a small distracting toy on the other side. The baby's eyes can frequently be seen to glance over to the audiometer when a sound is produced. The levels of intensity at various frequencies are altered and an estimate of the binaural free field level of hearing can often be obtained by this method, particularly if the tester acknowledges the responses, thereby encouraging the child's continued co-operation.

Some children will give a 'conditioned' response by holding a miniature animal toy to the audiometer and will wait for the noise to be produced (see Fig. 25.7); they are taught to withdraw the toy on hearing the sound. After one or two demonstrations it is frequently possible to obtain a useful threshold estimate in the free-field situation in the case of a 2–3-year-old child

Spoken voice tests

When testing children of over $2\frac{1}{2}$ years it is most helpful initially to do free-field speech tests so that there is a rough guide to the child's level of hearing prior to audiometry. The child is placed at one end of the room and allowed to watch the tester whose mouth is covered by a sheet of paper to prevent lip-reading: the conversational voice and whispered voice are used at increasing distances from the child. Each ear can be tested individually in the older child if the non-test ear is masked by rubbing with a sheet of paper, but children under 5 years old usually object to masking. The tester who is familiar with the results of his voice in a particular room, and the various types of hearing losses, will have a fair idea of the expected audiometric hearing threshold. A child with non-organic hearing loss can often be

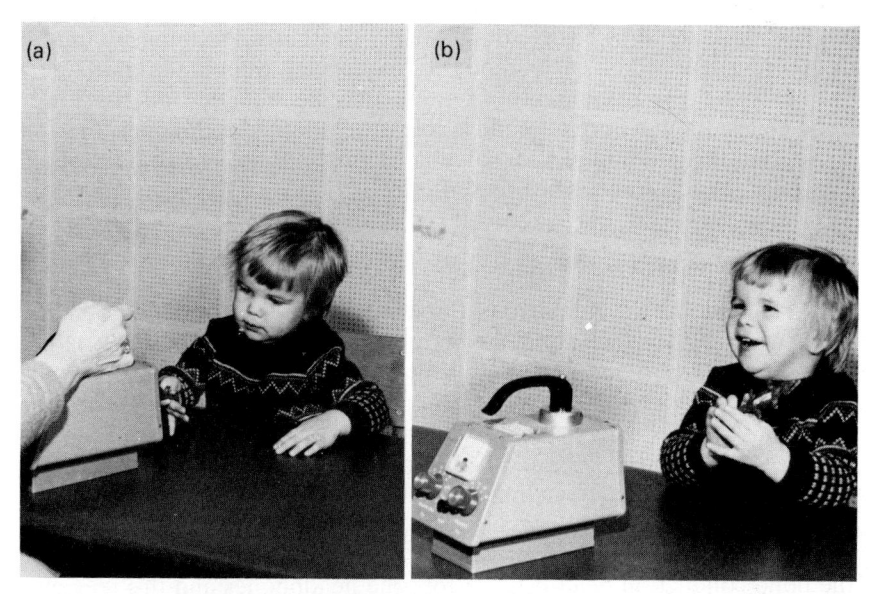

Fig. 25.7. (a). This infant is looking intently at the portable audiometer in the left-hand lower corner of the picture and is holding a plastic toy up to the audiometer. (b). On hearing the test tone he quickly withdraws the toy from the audiometer. This response is reinforced by the approval of the tester. In this way the approximate binaural free-field threshold can be estimated.

detected by this method (see Chapter 27). Parents watching these tests are often surprised to find the degree of handicap present, particularly in cases of good lip-readers who have largely compensated for their hearing disability. Young children can be tested by giving them a selection of small toys or picture cards each with monosyllabic names which must be known to him. He is requested to point to the objects named and the greatest distance at which he responds is noted. Children over the age of 6 years can usually be asked to repeat sentences or spondee words such as 'arm chair', 'eye brow', etc., and these simple tests give a general idea of his hearing capability. It is a good idea to have a typed list of spondees available for testing, otherwise the tester may repeat himself if using the words from memory. Inexperienced testers should practise with a Volume-Unit meter in order to keep the voice intensity steady.

'Conditioning' for audiometry

In order to obtain an audiogram at the earliest possible age, the 'conditioned' response can be taught with the portable free-field audiometer. This is an adaptation of the 'go-game' described by Lady Ewing, but working with the portable audiometer instead of the voice. The child is shown how to remove a ball from a 15-ball abacus, and to hold it in front of but not touching the audiometer, and to listen. When a sound is heard the child places the ball in a basket or a box, and another ball is taken. One usually starts with a sound of 80 dB and gradually decreases the intensity until a threshold is reached on each of the five frequencies. Should the child touch the audiometer a response to vibration may be obtained on the lower frequencies. Even before the child is able to accept the headphones for a full audiogram this method gives a valuable estimate of the binaural free-field threshold for the frequencies presented.

Pure-tone audiometry

When a child has a mental age of three years and over he should be able, when using a play technique, to perform conventional pure-tone audiometry (Fig. 25.8(a) and (b)). Occasionally, however, it is difficult to persuade a very shy child to wear the headphones and such a problem may be overcome by holding a single headphone to the ear, although this usually raises the threshold by 5–10 dB and this manoeuvre should only be regarded as an interim step in persuading the child to accept the headphones in the orthodox manner. It is important at as young an age as possible to obtain both the air and bone conduction thresholds. Occasionally a child will accept the bone conduction head-piece before the headphones and this may give valuable information. An air-bone gap is suggestive of a conductive loss and its absence suggests a sensorineural loss. The masking of one ear, which allows each ear to be tested individually when there is an appreciable difference (40 dB or more) between the threshold of the two ears, may be introduced at about 4–5 years of age, but in practice the ability of the child to produce a reliable response with masking can be a limiting factor.

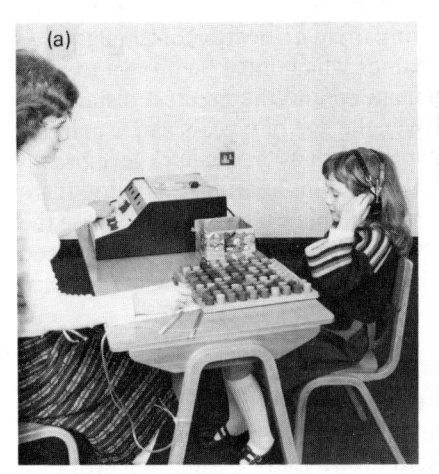

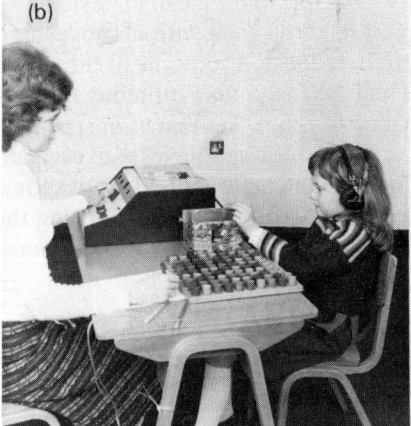

Fig. 25.8 (a). Pure-tone audiometry on a young child. The patient holds one of the pegs from the peg-board to her left ear, waiting for the tone to be presented. (b). On hearing the tone she drops the peg into a cardboard box. An audiology technician skilled in testing young children can obtain audiograms with a very satisfactory degree of accuracy by this method.

Many forms of play technique can be devised for this test and the resourceful technician will be able to improvise games which will catch the child's imagination. A choice of toys should be available for the tests and there should be multiple piece toys such as a peg-board with 100 coloured pegs, a stepped abacus or plastic discs on sticks so that should the child become bored the toys can be changed. Older children may be asked to indicate when they hear a sound by tapping gently on the table with a stick. Children should not be requested to say 'yes' when they hear a sound as this is so often found to give unreliable results; the shy child may not speak at all and those anxious to please may answer 'yes' quite inappropriately. When testing, the sound stimuli each lasting about two seconds, should be given at irregular intervals so that the child does not anticipate the responses. Throughout the test the child should be encouraged in order to maintain his co-operation. However, the tester should not give any facial indication when the test sound is produced, nor should the child be able to see the tester's hands.

Impedance audiometry

This objective test is a valuable adjunct to the other tests of hearing (see Chapter 29) and it is recommended that whenever possible every child attending an audiology clinic should have routine tympanometry and acoustic reflex threshold measurements. On account of their speed and ease of operation the automatic graph impedance meters are particularly useful in young children who cannot be persuaded to remain still for a longer test. However, problems are sometimes encountered, the most frequent being that the child objects to the probe being placed firmly in the ear, and if so, the test has to be abandoned. There can be a distorted graph pattern owing to the child moving or swallowing during the test, and the operator must watch out for the child sucking a sweet! In order to keep general movements to a minimum, older children can be asked to watch the graph or a younger child can be amused by the parent showing him a toy—the glove puppet has been found to be very useful. Occasionally another problem is that some children have a soft pinna and meatus and the probe is obstructed by lying against the meatal wall thereby giving a reading which suggests, falsely, a greatly reduced compliance. Blocking the orifices in the sound probe with cerumen gives a similar false result.

Electrophysiological tests of hearing

Before the electrophysiological tests of hearing were introduced an estimate of the hearing level of most children was made by subjective methods, but there were a few children who were difficult to diagnose, many of these having dual handicaps, e.g. blindness or retardation with a possible hearing loss. A great deal of time was sometimes wasted in these cases before the diagnosis was settled and satisfactory auditory training commenced because of the uncertainty of the hearing levels. Electrophysiological tests can now be performed and the diagnosis of a hearing loss confirmed so that the necessary treatment and training can be instigated without further delay.

At the Nuffield Hearing and Speech Centre the most satisfactory methods for infants are the transtympanic electrocochleogram (ECochG) and the brainstem electric responses (BSER) (see Chapter 31). This method is now not only used on the multiply handicapped children, but also quite to verify the presence of a suspected severe hearing loss in infants under three years old. It is often found that when a hearing loss in a baby has been confirmed by this method the hitherto reluctant parents are better able to accept the handicap and hence are prepared to give the necessary help in order to train their child. In cases where adoption is being considered long periods of delay have been avoided by using this sort of test for babies with a suspected hearing loss.

The brainstem response has been found useful because it can often be performed on babies sleeping after a feed or on older children without sedation or anaesthetic, whereas the transtympanic electrocochleogram requires anaesthesia. However, anaesthesia is, of itself, a great advantage when testing some very difficult, multiply-handicapped children.

FURTHER INVESTIGATIONS IN THE OLDER CHILD

The older school-age child who has developed language and understanding is gradually able to do more of the adult type audiological tests. These include speech audiometry, Békésy audiometry, tone decay, and loudness balance tests or the delayed feedback tests. These tests may help in discovering the cause of the hearing loss and later in the prescribing of hearing aids (see Chapters 15, 16 and 10).

Radiological diagnosis

An audiology centre should have access to radiography both for conventional radiography and polytomography either linear or hypocloidal (see Chapter 35). In cases of deafness there may be a need for radiological diagnosis of sinus infections, enlarged adenoids or chronic middle ear infections and tomography is of great value where congenital, infective, traumatic, or neoplastic abnormalities of the external, middle, or inner ears, or internal auditory meati, are suspected. Computerized axial tomography (CAT or CT-scan) can be of value in children being investigated for hearing loss, especially where ossicular anomalies are likely.

Pathological investigations

All babies suspected of having a sensorineural hearing loss, and their mothers, require a routine rubella antibody test to exclude or confirm rubella of pregnancy, and to determine their immune status in respect of this infection. This blood test should be done as early as possible in order to decrease the risk of subsequent spontaneous subclinical rubella infection, which will confound the result. It should be remembered that the child may have passively transferred maternal antibody in his blood for the first six months of life, and many four year olds have, themselves, acquired rubella antibodies owing to contracting rubella clinically or subclinically. Occasionally other haematological, biochemical, bacteriological, or virological tests are required according to general medical background in the fuller investigation of the individual cases of hearing loss.

Other specialized examinations

When investigating the hearing of an infant suspected of a hearing loss, in whom there is a complicated medical background it often is useful to call on the help of other medical specialists. A major audiological assessment centre, or an audiology clinic in a general hospital should have access to the services of a general paediatrician, developmental paediatrician, virologist, neurologist, ophthalmologist, psychiatrist, psychologist, geneticist and allergist.

Currently, all of the specialists mentioned, except for a geneticist, are available for consultation at the Nuffield Centre. Audiology centres which do not have the services of such specialists should refer the child and his parents to another hospital or clinic for consultation by the particular specialist whenever this is considered appropriate for the full evaluation of his hearing and other handicaps.

APPENDIX. QUESTIONNAIRE USED BY THE NUFFIELD HEARING AND SPEECH CENTRE, LONDON

CONFIDENTIAL

The Royal National Throat, Nose & Ear Hospital

NUFFIELD HEARING AND SPEECH CENTRE

(If there is a choice of answer, please circle the correct one:
e.g. (NO)   YES.   SOMETIMES).

SURNAME OF CHILD: FIRST NAMES: Date of Birth:
                                   Sex:
ADDRESS: TELEPHONE No.:   Religion:

NAME AND ADDRESS OF FAMILY DOCTOR: N.H.S. Number:

By whom were you referred to the Nuffield Centre? Please give name and address:

Is your child attending (or has he attended) any of the following:—

	Date first went there	For how long each day?	If residential
Play Group			
Nursery School			
Normal School			
School for the Deaf			
Partially Hearing Unit			
Other Special Unit (Please give details)			

IF OVER 16, STATE HOW EMPLOYED:

PARENTS

Father's Occupation:—

Mother's Occupation:—   At home all day.
                        Goes out to work.   If so, how many hours a day?

Father's Place of Birth and Nationality:—

Mother's Place of Birth and Nationality:—

Language normally spoken at home:—

P.T.O.

2.

What is your own main worry about your child and in what way do you most want help?

Are there any other problems and difficulties which may be relevant?

PRESENT COMPLAINT

Do you think your child is deaf?　　　NO.　　　YES.　　　Since when?

Does he respond to:—　　　NORMAL SOUNDS?　　　　　LOUD NOISES?
　　　　　　　　　　　　　YES.　　　　　　　　　　　YES.
　　　　　　　　　　　　　NO.　　　　　　　　　　　　NO.
　　　　　　　　　　　　　SOMETIMES.　　　　　　　　SOMETIMES.

Have there been any other hearing tests?　　　NO.　　　YES.
　　Where and approximate dates:—

Is your child wearing or has he ever worn a hearing aid?　　　NO.　　　YES.
　　If so, what type?

Do you think your child is:—　Late in talking?　　　　　NO.　　YES.
　　　　　　　　　　　　　　　Difficult to understand?　NO.　　YES.　　SOMETIMES.

Did he start to talk and then leave off?　　　NO.　　　YES.　　　At what age?

Can you think of any cause for these troubles?

Has he suffered from:　　Frequent colds?
　　　　　　　　　　　　Sore throats?
　　　　　　　　　　　　Earache?
　　　　　　　　　　　　Running ears?

3.

FAMILY HISTORY

Have you any other children? Please give age of each one and say whether Boy or Girl:—

Are any of them deaf?

Do any of them suffer from trouble dating from birth such as cleft palate or heart abnormality?

Is there any history of deafness in the family?
        On Father's side:—
        On Mother's side:—

Were any of the other children late talkers?

Is there any family history of late talking?
        On Father's side:—
        On Mother's side:—

Is the child   Adopted?   To be adopted?   Fostered?
        Please give names of foster parents and Authority responsible:—

MOTHER'S HEALTH DURING PREGNANCY OF THIS CHILD

Did you have:—

German measles (Rubella)?	If so, how many weeks pregnant?	
	It not, were you a contact?	
Any other infectious disease?	NO.	YES.
Toxaemia?	NO.	YES.
Blood pressure?	NO.	YES.
Excessive vomiting?	NO.	YES.
Episodes of bleeding before the baby was due?	NO.	YES.

Did you take any medicines or pills? If so, what were they?

Did you have any other illness or accident whilst you were expecting this child?

DETAILS OF BIRTH

Labour:—	Normal.	Unduly rapid.	Prolonged.		
Delivery:—	Normal.	Forceps.	Breech.	Twin.	Caesarian.

Baby born:— 33 weeks or less.   34-36 weeks.   37-39 weeks.   Full term.   41 weeks or more.

Birth weight:— ,....................lb.   ....oz.

Age of parents at birth of baby:—   Mother:—   Father:—

Condition of baby at birth:—   Normal.   Had difficulty with breathing.   Had jaundice.

At birth did baby require:—   Blood transfusion?
                            Nursing in an incubator?   How long?
                            Other treatment?

P.T.O.

PROGRESS AFTER BIRTH

Feeding habits in early months:—   Normal.   Slow.   Difficult.

Sleeping habits, first year:—   Normal.   Drowsy.   Cried a lot.

Has your child:—   Been vaccinated or immunised?   NO.   YES.   Please give details.

Had any infectious diseases?   NO.   YES.

Had any other illnesses, accidents or injuries?

Been admitted to hospital?   NO.   YES.
Which hospital and for what reason?

If your child has been under any other Doctors for investigation, would you please give details:—

Has your child been away from you for more than a few days?

GENERAL DEVELOPMENT

At what age did your child: Sit up?   Walk?

When did he:—   Start to babble, saying "Dad-dad-dad-dad", "Ba-ba-ba"?
Start to say first words?
Use hand to hold a spoon to feed?

Which hand does he prefer to use?   Right.   Left.   Either.

Are movements:—   Normal?   Is he clumsy with:—   Hands?
Unsteady?   Feet?

At what age was he dry during the day?

Have you any worries about your child's behaviour?

If attending school, do you consider he is:—   Having difficulties?
Getting on well?
Ahead of others in class?

Are there any subjects in which he:—   Is outstanding?
Finds particular difficulty?

Has he had an intelligence test?   NO.   YES.   If so, where?

Has he had his eyes tested?   NO.   YES.   What was the result?

REFERENCES

BOARD OF EDUCATION (1911). Annual report for 1910 of the Chief Medical Officer, London, p. 195. HMSO, London.

—— (1931). Annual report for 1930 of the Chief Medical Officer, London, p. 20. HMSO, London.

CONWAY, N. and BIRT, B. D. (1965). Streptomycin in pregnancy—effect on the foetal ear. *Br. med. J.* **ii**, 260–3.

DEPARTMENT OF EDUCATION AND SCIENCE (1975). Report of the Chief Medical Officer, the School Health Service 1908–74, p. 16. HMSO, London.

EWING, I. R. (1957). Screening tests and guidance clinics for babies and young children. In *Educational guidance of the deaf child* (ed. A. W. G. Ewing) p. 21. Manchester University Press.

FROST, M., KNIGHT, M., and SHARP, M. (1976). Evaluation of routine hearing tests in children under one year. (Unpublished.)

MCKINNA, A. J. (1966). Quinine induced hypoplasia of the optic nerve. *Can. J. Ophthal.* **1**, 261–6.

NOONE, P. (1978). Use of antibiotics. Aminoglycosides. *Br. med. J.* **ii**, 549–52.

PECKHAM, C. S., MARTIN, J. A. M., MARSHALL, W. C., and DUDGEON, J. A. (1979). Congenital rubella: a preventable disease. *Lancet* **i**, 258–61.

ROBINSON, C. G. and CAMBON, K. G. (1964). Hearing loss in infants of tuberculous mothers treated with streptomycin during pregnancy. *New Engl. J. Med.* **271**, 949–51.

SHEPPARD, S., SMITHELLS, R. W., PECKHAM, C. S., DUDGEON, J. A., and MARSHALL, W. C. (1977). National Congenital Rubella Surveillance, 1971–75. *Hlth Trends* **9**, 38–41.

SHERIDAN, M. D. (1968). Manual for Stycar tests of vision and hearing. NFER, Windsor, England.

VUORI, M., LAHIKAINEN, E. A., and PELTOREN T. (1962). Perceptive deafness in connection with mumps. *Acta oto-lar.* **55**, 231–6.

26 Education of the hearing-handicapped child

H. KERNOHAN, G. LUCAS, and V. MUTER

GENERAL EDUCATIONAL MANAGEMENT (HK)

Introductory outline

Of the 555 pages of the Plowden Report (1967) only 3½ pages are devoted to a discussion of *aims* in education; a substantial part of even that tiny proportion is devoted to doubts, not quite about whether it is actually worth having any aims but about whether there is any point in trying to state them. General statement of aims tends to be little more than expressions of benevolent aspiration which may provide a rough guide to the general climate of a school, but which may have a rather tenuous relationship to the educational practices that actually go on there.

The Lewis Report (1968) makes a specific reference to the hearing handicapped child and recommends as follows: 'The aim of educating children with impaired hearing should be to enable them to realise their full potential and as far as possible take their place in society as literate adults with whole personalities which they can express through generally understood media of communication.' Our aims must not be less than those for the hearing child.

Assessment of a hearing loss in a child is the first part in a programme of co-operation between the parents and a group of professionals including teachers, psychologists, audiologists, and others in order to assist the child to achieve his full potential as an active member of the community.

It is essential that parents are provided with the maximum of assistance from the earliest stages of diagnosis. Such help will take the form of: (i) pre-school advice and demonstration in the effective use of the child's residual hearing, (ii) advice on how a child acquires language, (iii) talks related to basic child development, and (iv) the setting up of realistic goals for achievement.

The Warnock Report (1978) quite rightly highlights the importance of parental involvement in the general management of the hearing-handicapped child. Since the family is primarily responsible for the educational treatment of the pre-school child, the parents of the hearing-impaired child must be provided with as much knowledge as possible in relation to the effects of the deafness. An exchange of information may take place both during short courses at a clinic or school, and during regular visits of the peripatetic teacher to the home.

Parents derive benefit from meeting other parents of pre-school children in a support programme of instruction devised and operated by teachers in local schools and units for the hearing handicapped. In such an environment, parents can experience the type of response expected of the nursery/infant pupil and are free to ask questions related to their own efforts before and during the school years.

Audiologists take great care in assessing the type and degree of hearing loss in the child. The assessment must be explained to the parents at the earliest opportunity. Perhaps such descriptions are best carried out over a period of time using practical situations to explore residual hearing.

It is not unknown for parents and some teachers in training to assume that amplification apparatus somehow permits a child to 'hear' frequencies which are not recorded as thresholds of hearing on the audiogram. Full but simple descriptions of acoustic phonetics are essential background knowledge for parents if they are to avoid early disappointments in the responses of the hearing-impaired child. The following points should be discussed and demonstrated regularly whilst emphasis must be placed on the positive aspects of the guidance programme:

1. Distinctions between vowel and consonant sounds in speech,
   (a) low and high frequency sounds,
   (b) loud and soft sounds,
   (c) the effect of raising the voice on vowels and consonants in connected speech.
2. The frequency range of the child's residual hearing in each ear.
3. The effect of amplification on speech and which parts of amplified speech the child is likely to perceive.
4. The disadvantage of ambient noise.
5. The importance of talking to the child.
6. Full information on the care and use of hearing aids. It is common knowledge among teachers that many secondary-age pupils cease to use their aids without supervision. This attitude may be the result of ineffective training in early life. The child must be taught the value of amplified sound.

Throughout the school life of the child, achievement of the child's full potential can be best ensured by setting out realistic goals or short-term objectives and the 'success stories' in this context have usually been the result of full family support for the teaching programme.

In order to focus attention on the principles and possible problems involved in the education of the hearing handicapped pupil, let us examine the topics as suggested by the mnemonic CHILD.

C Communication and Curriculum
H Hearing loss and use of residual hearing.
I   Integration and the Individual.
L Language.
D Development and Discipline.

Communication and curriculum

The hearing-impaired child must be thought of as a child first and second as a child with a learning difficulty. For the severely or profoundly deaf child with restricted frequency range in the residual hearing, the learning difficulty must not be minimized, but the child still requires the same experience as the normal-hearing child. Before the child can express himself, he must have the relevant experience of the environment. Visits and outings to places of interest, toys and games can be used to provide the experiences and the materials for language encouragement. One of the greatest weaknesses in the child's language development is his over-dependence on vocabulary without the necessary syntax to link the words together. Education in the true sense is not simply that which takes place in the class room. The work in the classroom is often quite artificial and may be only vaguely connected with the world outside. Language is a creative art. Language teaching must reflect the language which is in use in the child's own environment.

Since the hearing-impaired child does not 'pick-up' language as the normal-hearing child does, it follows that teaching programmes must provide for a classroom-based assessment and recording of the child's progress.

DEAFNESS HANDICAPS IN COMMUNICATION
Our aim is to encourage intelligent oral communication since that is the most efficient means by which we learn and communicate with others. Many profoundly deaf children fail to attain intelligible speech and rely heavily upon lip-reading for comprehension. However, lip-reading has its own limitations because a child cannot lip-read a word he does not know and many sounds will look the same on the speaker's lips. Many people with whom the deaf child will come into contact are very difficult to lip-read and lighting conditions are not always as ideal as the classroom situation. A non-oral child is not a failure. Hearing-handicapped children vary in many respects and one or more of these differences will affect the child's attitude to communication; for example, the children differ in hearing loss, ability to use residual hearing, personality characteristics, motivation, and mental abilities.

A child with no means of communication reflects a total lack of flexibility in educational provision. Cued speech, Paget–Gorman sign system, and the British Sign Language are major additions to the oral/aural method. The chief problems encountered in using additional means of communication are: (i) different methods are applied to different children, (ii) few workers including teachers have in-depth knowledge of all the systems, (iii) different systems are operated in different schools and areas of the country, (iv) teacher training courses are too short to enable teachers to acquire more than a superficial view of any or all of the systems, (v) parents and relatives need to learn the system, and (vi) changes of staff make it difficult to have consistent teaching programmes.

The major reason for language retardation in so many deaf children is the inadequate communication in the early years. The primary language-learning years are the pre-school years and an inability to communicate with parents and peers at this early age has a profound effect on development and adjustment. The hearing-handicapped child needs normal, idiomatic language patterns and needs the general education to go with them.

Cueing is a method of communication designed for use with and among the deaf, in which eight shapes of one hand are used in four positions near the face to supplement the information in the oral area. Cueing provides a complete, morpheme-by-morpheme representation of verbal language. Cued speech is in use in two primary schools and some units in England and has the following advantages:

1. The spoken message is clear to the deaf child—he is not subjected to the confusion of trying to understand through lip-reading alone.
2. Hearing parents of a young deaf child can develop communication at an early age without recourse to a new vocabulary.
3. The learning of verbal language does not have to wait on the development of expressive speech.

The Paget–Gorman sign system has a limited vocabulary of about 2500–3000 words. These include all the functional words likely to be used by children, i.e. all the pronouns, prepositions, conjunctions, and words which carry little meaning in isolation. It is therefore possible to sign full English sentences by means of this system. However, the signs are described in words and are written down and it requires a great deal of time and patience to become proficient.

Hearing loss and the use of residual hearing

The terms 'hearing handicapped' and 'hearing impaired' are blanket terms which cover a wide variety of children with hearing losses. The terms are inappropriate when discussing a particular child's hearing loss with a teacher, parent, or other professional worker. The terms cover hearing losses which may be slight (less than 30 dB) to one which is profound (greater than 90 dB). Hearing loss on each ear is usually described by teachers as the average loss for the three frequencies 500 Hz, 1 kHz, and 2 kHz. These three frequencies are often regarded as being the central speech frequencies. The hearing loss must be examined in terms of what the child will be likely to hear with amplification. In other words, the loss is seen in relation to the acoustics of speech sounds, particularly in vowel and consonant discrimination.

For older children, in addition to the pure-tone audiogram which should indicate air and bone conduction thresholds, speech audiometry may be used to demonstrate the child's ability to hear and comprehend speech. Speech and hearing are inseparable. From an early age, the child must be assessed on his ability to discriminate speech at supraliminal levels.

Management of the child for teachers and parents means an understanding of the consequences of impaired hearing. An appreciation of what a child is likely to 'hear' by means of amplification through hearing-aid apparatus and a knowledge of the possible effects of a limitation in the frequency range of hearing on speech perception are two important considerations. Since consonants provide the intelligibility of speech, a decrease in hearing for the higher frequencies is sure to create greater difficulty in a child's comprehension. This problem is further aggravated by the fact that consonants have less energy than vowels in connected speech. This is one reason for not shouting or raising one's voice to the hearing-handicapped child.

Unless optimum levels are maintained, the child will not achieve maximum benefit from amplification. Pupils under teacher supervision in acoustically treated classrooms are in ideal condition for the use of hearing aids. However, even in such ideal situations, the following factors are crucial and require careful consideration at all times:

1. Input levels to the microphone. Input plus the gain of the aid equals the output at the ear. A sensible speech level of 60 dB directed towards the microphone of the amplification equipment provides a good basis for the above equation. Research and experience has shown that a 90° turn of the head from the microphone can reduce the input by up to 15 dB. This procedure applies to the microphones of all wearable and classroom-based amplifying equipment and particularly to aids without automatic volume control.
2. Environmental noise levels. Hearing aids amplify all sound energy in the environment so it is essential that the signal-to-noise ratio is as high as possible. 'Environmental noise' includes unwanted noise, such as a noisy class, traffic, and radio or television sound as background noise.
3. Auditory feedback. The chief reason for the constant use of a hearing aid by hearing-handicapped children is to provide the opportunity for them to hear their own voices as well as the speech of others.

Children need to practise the use of the hearing aid. We need lots of practise in the skills of driving a car or playing golf and in the same way the hearing-handicapped child needs to experience the use of amplified sound. It is my own view that many secondary-age pupils cease to make use of their residual hearing because they have not had sufficient practise and training in making sense of the sounds which they are able to hear through amplification. Children from an early age require regular training in hearing aid use in a wide variety of everyday situations as opposed to the acoustically treated classrooms. Records should be kept of all hearing aid tests or experimental results and an attempt made to encourage the child to identify sounds.

Do we pay lip-service to lip-reading as an important medium of communication? Few adults with whom the child will come into contact are easy to lip-read. School-age children practise lip-reading to varying degrees as an addition to the use of residual hearing. However, the value of lip-reading is based upon a suitable distance from the speaker (1–1.25 m), the ability of the speaker to speak clearly and create slight differences in the lip patterns, lighting conditions, and face level with the speaker. The deaf child will seldom experience this ideal combination of conditions outside the classroom.

The use of residual hearing requires also the addition of contextual clues for effective understanding by the hearing-handicapped child. Contextual information is just as important to the child with the slight loss as to the child with the severe or profound loss. This information may take the form of background information or explanation, gesture or other visual information. Educationists usually categorize hearing losses according to the following table:

Degree of handicap	Average hearing level (dB)
Less than 25	Not significant
Slight	25 to less than 40
Mild	40 to less than 55
Marked	55 to less than 70
Severe	70 to less than 90
Profound	Greater than 90

The hearing levels, in dB, apply to the better ear and are based on the average value of hearing levels at 500, 1000, and 2000 Hz.

Many parents and teachers feel disappointed with the slow rate of development in communication and attainment by the child. I feel strongly that whatever the circumstances relating to the child's hearing loss and intellectual capacities, the educational treatment of the child must evolve around the following three factors: (i) consistent treatment in communication method, (ii) commitment by teachers and parents to work schedules geared to the individual needs of the child, and (iii) regular experience of the value of using the residual hearing.

The nursery/infant schoolchild will soon begin to rely on lip-reading or 'face-reading', since he cannot lip-read words which he does not know, because he will find it difficult to understand through hearing. There are many schools in the United Kingdom where listening experience is given. However, in my opinion, the best example of the regular experience of residual hearing is carried out at the St Michielsgestel School near Eindhoven in Holland. In the Dutch school, the pupils are offered a programme of listening practise involving amplified music which is supported by regular speech teaching sessions.

Obviously, a programme based on listening will demand tremendous expertise on behalf of the teachers and parents. Emphasis should be placed on voice quality, rhythm, and rate of speaking. In addition to articulation practise we require a scheme of integrated listening whereby the child experiments with and without lip-reading, gestures, or visual cues. We must endeavour to reduce listening strain without overlooking the value of the hearing which remains. Of course, some pupils are better than others and factors of attention, mental attitudes, motivation, and interest are major contributions to the success of such a programme.

The experience and use of residual hearing calls for the *imaginative* use of the equipment by the teacher and should result in recording the responses for future planning. Since the child uses the wearable aid for the majority of his waking hours, one should begin with its use. Thus, over a period of time, a working knowledge of aid settings, including tone and AVC settings, can be acquired by the child, parent, and teacher. Regular checks by children, parents and teachers can ensure that the hearing aid has not got a high level of distortion, the battery is efficient, and that the aid is providing an optimum listening level for the child.

Integration and the individual

Placement of the hearing handicapped child within existing educational provision is of the utmost concern to parents and educationists. The ever increasing trend to accommodate the hearing impaired pupil in the ordinary school places enormous demands on school resources. Recent work, the Haringey Project (Dale 1979), has indicated that hearing impaired pupils can be successfully integrated with their normal hearing peers provided the necessary teaching personnel is available to supervise their abilities.

The Education Act 1976 (Paragraph 10), not implemented at the time of writing, amends Section 33 (2) of the 1944 Education Act in that arrangements made by a Local Education Authority for the special educational treatment of pupils of any category shall provide for the education of the pupils in county or voluntary schools. There are exceptions in the Act related to inconvenience and finance.

A reduced normal-hearing school population should provide empty places in classrooms or empty classrooms in some schools and since the training establishments are producing about 230 newly qualified teachers of the deaf each year, the time is right for an expansion of educational provision in ordinary schools for many types of handicapped pupils including the hearing impaired. The Warnock Report (1978) in its comprehensive overview of existing provision and proposals for future policy has added incentive to the notion of treating the handicapped child as one having a learning difficulty which need not necessarily follow him for the rest of his life.

Local education authorities provide for the educational treatment of the hearing handicapped in one or more of the following ways: (i) pupils educated in the regular classroom with the use of a hearing aid, (ii) pupils placed in the normal classroom with regular assistance by peripatetic teachers of the deaf, (iii) pupils in a unit for hearing handicapped children. The unit is in the charge of a qualified teacher of the deaf and the pupil may spend a proportion of each day attending classes of peer groups in the normal school, (iv) pupils attending a school for the partially-hearing on a day or boarding basis, (v) pupils attending a school for profoundly deaf children on a day or boarding basis, or (vi) pupils may be enrolled in classes or schools catering for pupils with additional problems to the hearing handicap.

A policy of integration of hearing handicapped children into the ordinary class requires planning and co-ordinated provision within the Local Education Authority with respect to: (i) in-service training programmes for all types of teachers, and (ii) the changed nature and use of resources including the expertise of the staffs of special schools. In-service training programmes must, in future, deal with such children as the language disordered child and the child with an additional or multiple handicap. The present one-year full-time post-graduate training course offered by Universities, Polytechnics, and Colleges is too short to deal adequately with the many aspects of the training required.

The fundamental task of the teacher is to educate the child and this implies a curriculum including most of the subjects to be found in any school for children with normal hearing. The principles of curriculum construction and innovation are concerned with defining objectives, learning experiences, and ways of teaching. The parameters which come to mind when considering the curriculum for the hearing handicapped child are shown in Fig. 26.1.

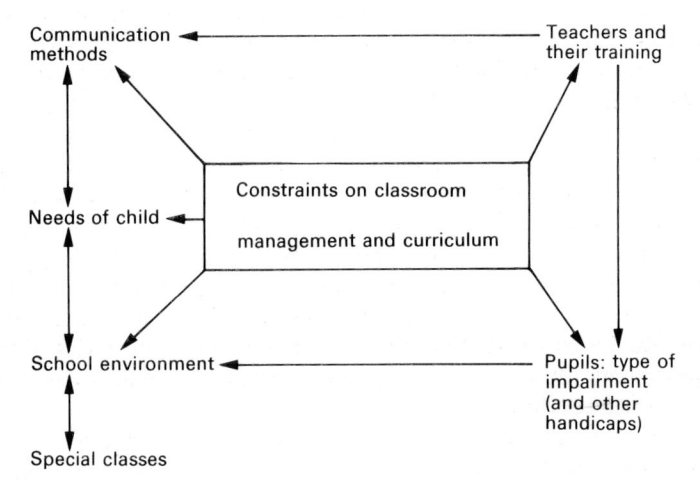

Fig. 26.1.

Placement of the hearing-impaired child in a particular school environment depends on many other factors as well as the hearing loss. These factors include: (i) the child's ability in communication; has the child got intelligible speech; does the child need additional means of communication? (ii) support from the home and parents, (iii) social development of the child, (iv) the personality of the child. Is the child well-behaved or is he disturbed or inattentive? (v) the intelligence of the child and his use of the hearing aid, and (vi) the possible school placements available to the child within a region, and, most important of all, we must consider the wishes of the parents and offer them the maximum amount of co-operation, information on schools, and support.

Language

Before he reaches school age, the normally hearing child will have achieved a substantial mastery of the language he hears spoken around him. Despite little or no conscious tuition by his parents, within three to four years he is able to produce and understand an endless variety of novel yet meaningful utterances. To do this he has resolved a stream of undifferentiated sound into meaningful segments which he can then use to help organize the stream of his experience. Moreover, from the beginning the child's speech shows regularities of construction and its development follows an orderly progression to more complex grammatical forms. This suggests that somehow the child is extracting grammatical rules from the patterns he hears and is applying them to his own speech. The achievement is surprising when one considers that the attention span and memory of a young child are short and his other cognitive abilities relatively limited.

In fact, it appears that, generally, a solid base of language has already been laid by three and a half years. The child's conversation is no longer tied to the 'here and now' and the child is able to distinguish these forms appropriate to his own language background from unfamiliar forms. Although all children share this tacit understanding of the underlying structure of their language, their linguistic abilities determined by such measures as size and variety of vocabulary, the complexity of their sentences, or their use of different structures, are found to show considerable variation within any age group. In Chomsky's (1965) terminology, there is a wide variation between individuals in the linguistic performance derived from their underlying competence.

Where a child's linguistic performance is markedly depressed he may be unable to function at a level appropriate to his capabilities within the school system. Success in school generally demands a familiarity with and ability to manipulate the more complex language structures and vocabulary that facilitates generalization and abstraction.

For the hearing impaired child, however, the handicap imposes far more fundamental barriers to his linguistic development. Impaired hearing reduces the quantity and quality of the sound input to the child to an extent dependent on the degree and type of hearing loss. The more severe the hearing loss the less the child's interest in language as a means of communication with others will be aroused, unless a conscious effort is made to teach him the vocabulary and structures of the language around him. Even a slight hearing loss will reduce the level of language input to the point where the child can no longer deduce the rules of his language from the patterns he hears and without help is unable to structure his own utterances correctly. With increasing hearing loss and consequent reduced auditory feed-back from his own voice the problems of producing speech sounds intelligible to others becomes greater, until the deafest children must rely only on sensorimotor and kinaesthetic feed-back.

Factors which have been found favourable to linguistic development in normally hearing children, such as the attention of responsive, caring adults and an encouraging, talking environment where language skills and books are valued, will in practice only prove to be so in the case of the hearing impaired children if special conditions are observed. A knowledge of how such factors interact with normal developmental process can provide a useful guide to the best ways to help language development of deaf children.

Early diagnosis of the child's deafness is certainly beneficial. As soon as the mother knows of her child's deafness, she can allow for the fact that he cannot hear the comforting sounds of her approach or of her continued existence when she is out of sight. Moreover she can begin to make a special effort to arouse his interest in her speech and encourage him to use his voice.

The warm relationship between mother and child, necessary for his optimum development, may be impaired if the mother finds it hard to accept his handicap. A prolonged period of doubt and conflicting opinions and advice may make the acceptance more difficult. Parents need good explanations of the nature and implications of their child's handicap and need support and guidance as to how they can help him overcome it. The knowledge that they are in the best position to help him in the early years and discussions with other parents similarly placed may encourage them to adopt the necessary positive approach to the handicap. It can be a strain caring for a young deaf child and the mother should not feel that she faces the task alone.

Fig. 26.2 illustrates the ways in which language acquisition, development, and use are linked to the child's experience in home and school life. The home affords many opportunities to engage the child's interest in language and there are many regular routines, such as bedtime and mealtimes when he can practise what he learns. Mrs Freddy Bloom (1979) recommends that the mother should make a habit of maintaining a running commentary on what she and the child are doing and of drawing the child's attention to the noises of everyday life. Instead of stopping talking when they learn their

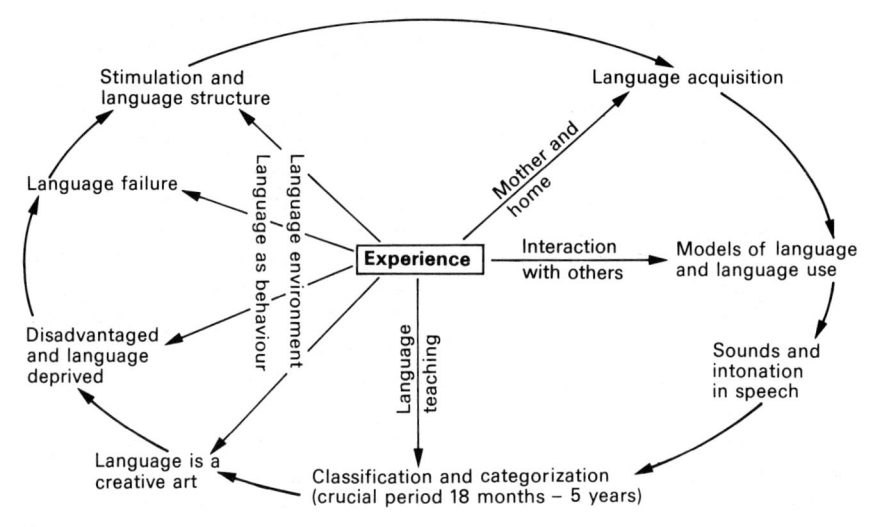

Fig. 26.2.

child is deaf, parents must be encouraged to talk even more. Fig. 26.2 illustrates the continuing process of language development. How people talk to the child is also important. As with the normally hearing child, short, simple, repetitive, and colloquial speech is found to be the most effective as long as it is spoken clearly and without destroying the normal rhythm. The model for the child's speech should be those patterns expected of a normal hearing child of the same age. There is a stage where learning separate names of objects is appropriate, but, whereas it is relatively easy to teach deaf children the 'open class' words, it is more difficult to explain the 'pivot' words which they will need to know if their speech is to be flexible and useful to them.

There is also a danger of stages being prolonged in the deaf child's development. Imitation of the child's language, rather than enhancing it, is rare with hearing children but can be a trap for deaf children. In the same way it should be remembered that normal hearing children acquire the use of the different structures in a certain order. It is no use trying to teach a child a particular structure unless he is master of those that should proceed it. For instance, children can use the negative form before questions even though they occur with equal frequency in the mother's speech.

Views differ as to what is the most advantageous approach to linguistic teaching and development and there is little in the way of empirical studies to distinguish the various claims on a more than qualitative basis. The first point of dissention centres around the need or advisability of providing the child with additional information beyond that which he can see and hear in the normal spoken form. Some teachers recommend that all early training should be given auditorily so that the children become auditorily minded. However, for those with a severe hearing loss this attitude gives even the most intelligent child very little language material to work with. On the other hand, the majority of teachers believe that the child should not only be encouraged to lip-read but that he should be offered the visual clues of the written form as early as possible. The written form will familiarize the child at an early stage with the awkward little words such as 'so' and 'but' that he tends to miss otherwise. It is only through reading that the arrears of language input of the hearing impaired child can be made up and he can achieve a flexibility of language use. I believe that the children's work should include a lot of reading, writing, and recording of *their* oral language from the age of four to five years. Cued speech is also aimed at providing the child with a clear model of the complete spoken language, with the aim of advancing linguistic development without detracting from lip-reading skills. Finger spelling is used to clarify the ambiguities left by lip-reading. Signing offers a totally visual representation of the 'speakers' meaning and provides a language readily usable among the deaf. However, its structure and vocabulary is so abbreviated compared to that of the spoken language that it may hinder the child in learning the spoken or written language of the wider community. The Paget–Gorman system was introduced to overcome this disadvantage but it is not widely used in the adult deaf community.

In recent years, we have seen the introduction of total communication into primary and secondary schools for the profoundly deaf. The basic principle of total communication is that several modes are presented at the same time and such a teaching strategy in schools is seen as a response to the needs of individual children or groups of children.

The other main point of difference seems to be whether language should be taught by a formal structured method or by a developmental approach based on the children's activities. The former can be accused of consisting of too many boring drills and inflexibility, while the latter can be accused of failing to provide sufficient practise of new language forms so that they become part of the child's active vocabulary. The first has the advantage of providing a clear statement of what the child should already know if the work has been properly covered and provides for a logical and gradual progression towards more complex language forms and uses. The second can always have the magic ingredients of relevance and interest that promote learning. It can be based on conversation which provides a natural situation for a balanced exchange of expressive and receptive language, with opportunity for using idiom, exclamations, questions involving attitudes, and the shifting of meanings that comes from interaction with the attitudes of others.

It seems to me that whatever method is used, and any method may be used imaginatively and well or boringly and badly, it is essential that the teacher should be clear as to the next step that he is aiming for in the child's linguistic development and that he later checks to see if the child has achieved it.

Development and discipline

A major reason for retardation of the general progress in so many deaf children is one of inadequate communication in the early years. The primary language learning years are pre-school years and an inability to communicate with parents and peers at this early age has a profound effect on general development and adjustment. Parents need to know how to deal with such things as temper tantrums but more important is the counselling and guidance on communication methods with the young deaf child. Boredom often creates secondary handicaps and the deaf child needs to feel secure in his relationships with adults. He needs to be taught. Great care must be taken in the presentation of material and in the teaching by example because we have little knowledge concerning perception processes and it is extremely difficult to unteach at a later stage.

Parents and teachers are concerned with the development of the whole child, including (i) physical development, (ii) linguistic and intellectual development, (iii) social and emotional development, and (iv) personality development. Therefore, the school curriculum must plan opportunities for the hearing-handicapped child to develop in a variety of ways and endeavour to create attitudes of initiative and independence.

Motor development and body control play major roles in the child's life and in his overall development, not only because motor action is important in its own right, but because it makes possible a wide variety of activities that are not ordinarily thought of as being motor behaviour. The failure of a child to achieve a reasonable level of body control as compared with others of his age can have great significance for the kind of personal adjustments he makes, for his interests, attitudes, feelings of achievement, and competence he holds towards himself and, in general, for his self-concept. A well co-ordinated child and one with an attitude of self-confidence is more accepted and sought after by his peers. Personality development is related to a degree of autonomy and self-directedness of behaviour. The hearing-handicapped child needs independence of action; he needs to feel capable of mastering and controlling various elements of the environment. For these and other reasons, it is essential that consideration of school placement for the hearing-handicapped child should be a team decision involving professionals who can report upon the following factors: (i) hearing loss, (ii) communication skills, including lip-reading skills, (iii) stage of linguistic development, (iv) intelligence, (v) educational attainments (other than language), (vi) social and emotional development, (vii) parental wishes, and (viii) the possibility of additional handicaps.

The Warnock Report (1978) (Chapter 5—'Children Under Five') points out that the assessment of a handicapped child is not a simple task and cannot be made with finality. It is a continuing process and because of the complexity of the task, both the process itself and the treatment of the total situation demands teamwork, in which teachers, doctors, psychologists, parents, and others must co-operate. Thus, as the Report rightly stresses, any arrangements made for the education of a handicapped child must be subject to constant review.

Intelligence tests are constructed in an attempt to assess the child's capacity for integrating and organizing material. However, ability in such tests depends on previous learning experiences. These come to the child through his senses and any impairment of the senses will seriously alter the learning experience. The hearing-handicapped child needs to hear and *see* the task presented to him. Only those tasks which minimize the use of language will accurately assess the deaf child's intellectual ability. Although language is useful for thinking, it is not a prerequisite and hearing-handicapped children are endowed with the same intellectual capacity as hearing children but the attainment of this reasoning capacity depends upon a good educational programme. In deaf education, if a child is to be helped to achieve his full potential, more curriculum emphasis must be placed on providing activities that challenge the child's thinking. The teaching of language in itself will not produce an intelligent thinking adult, unless we provide the child with the stimulus and opportunity to use language as the sophisticated vehicle of thought it is considered to be.

Relevant experience, intelligence, motivation and observation are considered to be the major factors which influence the learning process in children. However, in the education of the hearing-handicapped child, reinforcement, repetition and the concept of transfer of learning have great importance.

1. We must reward the good efforts of the child but never reinforce the bad habits.
2. Repetition helps the learning process considerably, especially the more complex activities.
3. The hearing-handicapped child needs to have his attention drawn to the fact that what is taught in one subject has value and applicability to another subject. The hearing-handicapped child tends to pigeon-hole ideas and consequences and not relate them to other learning situations. For example, secondary school age profoundly deaf pupils in my own science class refused to accept my explanations on heat transference because I related them to cooking utensils and the pupils considered that subject to be solely one of home economics. Teachers make tremendous efforts to create a programme of language across the curriculum in an effort to facilitate transfer of learning from one subject to another.

In my own view, the learning difficulties for the child and the teaching difficulties for the teacher are so great in themselves that problems related to discipline in the classroom should not arise. Standards of discipline, outside as well as inside the school, should be the results of group discussions with the parents when all are made aware of the child's maturity, emotional stability, and level of confidence. Illogical consequences such as punishment for poor behaviour can be bewildering to a hearing-handicapped child. It is wasted effort to try to teach during a child's emotional outburst; effective discipline can be best achieved in the following ways:

1. The same standard for everyone. This attitude applies to homelife as well as the classroom and should be applicable to hearing as well as deaf children.
2. Good examples of behaviour by parents and teachers.
3. The formation of simple rules which are easily understood and can be obeyed by everyone.
4. Recognized and accepted consequences for bad behaviour.
5. Adequate supervision at all times.

In 1979, there are over 2000 teachers working with approximately 12 000 hearing-handicapped children throughout England and Wales. One of the major concerns of the teacher-training establishments is that the one year full-time course of training for qualified teachers of normally hearing children is too short for inclusion of all the necessary subjects of study and yet provide adequate practical training in the classroom. Over the past decade, there has been a growing tendency for severely hearing-handicapped pupils to be placed in a unit or class attached to the ordinary school and for the children to be integrated in the normal classroom and receive their education with their hearing peers. Such placements require teachers of normal hearing pupils to know and understand how to deal with the hearing handicap. A recent survey in Scotland of the views of newly qualified teachers indicated that 28 per cent of the teachers felt inadequately prepared for teaching handicapped children and 61 per cent said that the topic had not been dealt with in the initial training course. Thus, the Warnock Report

(Chapter 12) correctly highlights the necessity for a Special Education element to be included in all initial teacher training programmes. Universities and Colleges which provide training in the education of the hearing-handicapped are already making efforts to cope with the massive in-service training programme for teachers of normally hearing children and micro-teaching techniques which make economical use of time both for students and for the school have been in use in the Hertfordshire College since 1975.

ROLE OF PSYCHOLOGICAL ASSESSMENTS (VM)

The effective diagnosis and management of the child with a hearing loss may frequently involve a psychological investigation of his abilities, attainments, and behaviour. An acceptably reliable and valid psychological assessment can be carried out on children of about three years and above, although the specific reasons for carrying out such an assessment will vary according to the age of the child. Psychological assessments usually go well beyond the administration of the ubiquitous intelligence test, although this generally marks the starting point and base reference point for any investigation. The administration of verbally-biased intelligence tests, including the well known Stanford Binet test, are deemed unsuitable for deaf and partially hearing children because they penalize the child for his lack of speech and language, and thereby result in a marked underestimate of the child's true learning ability. On verbally-biased tests, children with a hearing loss frequently score within the 'mentally subnormal' range, whereas it may be apparent from other sources of information that the child is not retarded but 'catches on' quickly. Fortunately, there are several Non-Verbal or Performance Scales of Intelligence which give a truer representation of the child's learning ability. These tests use minimal verbal instructions (if any); test requirements are transmitted to the child with a combination of simple mime and gesture, together with demonstration items. In addition, no speech and language response is required from the child. The Merrill–Palmer Scale (with verbal items omitted *a priori*) and the Wechsler Performance Scales are examples of Non-Verbal IQ tests which do not penalize children with a hearing loss for their lack of speech and language. Such children obtain scores similar to those of normally hearing children. Some IQ Scales have been designed specifically for use with deaf children and, therefore, provide norms and standardization data for the deaf, e.g. Hiskey–Nebraska and Snijders–Oomen Scales, and the Leiter International Performance Scales. In addition to IQ testing, psychological assessments frequently employ verbal attainment tests, specific ability tests (e.g. memory tests such as the Benton Visual Retention Test, tests of visual perception such as the Frostig), and educational attainment tests (reading and arithmetic tests). The resultant test scores are interpreted in the light of knowledge of the child's medical history, reports from parents and teachers, and observations of the child's social and cognitive behaviour (the latter refers to attention span, cooperativeness, motivation, etc. during the course of the assessment).

The information derived from a psychological assessment may, according to the age of the child, be used to:

1. Assist in diagnosis. A child being investigated for a hearing loss has usually been referred because of apparent lack of responsiveness to sounds, with or without delayed speech development. Such symptoms need not necessarily arise from lack of hearing, but may be a result of the child being mentally retarded (the commonest cause of speech delay in young children is mental retardation). A further, not uncommon, cause of delayed speech is the specific learning disability usually simply referred to as 'developmental language delay' which affects young children of normal hearing and intelligence. A psychological assessment is frequently essential in cases of difficult diagnosis to tease out the relevant cause or causes of the presenting symptoms. A minority of children with a hearing loss are multiply-handicapped, e.g. suffer from hearing loss in addition to being mentally retarded. Once again a psychological assessment is essential in clarifying the precise nature of the multiple handicap.

2. Assist in school placement plans. The appropriate school placement of a deaf or partially hearing child is not wholly dependent on the extent of his hearing loss, but is strongly determined by other factors including his intelligence level, his language attainment, pre-educational skills, and cognitive behaviour. The information derived from the assessment is considered together with the medical history and family circumstances in making specific recommendations regarding the kind of school which would cater most satisfactorily for the child's individual needs. In comparatively straightforward cases of hearing loss, i.e. children not severely multiply handicapped, the school choices available (excluding the private sector) are: (i) a residential or day school for the deaf, reserved for the most handicapped of deaf children; (ii) a partially hearing unit attached to a normal primary school for children who are capable of acquiring spoken language to such a degree that at least partial integration into the normal school will be possible, and; (iii) normal school with regular visitation by a peripatetic teacher of the deaf for children minimally handicapped, who are able to cope with the language and educational expectations of the normal classroom.

3. Provide practical advice in cases where there is marked lack of progress in developing language, or lack of educational progress at school. A psychological assessment, in which tests of language and educational attainment and tests of specific abilities are administered, may be able to identify areas of relative deficit (perhaps specific learning disabilities) and areas of relative competence in the child's pattern of intellectual and educational functioning. Recommendations can then be made regarding future school placement and management, the need for remediation, and the nature of any remedial therapy.

4. Assist in the understanding of, and therapy for, behaviour problems and emotional and social maladjustment in children with a hearing loss. A recent study by Ives (1976) found that of over 2000 deaf and partially hearing children, $12\frac{1}{2}$ per cent were judged to be severely maladjusted, twice the maladjustment rate found among normally hearing children. The deaf child's difficulty in adjusting to his handicap and his behavioural reaction to this may stem from a number of causes including frustration arising from an inability to communicate, debilitating motivation in learning situations arising as a reaction to repeated failure in learning to speak or read, parental mismanagement and spoiling. Parent counsell-

ing in order to prepare families for the adjustment problems and behaviour difficulties which are commonplace is an increasingly important role for the clinical or educational psychologist working with hearing-handicapped children. It may be necessary in individual cases to provide specific forms of therapy to enable children with marked adjustment problems and their families to overcome these difficulties, e.g. behaviour modification techniques have proved effective in eliminating problem behaviours while developing more appropriate behaviours in many handicapped children.

Clinical and educational psychology is increasingly extending its service to hearing-handicapped children, beyond the limited provision of IQ test results to the understanding and management of the child's learning and educational problems together with his social adjustment and behavioural reactions to his disability.

SOME PROBLEMS ASSOCIATED WITH THE CHOICE OF HEARING AIDS (GL)

This is inherently a difficult problem as much of the evidence in favour of one or other type of aid, as it is applied to a certain hearing-impaired child, is subjective and individualistic. One of the problems is the need to provide adequate amplification for a young hearing impaired infant when the true extent of his hearing loss may be incompletely known.

Even with a young infant it is usually possible to say whether his hearing is probably normal, or only slightly impaired; or that it is considerably impaired, or profoundly affected with only a little residual hearing. In the case of older children and adolescents, there will be one or more audiograms available. This will ease the task of selecting a suitable aid for the child, but as will be shown later, reliance solely on audiograms can produce some paradoxical results. Generally speaking, children with a mild or moderate hearing loss present few problems when choosing a hearing aid. These children have substantial residual hearing and virtually any amplification system will be beneficial. On the other hand those with profound hearing losses and only small vestiges of residual hearing pose the most difficult problems of choice. The reasons for this of course are obvious; much of the residual hearing may be of questionable value in the discrimination of speech, there may be tolerance problems owing to recruitment and the audiometric curve may be steeply sloping (high-tone loss), or in many profound losses, the bulk of the residual hearing may be concentrated in the lower frequencies with little or no useful hearing in the high frequencies. These are the most difficult cases when it comes to hearing aid selection.

It is evident from the foregoing that the choice of an aid for a young infant who is too young to be assessed by an audiogram, is a somewhat empirical process. In cases with a modest loss it is quite easy to fit the child with a suitable aid and get his teaching programme underway without delay. Reappraisal from time to time as his teaching proceeds will enable modifications in the gain settings to be made and the child will be encouraged to co-operate in attempts at audiometry until eventually a stable audiogram is available which may influence the audiologist to revise the choice of aid. His progress in acquiring speech, however, is probably of greater significance. For this group of children in the United Kingdom the Medresco range of aids is available at NHS* hearing aid dispensaries, while contract arrangements exist whereby the consultant (otologist or audiological physician) can order one of the many commercially available aids if the regular NHS model is considered insufficient. The availability of 'free' NHS aids has some distinct advantages, especially with young children, because the audiologist will not feel inhibited from ordering one of these aids on a tentative basis so that the child can have a trial of diagnostic teaching with the aid. Should it later emerge that the child can manage without an aid (the loss being too slight to matter much) or if a conductive hearing loss should clear (spontaneously, or as a result of surgical treatment) the aid is simply taken back into stock.

In a young child who clearly has a severe or profound loss, but who is too young for adequate audiometry, it is essential to provide a realistically powerful aid. Initially there may be some problems in inducing the young child to accept a strong aid and it may be wise to use a less powerful one, e.g. a conventional NHS model, initially before attempting to fit a really powerful aid. It would seem reasonable to try fitting him with an aid which will give an output 40 dB above his presumed threshold. One has to look for signs of awareness to sound as a result of wearing the aid and at the same time be on the lookout for evidence of intolerance to sounds (possibly the result of recruitment) which may lead to the child wincing, or protesting bitterly and refusing to wear the aid. Most aids chosen for such children would incorporate some form of dynamic range compression, either peak limiting, or better, automatic volume control which operates without distorting the input signal. Regular supervision of a young infant fitted with a powerful aid together with regular consultations with the teacher of the deaf will usually permit the efficacy of the aid to be estimated. A Y-lead configuration is often employed initially with aid supplying amplified sound to both ears. If asymmetry in the loss on the two sides is suspected a pair of aids may be provided. It is of course essential to ensure that well fitting earmoulds are supplied and replaced as often as necessary to maintain a good fit in the meatus so preventing oscillation. Adjustments of the frequency response may be made on a trial basis.

When a stable audiogram has been obtained from a profoundly deaf child there may be grounds for revising the choice of aid if it is felt that the initial choice was not the ideal one. Audiometric thresholds, however, are not the ultimate arbiter of hearing aid selection, as many anomalous results are observed.

In choosing aids school age children who can do audiograms and have some language there are at least two differing approaches.
1. One is the method of Byrne (1978) and Gengel, Pascoe, and Shore (1971)—*inter alia*—where audiometric thresholds are established (in dB SPL) using a calibrated hearing aid receiver and earmould especially made for the child, with a length of plastic tubing as in an ear level aid if

* National Health Service.

such is envisaged. These measurements are then used as a basis for the choice of aid according to its maximum output and its frequency response. This method relates the aided threshold to a speech spectral profile so as to select the aid with the most suitable gain, output and response characteristic. These commendable efforts, however, still leave a number of uncertain or even empirical steps in the choice process and the Nuffield Centre of the Royal National Throat, Nose, and Ear Hospital a slightly simpler method is used for deciding between the merits of one aid as opposed to others.

2. The method used at the Nuffield Centre consists of finding unaided and aided thresholds using ⅓ octave noise bands in a free field, so as to establish the effective gain of the aid in the ear. This permits the gain to be plotted on the conventional audiogram and allows the uncomfortable loudness level (UCL) to be measured and thus the dynamic range of the ear to be estimated. A restricted dynamic range would support the likelihood of sound intolerance. (Evidence of recruitment based on the stapedial reflex thresholds—if available—can also be helpful in this context.)

In addition, aided speech discrimination scores using suitable recorded material (Fry or Boothroyd word list) give some measure of the efficiency of one aid as opposed to another, bearing in mind the inherent variability of these measures. An improvement of 10 per cent in the discrimination score is the least that is considered meaningful in this context. Adjustments to an aid, e.g. alterations of frequency response, can also be monitored by these methods. In addition, simulated environmental noise can be added to the test sounds.

As well as choosing the most suitable aid for a profoundly deaf child, these methods can be used in assessing the relative performance of ear-level versus body-worn aids. It is well known that most older children become restive about wearing body-worn aids and at puberty many simply throw off their aids altogether. An ear-level hearing aid is often the only way out of this situation even in some profoundly deaf children whether the ear-level aid is equally effective (or even a little less effective) than the body-worn, if the alternative is a stubborn refusal of the child to co-operate in use of any form of amplification.

The use of narrow-band free-field (NBFF) noise and free-field speech testing has proved very helpful in hearing aid selection at the Royal National Hospital. It has also demonstrated some unexpected tolerance difficulties in a number of cases which would have gone unsuspected if the choice of aid had been based primarily on inspection of pure-tone audiometric thresholds.

Fig. 26.3 shows NBFF charts used at the Nuffield Hearing and Speech Centre. Figs. 26.4–26.6 show charts from selected patients.

This selection of audiometric tests indicate the fact that slavish attention to details of the pure-tone audiogram does not always produce the best results when fitting a hearing aid to a severely deaf child. In such cases the

(a) Free-field narrow-band results

	Unaided	Using Aid A		Using Aid B	
Frequency (Hz)	Threshold (dB)	Threshold (dB)	Gain (dB)	Threshold (dB)	Gain (dB)
250	90	70	20	85	5
500	85	50	35	50	35
1000	85	45	40	40	45
2000	80	45	35	40	40
3000	90	70	20	55	35
4000	90	75	15	60	30

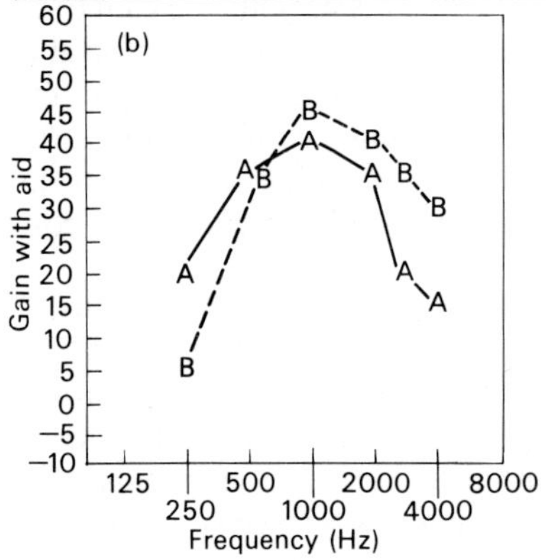

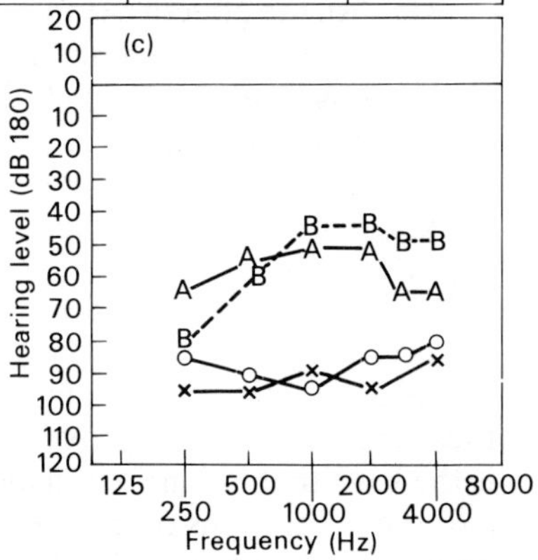

Fig. 26.3. NBFF charts used at the Nuffield Hearing and Speech Centre. (a). The hearing threshold results are charted according to the frequency used and the type of aid worn at the time. The volume setting, type of receiver, and whether worn monaurally or binaurally are noted. (b). The gain used is then plotted direct on to charts for each aid used, A and B. (c). The gain obtained is then added on to the PTA for the respective ear, or a combination of both to give the level at which the child is perceiving amplified sound.

NB Frequency (Hz)	UCL (Δ) with aid E (dB)	Threshold with aid E (dB)	Dynamic range = aid E (dB)
250	none	↓ 90	–
500	80	65	15
1000	75	60	15
2000	75	70	5
3000	none	↓ 90	–
4000	none	↓ 90	–

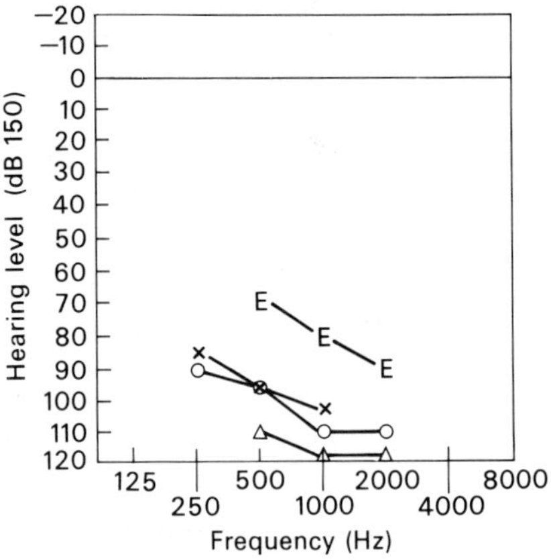

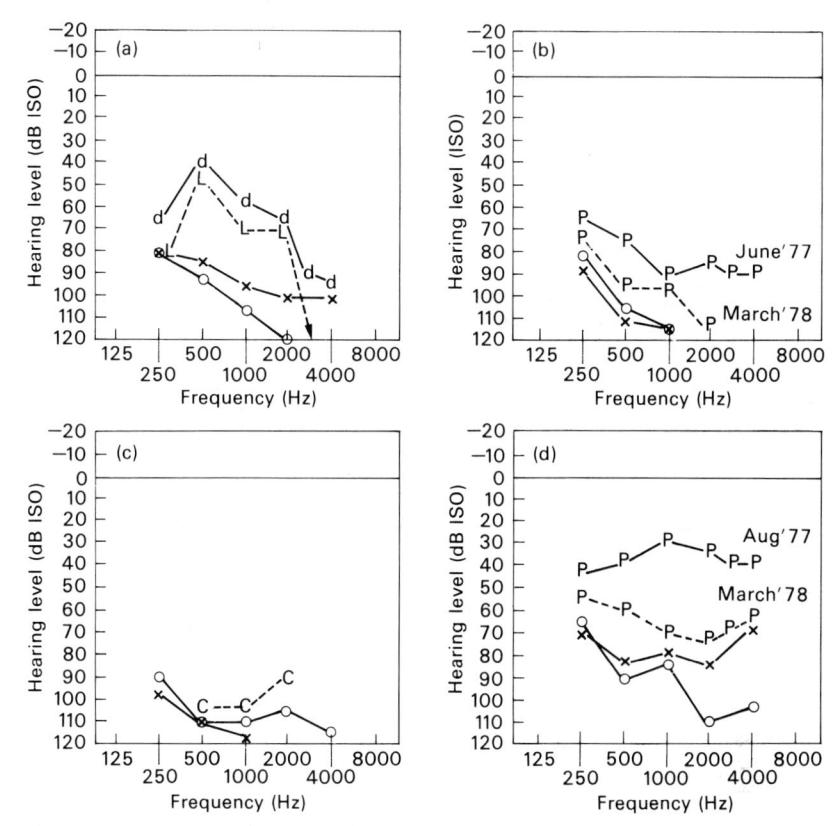

Fig. 26.5. Four different problems which have been elucidated by NBFF testing. (1). Boy with good auditory awareness but with poor speech discrimination. He preferred aid (L) to aid (d) on first visit but accepted the latter after six weeks of intensive auditory training. (2). Girl of 14 years who, on testing in June 1977 showed loudness intolerance and has a good gain with aid (P). In March 1978 the same aid showed a marked decrease in gain and loudness intolerance was now very noticeable. (3). Girl of 9 years with such severe loudness intolerance that even a compression aid (C) gives minimal gain and the girl refuses amplification. (4). Boy showing a decrease in auditory awareness over a six-month period of using post aural aids (P) owing to poor motivation to use amplification in the absence of any loudness (in)tolerance problem.

◁ Fig. 26.4. Results of the NBFF test in a profoundly deaf boy whose ears have a very restricted dynamic range which caused severe tolerance problems. The table on the left shows the restriction of the dynamic range (in relative dB) while the audiogram on the right shows the gain using aid E that could be achieved. Such a gain however would exceed his uncomfortable loudness level (U). During this test the boy showed no intolerance to loud sounds until the NB frequency centred on 2 kHz was introduced. This noise band initiated intolerance which was noticeable at all other frequencies tested. These symptoms of intolerance persisted on retesting for at least two hours. (NB = narrow band, UCL = uncomfortable loudness level.)

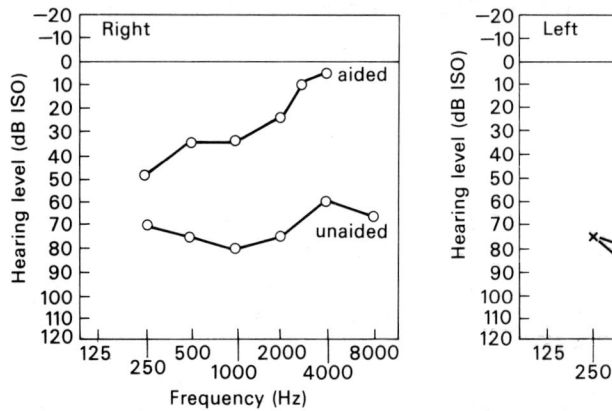

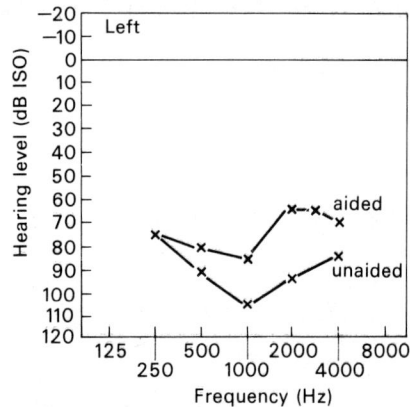

Fig. 26.6. Patient with unilateral distortion of the hearing in the left ear which was confirmed by NBFF and speech discrimination tests. It can be seen that the aided threshold is much lower in the right ear than in the left ear when tested by NBFF sounds. Fry word lists were presented wearing the aid: (i) right ear, aided, at 65 dB dial settings = 94 per cent; (b) left ear, aided, at *any* intensity, the right ear being blocked = 6 per cent; (c) right and left ears both aided, at dial settings of 65 dB = 69 per cent. This shows amplification applied to the left ear actually *decreases* the child's overall binaural performance.

NBFF and speech discrimination scores often give additional information which allows a suitable hearing aid to be chosen and fitted successfully, thereby enhancing the child's educational progress.

REFERENCES

BLOOM, F. (1979). Our deaf children—into the 80s. National Deaf Children's Society, London.
BYRNE, D. (1978). Selection of hearing aids for severely deaf children. *Br. J. Audiol.* **12**, 9–22.
CHOMSKY, N. (1965). *Aspects of a theory of syntax.* MIT Press, Massachusetts.
DALE, D. M. C. (1979). Educating deaf and partially hearing children individually in ordinary schools. *Talk* **91**, 20–3.
GENGEL, R. W., PASCOE, D., and SHORE, I. (1971). A frequency response procedure for evaluating and selecting hearing aids for severely hearing-impaired children. *J. Speech Hear. Dis.* **36**, 341–53.
IVES, L. (1976). Conclusions and recommendations from a screening survey of 2060 hearing-impaired children in the Midlands and North of England. Royal Schools for the Deaf (Manchester), Occasional Publications.
KERNOHAN, H. and JONES, H. (1979). Micro-teaching techniques in teacher training. *Br. J. In-service Educat.* **5**, 53–4.
PLOWDEN REPORT (1967). Children and their primary schools. Central Advisory Council for Education (England). HMSO, London.
ROBSON, P. I. (1979). Total communication. A description of work undertaken at the Jack Ashley School between Nov. 1976 and Jan. 1979. (Limited publication.)
WARNOCK, H. M. (1978). Chairman: Report of the committee of enquiry into the education of handicapped children and young people. HMSO, London.

27 Non-organic hearing loss in children

H. A. BEAGLEY

Non-organic hearing loss (NOHL) has come into prominence in recent years mainly because of the availability of various 'objective' tests by which the diagnosis can be verified. Prior to this the clinician often suspected NOHL but had no means of identifying it with certainty, and it was usually only in retrospect, when the hearing loss simply seemed to have disappeared, that NOHL was considered to have been the likely cause.

Disappearance of the apparent hearing loss is one of the key features of NOHL, especially in children where the condition is essentially transient in nature, rarely lasting more than a few weeks or months. In a series of many scores of these cases, all were of relatively short duration except for one which lasted for a whole year and that case had a strong psychiatric element. But even in this example the apparent hearing loss eventually disappeared completely.

Some years ago the scheme shown in Table 27.1, was proposed (Beagley 1973) to indicate the various organic and non-organic hearing losses and how one is related to the other. This scheme is still valid except that (4) tends to be seen in adult mediological cases rather than in children (Fig. 27.1). These various combinations are met when investigating cases of suspected NOHL.

TABLE 27.1. *Scheme indicating the continuum of hearing losses encountered when investigating cases of suspected NOHL (from Beagley 1973)*

1. Pure simulated hearing loss
2. Organic hearing loss and simulation
3. Organic hearing loss and dissimulation
4. Complete unilateral hearing loss and simulation
5. Apparent simulation
6. Pure organic hearing loss

In the past, clinicians who suspected NOHL had to use various subterfuges to uncover the patient's deception, but today the diagnosis presents no serious problems by virtue of the powerful tests now at the disposal of the audiologist. But these important modern diagnostic aids would be quite useless if the clinician did not in the first instance *suspect* that the hearing loss that he detected in the patient might possibly be non-organic, for if he did not suspect NOHL the diagnosis procedures to prove or disprove it would not be instituted. In fact the audiogram shown in Fig. 27.2 presents such a case. The patient, a 9-year-old girl, appeared to have a sensorineural hearing loss of 40–50 dB which had largely disappeared after 21 months. Indeed it *may* have been a true hearing loss which recovered; but equally, or perhaps more likely, it could have been a case of NOHL. Unfortunately the appropriate tests were not carried out to confirm or disprove NOHL which in retrospect, is the probable diagnosis, especially as stress within the family (the father had recently died of leukaemia) was a notable feature of the case history.

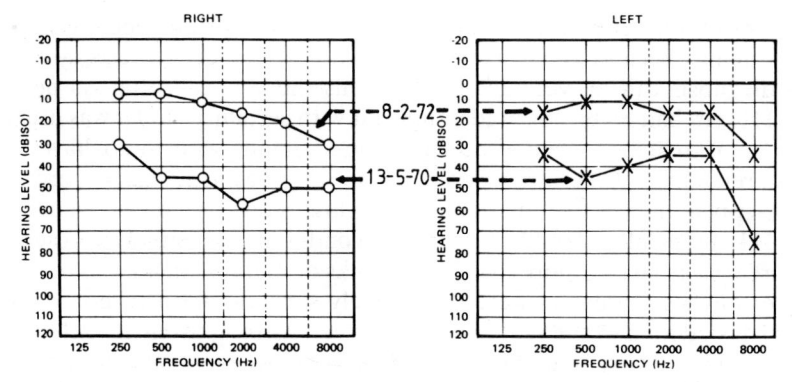

Fig. 27.1. This shows the pure-tone audiograms of a 9-year-old girl thought to have a moderate sensorineural hearing loss, but this apparently cleared up spontaneously in less than two years. In retrospect, this was almost certainly a case of non-organic hearing loss which was not suspected initially and not therefore investigated sufficiently to clarify the diagnosis. (From Beagley 1973.)

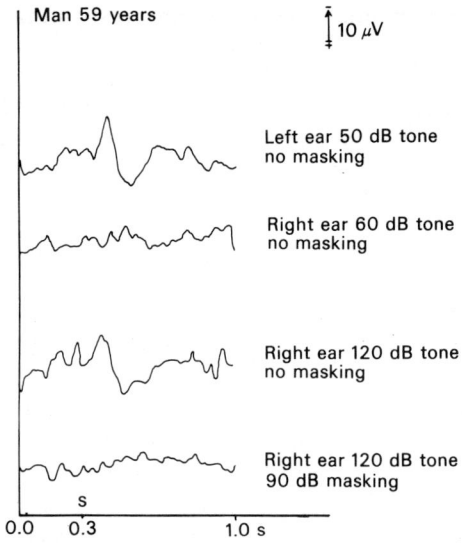

Fig. 27.2. This shows a patient with a total hearing loss in one ear. He refused to acknowledge cross-over hearing to the deaf ear at high levels of stimulation, although the cortical-evoked potential revealed that cross-over was in fact occurring in the normal way. This effect is more likely to be seen in an adult patient in a medico-legal context. (From Beagley 1973.)

Simulated hearing loss and malingering in adults and the medico-legal consequences of these are dealt with by Alberti in Chapter 41 (see also Coles and Priede 1971). Malingering is rare in children but some of the relevant aspects of NOHL in children will now be considered. What most alerts the clinician to the possibility of NOHL in a child is the discordance between the various clinical tests, and the patient's performance. The child may claim that he cannot hear well, and a formal voice test where he is asked to repeat words delivered by the clinician in a normal conversational voice may seem to confirm this. The pure-tone audiogram similarly indicates a hearing loss. Nevertheless, the clinician may still be unconvinced because in a less formal situation the child seems to communicate remarkably well, answering questions normally and obeying verbal instructions. He may, however, claim or give the impression that he needs to lip read to be able to communicate with the examiner.

Faced with this inconclusive situation the clinician can do a number of things:
1. The stapedial reflex threshold can be obtained and if it is normal it means either normal hearing, or hearing loss with recruitment.
2. A speech audiogram can be very helpful as occasionally it is quite normal, and if such is the case, the diagnostic efforts can be discontinued and the patient reassured and his case simply kept under review.
3. If the speech audiogram (or the live voice test) is not entirely normal then some form of electrophysiological test of hearing should be employed to clarify the situation. Testing by Békésy audiometry can be revealing but young children are often unable to cope with the task. The Type V curve described by Jerger and Herer (1961) is an indication of stimulation.

UNILATERAL NOHL

Sometimes a patient will complain that one ear has a substantial hearing loss, say 70–80 dB or even more, yet on audiometry without masking there appears to be no transcranial transmission of sound to the opposite, normally hearing ear. Sometimes even when bone-conduction testing is being carried out the same thing is noted. As the transcranial attenuation by bone conduction is close to zero any reluctance to admit hearing the bone-conducted sound in the normal ear is extremely suspicious and the clinician will rightly suspect NOHL.

Reference was made above to complete unilateral hearing loss with (simulation condition 4 in Table 27.1). This is generally seen in adult cases in a medico-legal context. The subject in this case has an indisputably deaf ear usually as the result of an accident but the opposite ear is normal. When tested the patient may similarly fail to acknowledge any cross-hearing at all. It is of course impossible for the sound not to be transmitted transcranially to the good ear when an adequate intensity level is employed. It seems that the patient does not acknowledge the sound in his good ear because he feels, presumably, that it will in some way weaken his case.

Figure 27.1 shows an example of unilateral total deafness with simulation in an adult. Cases of this sort are unusual in children. The Doerfler–Stewart and Stenger tests can be very useful in elucidating cases of unilateral NOHL but in general they are more appropriate to adults than to children.

The most satisfactory test for elucidating NOHL is the ERA based on the V-potential (see Chapters 31 and 33). By this means a full audiogram can be obtained from either ear at any of the desired audiometric frequencies (Fig. 27.3). As the ERA is always a little less sensitive than the subjective ERA there is a built-in safeguard in using this test. That is to say, it is difficult to envisage the situation where the ERA would over-estimate the patient's ability to hear; usually it will be about 10 dB less sensitive, sometimes more.

Although ERA using the V-potential is the most desirable test for elucidating NOHL there are many cases where it cannot be used satisfactorily in children, even reasonably co-operative children, as co-operation can deteriorate during the lengthy ERA test procedure. In addition, young children's ERA traces are sometimes equivocal due to the large slow EEG

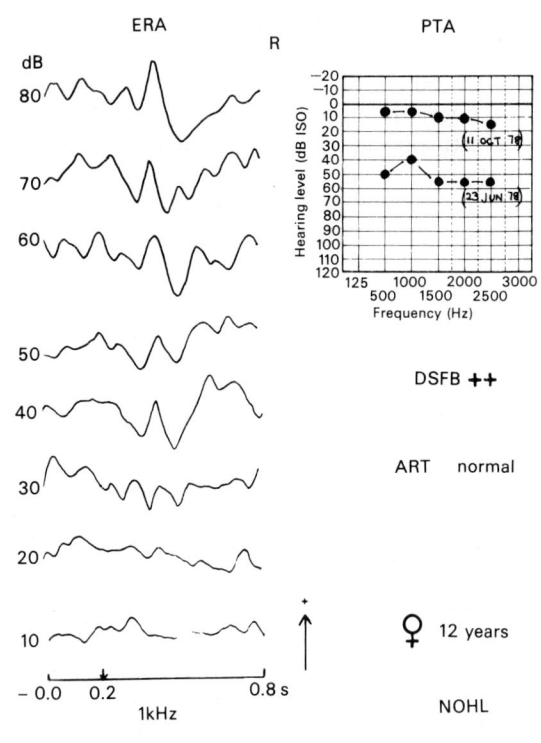

Fig. 27.3. This 12-year-old girl was simulating a hearing loss of about 50 dB, apparently the result of emotional stress. The ERA shows a positive response to at least 20 dB, the DSFB effect was strongly positive, and the acoustic stapedial reflex threshold was normal. The symptoms of hearing loss passed off spontaneously in a few months following reassurance.

Unilateral NOHL 689

waves which are not well handled by the averager while conditions such as epilepsy, habit-spasms, athetoid movements, or just plain fidgeting or frank non-co-operation can render the test impracticable.

In a reasonably co-operative infant the brain-stem electric response (BSER) can be obtained easily and quickly using clicks or high-frequency tone bursts. Unfortunately this very useful procedure gives little frequency information, but it does indicate the hearing level in the 2–8 kHz frequency range which can be compared with the subjective audiogram (Fig. 27.4).

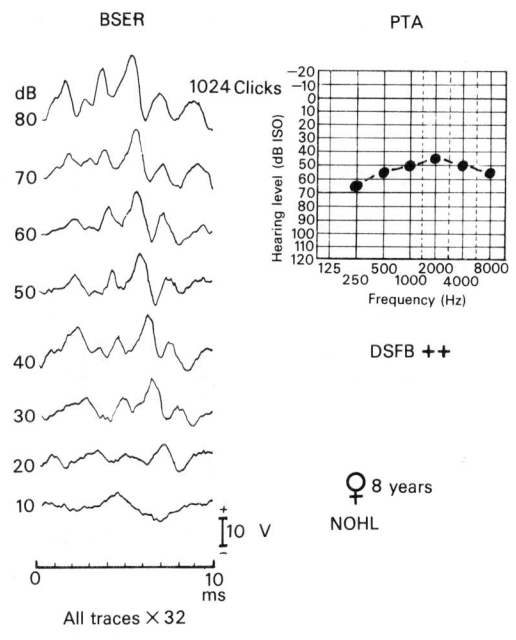

Fig. 27.4. This 8-year-old girl appeared, clinically, to be simulating a hearing loss of about 50 dB. However, the BSER and the delayed speed feedback test suggested that the hearing was normal. The apparent hearing loss subsequently disappeared spontaneously.

Rarely a child may be so unco-operative as to make BSER unsuitable even with mild sedation. In that case the BSER can be carried out using heavy sedation or even general anaesthesia (Hutton 1976; and Chapter 34). In such a case some audiologists, especially those trained basically in otology would proceed to carry out a transtympanic electrocochleogram as shown in Fig. 27.5. Fortunately it is very unusual to be faced with difficulties of this sort when investigating NOHL.

The clinical examination, pure-tone and speech audiometry, together with some form of electrophysiological assessment will permit NOHL, if present, to be identified, or if not present, to be eliminated diagnostically (Fig. 27.6).

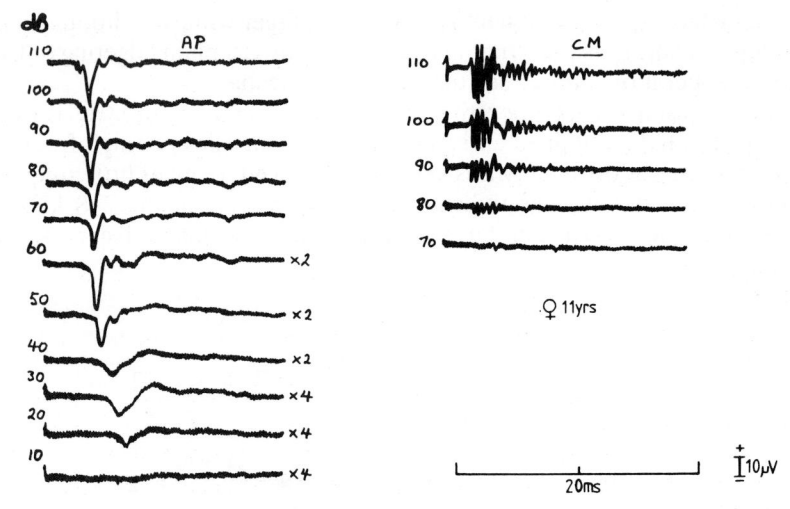

Fig. 27.5. This 11-year-old girl presented with many bizarre symptoms including an apparent hearing loss. ERA was unsatisfactory on account of inadequate cooperation. Electrocochleography under anaesthesia indicated that this was an example of NOHL. (From Beagley 1978.)

According to the results of the various tests the clinician can decide whether he is dealing with a pure NOHL, i.e. pure simulation, the true hearing being demonstrated to be within the normal range. More often the picture is mixed. One then finds that there is a certain level of organic hearing loss with an overlay of simulation which makes the loss appear greater than it really is. Finally, the tests may confirm that the hearing loss is entirely organic in which case the clinician's suspicion of a non-organic component cannot be sustained.

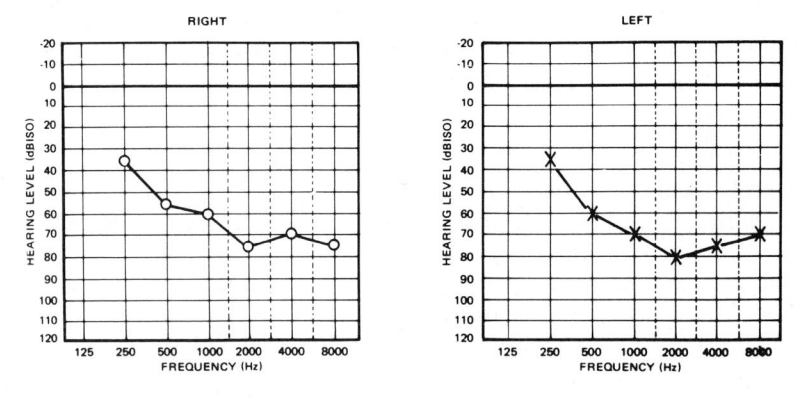

Fig. 27.6. Pure-tone audiogram of an 8-year-old child suspected of a non-organic hearing loss. However, the thresholds established by Békésy audiometry and ERA were in good agreement. A positive DSFB effect and normal acoustic stapedial reflex thresholds were attributed to recruitment, and the hearing loss was considered to be organic in nature and not an example of simulation. (From Beagley 1973.)

Once the presence of NOHL either complete or partial, has been discovered as a result of electrophysiological testing it is highly desirable to use a different test method by way of confirmation and many clinicians make use of the delayed speech feedback (DSFB) test. In this test the patient's voice is played back either to his right or his left ear with a delay of 200 ms, generally by using a specially adapted twin-track tape recorder. The delay in the voice-sounds that the patient hears disturbs the timing of his speech (as he reads a passage of simple prose) with the result that his speech becomes slurred and clear articulation of words is often quite difficult to achieve. This is known as a positive DSFB effect. Although the test has some disadvantages being somewhat qualitative, it nevertheless has the great advantage that a positive DSFB effect means only one thing, namely *that the patient has heard his own voice.* If he fails to hear his own voice owing to hearing loss then the characteristic voice changes will not be observed. Other disadvantages of the DSFB test is that a small minority of people are such fluent speakers that they are not noticeably affected by the delayed feedback and yet others are so semi-literate that their halting mode of reading a passage of simple prose means that there is no real fluency of speech against which the delayed feedback effects can be assessed.

To establish the norms for this test it is advisable to induce the speech changes by the DSFB method in a group of normal listeners and find the decibel level at which the effects are just observable. The tester should then listen to the tape and determine the decibel level at which the presence of the speech-sounds are just discernible in the taped recording and the difference between this value and the lowest level at which the subject showed speech slurring gives a measure of the DSFB effect. Commonly this is between 25 and 45 dB and this gives some basis for estimating whether or not the DSFB effect noted in a patient simulating a hearing loss is consistent with normal hearing. Absolute quantification of the method is impossible, but despite this it remains a valuable confirmatory test in cases of NOHL. But, as with the acoustic stapedial reflex, hearing loss with strong recruitment occasionally leads to a positive result (Fig. 27.6).

CONCEALMENT OF HEARING LOSS

This is the converse of NOHL, being the attempt by the patient to conceal a hearing loss, shown as item (3) in Table 27.1. A child may try to do this in order to avoid wearing a hearing aid. Careful audiometric technique will prevent such concealment as the latter is possible only by correctly guessing when the audiometric tone is presented sufficiently often to deceive the tester. Only rarely are special tests required to clarify the position. If it is suspected, all that is required is to repeat the audiogram under more rigorous conditions so as to avoid being deceived by the patient.

APPARENT SIMULATION

This includes those children frequently seen in audiology clinics who are referred following a school hearing survey and who have failed the audiometric test. On retesting in the clinic they may again produce an audiogram which suggests a hearing loss. But despite this they seem to hear and converse easily. Some even deny any suggestion that their hearing is other than quite normal. Spoken voice tests reveal no abnormality and a speech audiogram will be normal. Some of these children, in the course of a series of hearing tests, begin to produce normal pure-tone audiograms while others persist in giving audiograms which seem to indicate a hearing loss.

It is clear that such children do in fact hear normally, but for some reason they seem unable or unwilling to respond normally on pure-tone audiometry possibly because they are too cautious to admit hearing the test sounds as they are reduced in intensity towards subjective threshold. Once again, this is a transient condition. The clinician, having obtained a normal result on live voice testing or formal speech audiometry will usually find on seeing the child again in a few weeks' or months' time that he will respond normally on audiometry. Such children can be regarded as simply being 'poor audiometric subjects' and this is the reason for their apparent simulation.

CONCLUSIONS

Non-organic hearing loss is by no means uncommon in children of school age and early adolescence. Several different forms have been described and it must be stressed that most are transient episodes, usually clearing up in a few months or weeks and indeed in some cases there is no real simulation at all, simply an inability or an apparent unwillingness to perform and produce a valid audiogram without other evidence of hearing loss.

The management of NOHL is fairly simple. It consists mainly of reassuring the child and his relatives that his hearing problem is not serious and that it will disappear spontaneously before very long. In cases where the loss, or apparent loss, is causing much distress to the child or parents, a hearing aid can be given as a relatively short-term expedient on account of its placebo effect. Psychological or psychiatric problems which sometimes precipitate the condition, of course require the appropriate counselling and management. It is unwise to adopt a censorious attitude towards a child who simulates a hearing loss, as the origin of the simulation may be complex and obscure in many cases, just as it is fairly obvious in others. A warm, reassuring attitude towards the child is more likely to cause this essentially transient condition to clear up rapidly than will any rebuke or overt disapproval.

REFERENCES

BEAGLEY, H. A. (1973). The role of electro-physiological tests in the diagnosis of non-organic hearing loss. *Audiology* **12**, 470–80.
—— (1978). Edith Whetnall's contribution to British audiology. *J. R. Soc. Med.* **71**, 870–8.
COLES, R. R. A. and PRIEDE, V. M. (1971). Non-organic overlay in noise induced hearing loss. *Proc. R. Soc. Med.* **64**, 194–5.
HUTTON, J. N. T. (1976). Anaesthesia for electrocochleography. *Clin. Otolar.* **1**, 39–44.
JERGER, J. and HERER, G. (1961). Unexpected dividend in Békésy audiometry. *J. Speech Hear. Dis.* **26**, 390–1.

28 Surgical treatment of conductive deafness in children

N. SHAH

Sound energy is conveyed from the external ear to the inner ear via the tympanic membrane and the ossicles. For the middle ear to function efficiently it must have the following: an intact mobile tympanic membrane; an intact mobile ossicular chain; phase difference of the oval and round window; and a physiologically functioning Eustachian tube. Dysfunction of any of the above four will result in conductive deafness. The types of conductive deafness amenable to surgery described here are: congenital atresia; ossicular abnormalities; perforation of the tympanic membrane; middle effusions; and chronic otitis media.

CONGENITAL ATRESIA

During embryonic development the middle ear arises from the branchial system, whereas the inner ear is derived from the ectodermal cyst. Therefore, it is rare to find congenital defects in both the middle and inner ear on the same side. Any deformity may be unilateral or bilateral and varies a great deal in individual cases. In the external ear there may be complete absence of the auricle, accessory auricles, or microtia with atresia of the meatus. Atresia is usually associated with a deformed middle-ear cavity, but usually the inner ear is normal. The incus and malleus are almost invariably deformed and often fused together. The facial nerve may take an abnormal course in the middle ear.

If any abnormality is suspected, a comprehensive developmental assessment of the child should be made and special attention paid to the upper respiratory tract. This assessment should include detailed X-ray studies including polytomography, under anaesthesia if necessary. These studies should reveal whether an auditory canal is present, and the condition of the ossicles, cochlea, and labyrinth. It is very important to know whether the mastoid is sclerotic, diploic, or well pneumatized.

Surgery is not indicated, in the author's view, when the deformity is unilateral. However, when deformities exist in both ears, surgery at an early date should be considered. If suitable, one ear should be operated on when the child is between three and five years old, before starting school. Although the cosmetic result may be imperfect, the creation of a new meatus, and ossicular reconstruction with restoration of partial hearing allows satisfactory use of a hearing aid (Fig. 28.1). However, surgery must only be performed by an otologist with experience in this field if disastrous results are to be avoided (Fig. 28.2).

Since the anomaly can vary from a simple deformity of the pinna to

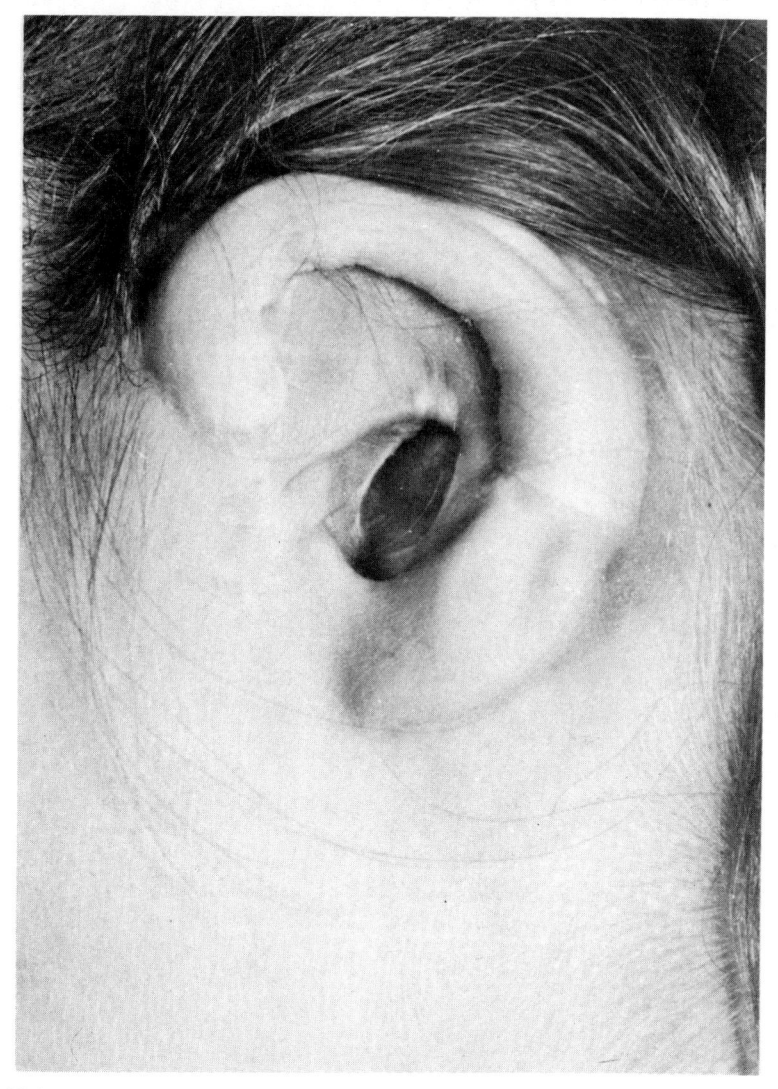

Fig. 28.1. New ear and new canal with a clean, dry cavity.

complete absence with stenosis, only the basic principles of surgery are described. If present, the deformed pinna is always situated forwards and downwards near the temporomandibular joint. Some form of Z plasty is always necessary to create a new external auditory meatus. After the skin incisions have been made, the bony landmarks can be identified. The triangular area between the linea temporalis and lateral sinus is explored with a drill and mastoid antrum is exposed. The aditus is followed upwards

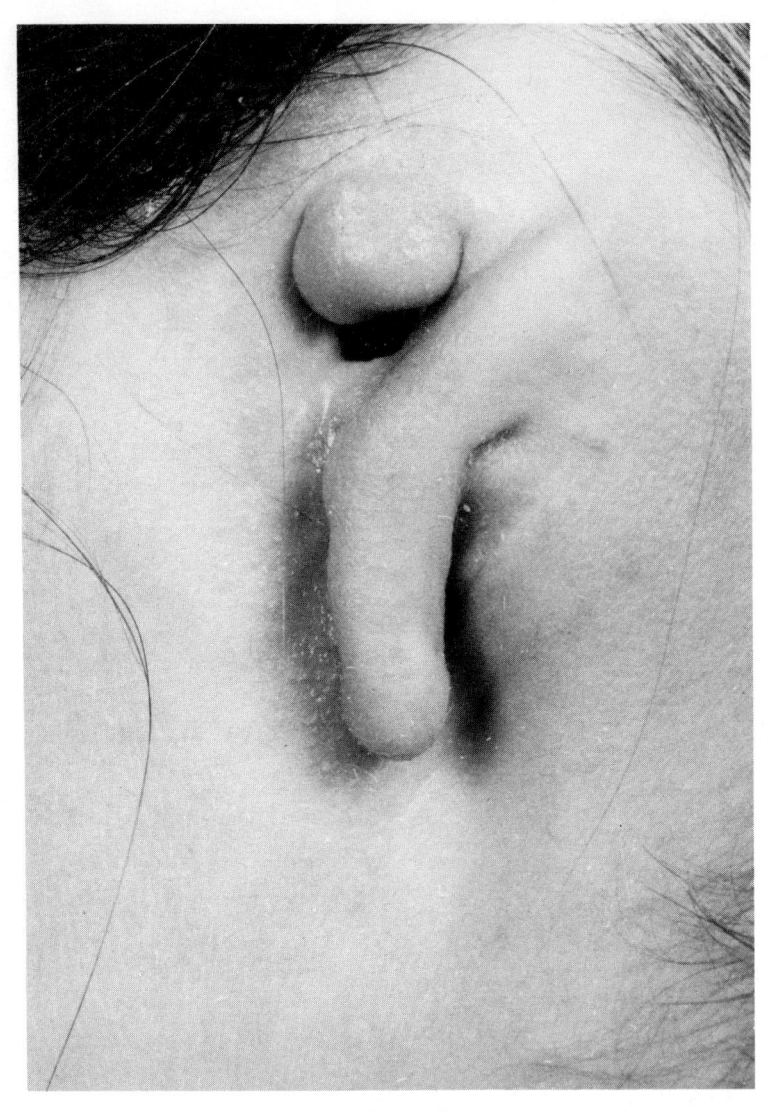

Fig. 28.2. Unsatisfactory surgical result. Discharging cavity and facial palsy.

and forwards until the ossicular chain is identified. A wide area of exenteration is required to create a sufficiently large canal. By using tympanoplastic techniques of reconstruction or using cadaveric homografts, a new sound energy transfer mechanism is established. The new canal is well prepared by skin grafts and adequate packing is applied. Meticulous post-operative care of the mastoid cavity and the meatus is essential if good results are to be achieved.

OSSICULAR ABNORMALITIES

Ossicular deformity with a normal external auditory meatus and pinna may be found. This may be of congenital, infective, or traumatic origin. The deformity may involve one or all ossicles and both the oval and round windows. The malleus and incus may be fused together or fixed in the attic, and there may be congenital fixation of the stapes. In cases of traumatic origin, there may be fracture or dislocation of the ossicles. If the deformity is bilateral, an exploratory tympanotomy should be considered. Reconstruction or reposition of the ossicular chain can be performed by using autologous or homologous grafts. However, in young children stapedectomy or opening of the vestibule should be postponed until the child is older.

TYMPANIC MEMBRANE PERFORATIONS

Following an acute infection in the middle ear, the tympanic membrane may rupture, resulting in a perforation which usually heals. If it fails to do so there may be secondary infection. A perforation that remains wet despite adequate local treatment is usually due to the presence of infection in the middle ear cleft. A careful assessment of the upper respiratory tract should be made and attention paid to adenoid, tonsil, and sinus disease before surgery is contemplated. Small or moderate sized central perforations may be freshened either with a caustic or a sharp instrument. In addition, the area may be covered with a thin paper or cellulose dressing.

Accidental head injuries or foreign bodies in the meatus may also cause the tympanic membrane to rupture. Usually perforations caused by such trauma close by themselves. However, careful inspection of the canal is mandatory and in some cases general anaesthesia may be necessary in order to remove foreign particles, debris, etc., if permanent damage is to be avoided.

The closure of a dry perforation of the tympanic membrane prevents recurrent discharge, may improve hearing, and enables the patient to swim. To close such a perforation, provided there is no disease in the middle ear or mastoid and the Eustachian tube is normal, the operation of myringoplasty should be performed. This procedure requires good exposure and is performed under general anaesthesia. Either the trans-meatal, endaural, or posterosuperior route may be used. The posterosuperior route (Fig. 28.3) is far more flexible and a temporalis fascia graft is obtained at the same time. To close the perforation, meatal skin, vein, periosteum, and more recently tympanic membrane homografts have been used. However, temporalis fascia is most widely used today. The graft may be placed outside (onlay) or inside (inlay) the remainder of the tympanic membrane but this depends upon the size and position of the perforation. In experienced hands, closure of the central perforation by this operation is achieved in over 90 per cent of cases.

The posterosuperior route is described here, as this is favoured by the

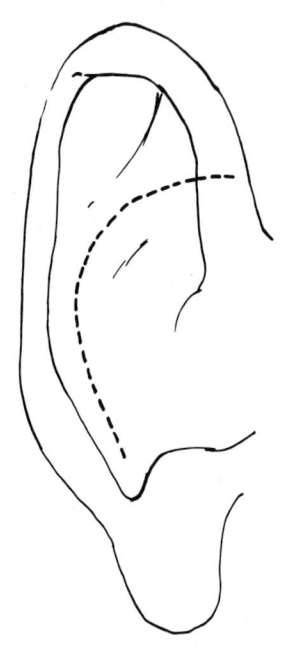

Fig. 28.3. Posterosuperior incision for mastoid surgery.

author. A posterosuperior incision a few millimetres behind the post-aural groove is made and the pinna is pushed forwards. The temporalis fascia and the mastoid are exposed. The skin at the top end is elevated by an angled retractor and the temporalis fascia is exposed further. A horizontal incision a few millimetres above the bony meatus is made through the fascia and it is separated from the muscle with a blunt elevator. A suitably sized piece of fascia is removed, cleaned, and dried for later use as a graft. The periosteum is incised and the meatal skin is elevated from the posterior meatal wall up to the tympanic annulus. An incision is made from the positions of twelve to six o'clock exposing the entire tympanic membrane. The retractors are positioned and the graft bed is prepared.

The posterior meatal skin and tympanic annulus is elevated and the graft is placed under the remnant of the tympanic membrane. If necessary the anterior bony canal wall is exposed and drilled to gain sufficient exposure. The condition of the ossicular chain is inspected at the same time. To support the graft, the middle ear may be filled with Sterispon soaked in an antibiotic–steroid preparation. The remnant of the tympanic membrane is replaced and the graft is covered by gelfoam pieces. The author uses a silicon disc on the lateral surface of the graft to maintain its position and for the prevention of adhesions between the graft and the packing material (Fig. 28.4). The previously elevated skin is replaced and the meatus is packed with half-inch BIPP (bismuth, idoform, and paraffin paste) ribbon gauze. The skin incision is closed with interrupted subcutaneous catgut sutures.

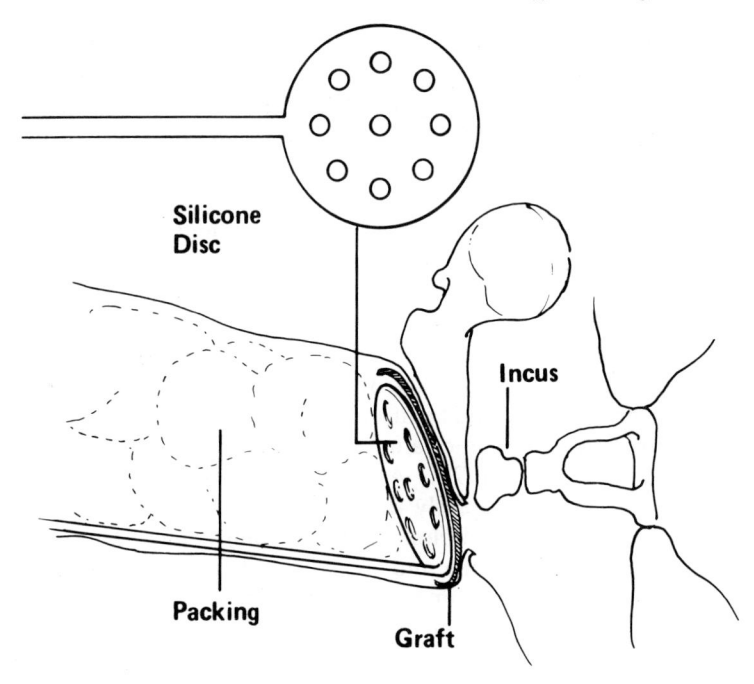

Fig. 28.4. Use of a silicone disc in myringoplasty.

MIDDLE EAR EFFUSION—GLUE EAR

Glue ear is the commonest cause of deafness in children in the western world. Approximately 10 per cent of all children are affected at some time in their early years. The incidence in infants and pre-school children is very much higher than generally recognized. In a recent survey of 'normal' nursery-school children in London, over 35 per cent had evidence of unsuspected fluid in their middle ears (Shah, unpublished observations). Between 1970 and 1977 at the Nuffield Hearing and Speech Centre, of 3472 children with impaired hearing, 1321 (38 per cent) had middle-ear problems. Of the total of 6049 in-patient admissions in 1977 at the Royal National, Throat, Nose, and Ear Hospital, London 1282 were for middle ear effusion.

Medical treatment should always be attempted before surgery. This usually consists of treatment with nasal decongestants. A combination of a solution of 0.9 per cent ephedrine hydrochloride and mild silver protein 1 per cent drops (Argotone drops) used twice a day seems to be more satisfactory than Ephedrine alone. Anitihistamines or specific treatment for a known allergy is advocated. However, long-term use of antihistamines should be avoided. If simple decongestant measures, for a period of six to eight weeks, are ineffective, surgery may be required.

The aim of the surgery is to remove the fluid and aerate the middle ear cleft. Under general anaesthesia, the ears are examined with an operating microscope. The external canal is irrigated and cleansed with normal saline, avoiding undue suction and trauma to the skin. With a sharp sickle knife a very small radial opening is made in the anterior or posterior inferior segment of the drum. The fluid, which is under pressure, soon appears through the incision, and is usually aspirated with a fine suction tip. If the fluid is viscous, the opening may be enlarged and aspiration using a larger bore suction tip can be continued until most of the fluid is removed. It may be necessary to make a counter incision to allow air into the middle ear in order to facilitate aspiration, and subsequently to insert the ventilating tube (grommet). Damage to the drum and consequent bleeding should be avoided. If there is excess bleeding it should be controlled by topical application of epinephrine solution. In all cases where the fluid is viscous ('glue'-like) a grommet should be inserted. Without this, myringotomy and aspiration are of no therapeutic value, and any initial hearing improvement is not maintained (Shah 1971). Although many varieties of tubes are available and function efficiently the 'Shah' tube (Fig. 28.5) has several advantages. It is firm, has an elongated triangular flange requiring only a small opening and slips readily under the incised drum margin like a shoe horn. After inserting the grommet, the procedure is completed by a gentle counter pressure on the opposite end of the tube which then slips inside the middle ear like a button. A few drops of oily antibiotic–steroid solution are put into the ear in order to prevent any blood clotting and secondary infection. A small pledget of cotton wool is placed in the meatus and removed the following day.

Adenoidectomy is also performed in most cases except in children with submucous or overt cleft palate. Tonsillectomy is only performed where there is a definite history of tonsillitis or where the tonsils are grossly enlarged, causing mechanical obstruction.

No special after care is required and there are usually no further complications. Parents are advised to place a plug of cotton wool covered with vaseline in the external meatus of their children's ears. This helps to prevent water from entering the ears, and, although children are not actively encouraged to go swimming, they are allowed to go in water provided the ears are covered by a bathing cap and they refrain from under-water swimming or diving. Surprisingly very few children develop secondary infection and any infection that does occur usually responds to local treatment. However, should such treatment fail the grommet tube should be removed.

After the operation, all children should be regularly examined and hearing tests performed. Usually they should be seen at intervals of three months. In most cases the tubes are extruded within six to nine months. However, if the tube is found to be migrating too rapidly or if there is marked evidence of tympanosclerosis the tube should be removed early.

Approximately 85 per cent of children respond if this treatment is carried out. However, where there is recurrence of glue ear, each case should be judged on its own merits and where necessary the child should be fitted with a hearing aid in preference to multiple operations. It is most important that

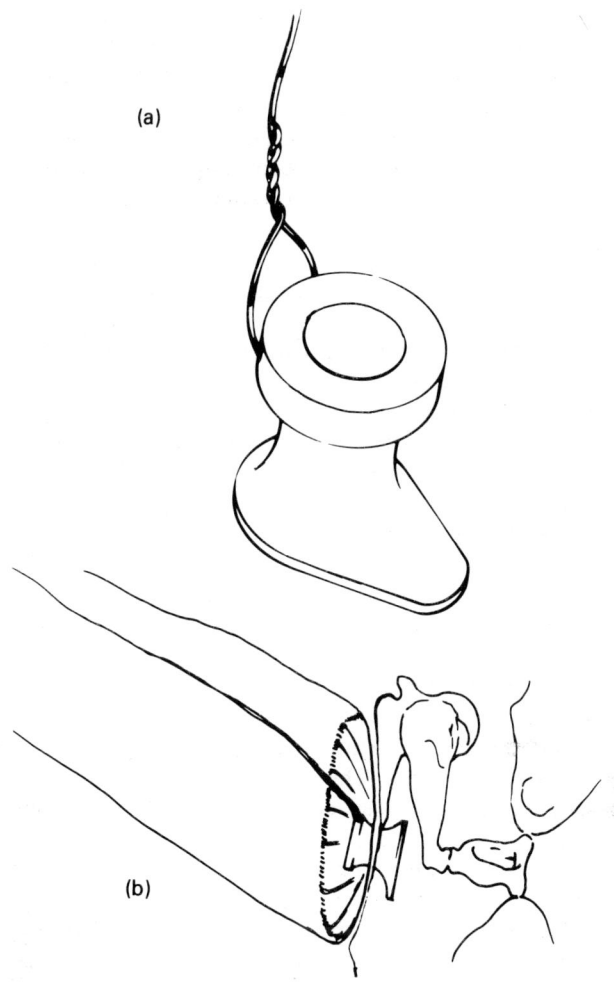

Fig. 28.5 (a). The 'Shah' grommet. (b). 'Shah' grommet shown in position in cross-section.

these children are followed closely and supervised by a qualified teacher of the deaf. Children with severe sensorineural hearing losses requiring grommets pose a considerable management problem. Ear moulds in the canal predispose the child to secondary infection, and where possible a vented mould should be used.

CHRONIC OTITIS MEDIA

Despite extensive use of antibiotics for treatment of upper respiratory tract infections, the incidence of acut middle-ear infection remains the same. However, early use of antibiotics has led to a dramatic fall in the complications of otitis media. It is now uncommon to see children with discharging ear or acute mastoid abscesses in hospital practice.

For many years the surgery of chronic otitis media was entirely concerned with eradication of diseased tissue to prevent serious complications. However, the development of microsurgical tympanoplastic techniques has made it possible to reconstruct a sound conducting apparatus in most cases. The very keen interest in combined-approach tympanoplasty over the last decade has not been maintained. Poor selection of cases, poor surgical technique, and resultant persistent residual cholesteatoma have led to multiple operations; this has resulted in some disenchantment with the procedure.

Difficult management problems are posed when surgical treatment of otitis media is attempted in younger children. Younger children are more prone to upper respiratory tract infections and attention must be paid to the tonsils, adenoids, and sinuses before embarking on surgical treatment. Radical mastoidectomy and similar open techniques require after-care which is both uncomfortable and painful. Unless necessary for fear of complications such operations should be postponed until the age of ten years or more.

The choice of surgical management is determined by the sharp distinction between two different forms of the disease.

Simple chronic otitis media—tubotympanic type

This is an acute suppurative otitis media resulting in a moist central or subtotal perforation. There is a mucous discharge which varies with the state of the upper respiratory tract. The middle-ear mucosa is red, oedematous, and thickened. The hearing loss may vary from 20 – 60 dB, being worse if the ossicular chain is affected.

The operation to be chosen for simple chronic otitis media is mastoidectomy with tympanoplasty using a closed technique. The technique is suitable for all types of simple chronic suppurative otitis media without cholesteatoma. The incision is almost identical to that described for a simple myringoplasty. The post-auricular incision is made and the pinna is pushed forwards. The periosteum is cut by two parallel incisions perpendicular to the posterior meatal wall through the muscular apponeurotic layers. When the two incisions are joined a wide periosteal flap is raised anteriorly. The piece of fascia for use as a graft is removed and retractors are positioned to expose the mastoid cortex. The posterior meatal skin is elevated and retracted forwards so as to expose the drum and its perforation. The bony landmarks are identified and the mastoid cortex is drilled using a large round burr. The mastoid antrum is opened and a complete mastoidectomy is performed. The middle ear is cleaned carefully and the ossicular chain is inspected and repaired if necessary. The temporalis fascia graft is placed in position over the perforation and the posterior meatal skin is replaced. The meatus is packed with ribbon gauze and the incision is closed in layers.

Chronic otitis media with cholesteatoma—attico-antral type

In this type of chronic otitis media it is possible to perform closed-technique tympanoplasty in selected cases, but most otologists agree that at least in children, open-technique radical mastoidectomy with tympanoplasty is the operation of choice.

The procedure consists of widely opening the cavities of the antrum, attic, and middle ear together with the removal the bony posterior canal wall. The so-called modified radical mastoidectomy involves leaving a bony bridge between the attic and the middle ear, and was designed to preserve function of the ear. However, this technique is unsatisfactory and is now replaced by the complete operation with some form of tympanoplasty.

The procedure is the same as for any ear operation—a posterosuperior incision is made in the skin and the pinna is pushed forwards. Haemostasis is completed by diathermy. The periosteum is incised close to the posterior canal wall and is elevated backwards to expose the mastoid cortex. The bony landmarks are identified and retractors are positioned. Bone removal is carried out by a drill with a round burr and the meatus is enlarged. Great care is taken to avoid exposing the dura or damaging the third portion of the facial nerve. The attic and antrum are opened with a drill with a small burr. The drilling is continued until the whole of the cholesteatoma matrix is exposed. All diseased tissue is removed and the facial ridge is sufficiently lowered to convert the bean-shaped cavity into a rounded one. Depending upon the size of the mastoid excavation, appropriate meatoplasty is performed for adequate ventilation of the eventual mastoid cavity. The cavity is cleaned with suction irrigation and in some cases a temporalis fascia graft may be placed to seal the middle ear. The cavity is packed with BIPP ribbon gauze and the wound is closed in layers. A mastoid dressing and bandages are applied. The immediate post-operative care of the mastoid cavity must be carefully performed if the life-long misery of a discharging mastoid cavity is to be avoided.

REFERENCE

SHAH, N. (1971). Use of grommets in glue ears. *J. Lar. Otol.* **85**, 283–7.

Section 6
Acoustic impedance and tubal function

29 Clinical use of acoustic impedance testing in audiological diagnosis

JAMES JERGER and DEBORAH HAYES

INTRODUCTION

The routine clinical use of impedance audiometry has substantially altered audiological evaluation and diagnosis. In the 30 years since Metz's (1946) initial report, the clinical value of impedance audiometry has become evident and its routine use is now widespread. Clinicians have long recognized the value of impedance audiometry in the identification of conductive hearing loss and the differentiation of middle-ear disorders. More recently, impedance audiometry has shown important diagnostic applications in the evaluation of sensorineural hearing loss and brainstem auditory pathway disorders. In addition to these significant diagnostic applications, clinical experience with impedance audiometry has shown that it makes an important contribution in the identification of conductive and sensorineural hearing loss in infants, young children, and the difficult-to-test patient.

In this chapter, we describe the components of the impedance test battery, their diagnostic applications in conductive, sensorineural, and brainstem auditory disorders, and discuss the application of impedance audiometry in the prediction of hearing sensitivity.

COMPONENTS OF THE IMPEDANCE TEST BATTERY

The impedance test battery consists of three measurements, the static compliance, the tympanogram, and the acoustic reflex test. Before discussing each of these measurements in detail, however, it is important to emphasize the distinct differences between individual impedance measurements, and the combination of these measurements into the impedance test battery.

Individually, the results of any single impedance measurement are usually ambiguous and have only limited diagnostic value. The patterns formed by the combinations of these different measurements, however, are usually unique to specific clinical conditions. This important point cannot be overemphasized. The search for diagnostic significance in any individual impedance measurement will lead inevitably to frustration and disappointment. The recognition of the diagnostic patterns formed by the individual impedance components, on the other hand, will lead to the definition of distinct clinical conditions. Herein lies the difference between impedance measurement and impedance audiometry. Impedance measurement is simply the gathering of data—the static compliance,† the tympanogram, and the acoustic reflex-threshold hearing level. Impedance audiometry, however, is the combination of the individual measurements into a test battery, the identification of the resulting pattern, and the recognition of this pattern as specific to a distinct clinical condition. With this important distinction in mind, we can first describe the individual impedance measurements, then examine the patterns of results formed by the complete test battery.

Static compliance

Static compliance is a single numerical value representing the acoustic impedance of the middle-ear system, in the plane of the tympanic membrane, at rest. It is typically measured as the equivalent volume, in cubic centimetres, of a column of air offering the same acoustic compliance as the middle-ear system under test.

Static compliance is derived from two measurements. First, a volume measurement is made with the tympanic membrane clamped in a position of low compliance, usually at $+200$ mm/H_2O air pressure. Next, a new volume measurement is made with the tympanic membrane at its point of maximum compliance (in normal ears, at, or around, 0 mm/H_2O). The second value is subtracted from the first, resulting in a numerical expression of the static compliance of the middle-ear system. In this manner, the volume of the external ear canal is subtracted out to yield the expression of the equivalent volume of air offering the same acoustic compliance as the middle-ear system under test.

The static compliance of the middle ear varies as a function of the frequency of the probe tone. For a probe-tone frequency of 220 Hz, for example, the average static compliance of normal middle ears is 0.67 cm^3 with a range of 0.30 to 1.60 cm^3 (Jerger, Jerger, and Mauldin 1972). As the probe-tone frequency is raised, the static compliance of normal middle ears also increases. A probe-tone frequency of 1000 Hz, for example, yields an average static compliance value of about 5.00 cm^3 (Dempsey 1975).

Usually middle-ear disorders will alter the acoustic compliance or impedance of the middle-ear system in a predictable manner. An increase in either mass or stiffness will result in a decrease in compliance (or, conversely, an increase in impedance). Thus, both otitis media and otosclerosis may result in static compliance values of less than 0.30 cm^3. Conversely, ossicular discontinuity increases the compliance of the middle-ear system, and in this condition static compliance values in excess of 1.60 cm^3 are frequently recorded.

Unfortunately, however, the static compliance values recorded in most middle-ear disorders tend to fall within the normal range of 0.30 to 1.60 cm^3,

† The term 'static compliance' is a widely used and useful term for discussing the acoustic impedance of the ear. Purists, however, may claim that with sound, which is a dynamic stimulus, there can be no true 'static' compliance. The term, of course, refers to the total middle-ear compliance as measured between the baseline and the highest point on the tympanogram.

and there is little diagnostic significance in the static compliance measurement in isolation (Jerger 1970). Even an abnormal static compliance value has little diagnostic significance since a condition such as a scarred tympanic membrane, which produces no loss in hearing sensitivity, may result in the same abnormal static compliance value as that of an ossicular discontinuity which produces a substantial hearing disorder.

Static compliance, therefore, represents the acoustic impedance of the middle-ear system at rest, expressed in terms of the equivalent volume of air. The static compliance values recorded in pathological conditions using a 220 Hz probe-tone, overlap into the normal range of 0.30 to 1.60 cm^3. This substantially reduces the value of the static compliance measurement in isolation. The principal diagnostic value of the static compliance measurement lies in the detection of tympanic membrane perforations.

Tympanometry

Tympanometry is the measurement of the effect of varying air pressure on the mobility of the middle-ear system. The tympanogram, the graphic result of tympanometry, shows the change in compliance of the middle-ear system as air pressure is varied in the external ear canal.

In normal ears, the tympanogram will show a sharply defined peak of maximum compliance at or around 0 mm/H_2O air pressure. This shape will vary somewhat depending on the frequency of the probe tone. For a probe tone frequency of 800 Hz, for example, many normal ears show a notched, 'W-shaped' tympanogram (Alberti and Jerger 1974).

Fig. 29.1 shows the three types of tympanograms frequently observed using a 220 Hz probe tone (Jerger 1970). As stated earlier, the normal type A tympanogram shows a sharp peak of maximum compliance at or around 0 mm/H_2O, indicating a middle-ear system which transmits sound maximally at normal atmospheric pressure.

The type B tympanogram is characterized by the lack of a sharply defined peak of maximum compliance. Graphically, this tympanogram exhibits a rounded or flat rather than a peaked curve. Typically, it represents a middle-ear system of low compliance or high impedance.

The type C tympanogram is characterized by a peak of maximum compliance below −100 mm/H_2O. Similar to the type A, this tympanogram shows a sharply peaked curve. The middle-ear system transmits sound energy maximally at a particular air pressure value, but this value is outside the range of normal (+50 to −100 mm/H_2O) peak air pressures. This tympanogram indicates a condition of negative pressure in the middle-ear space.

Like the static compliance, the tympanogram has little diagnostic significance in isolation. The type A tympanogram, for example, is usually observed in normal middle ears, but in two important categories of middle-ear disorder, otosclerosis and ossicular discontinuity, a type A tympanogram is also seen. The type B tympanogram is typically associated with fluid-filled ears, as in secretory otitis media. It may also be observed in cases of cholesteatoma, or any other condition of mass-loading of the ossicular chain.

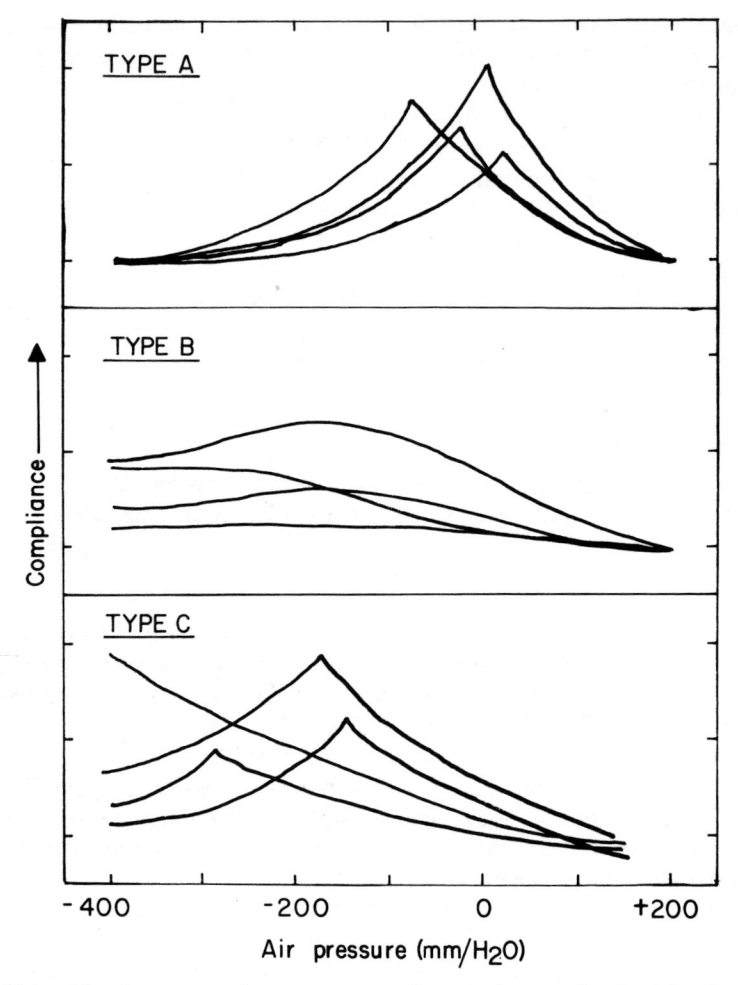

Fig. 29.1. The three types of tympanograms. Type A shows a sharply defined point of maximum compliance at or around 0 mm/H$_2$O air pressure; type B shows no maximum compliance point; type C shows a point of maximum compliance in the range below −100 mm/H$_2$O air pressure.

Therefore, the tympanogram is the graphic representation of the mobility of the middle-ear system under varying air pressure. In general, three basic shapes emerge depending on the mobility of the tympanic membrane, the status of the ossicular chain, and the air cushion in the middle-ear space. Although the three basic tympanograms are associated with several middle-ear disorders, they only grossly delineate these pathological conditions.

Acoustic reflex

The acoustic reflex is a much more complex measurement than either the static compliance or the tympanogram because it requires, simultaneously, sufficient sound intensity in the sound-stimulated ear, intact motor pathways in the brainstem and seventh (facial) nerve, and a normal middle ear on the recording (probe) ear.

The stapedius muscle typically shows a reflex contraction to sounds of sufficient intensity. Pure-tone signals (500 to 4000 Hz) in the range of 75 to 95 dB will usually produce the stapedius reflex. The reflex contraction is bilateral even with unilateral stimulation. Therefore it is possible to record both ipsilateral (uncrossed) and contralateral (crossed) acoustic reflexes. The ipsilateral acoustic reflex is elicited and recorded in the same ear. The contralateral acoustic reflex is elicited in one ear and recorded in the other ear.

The importance of ipsilateral acoustic reflex testing cannot be overemphasized. Certain ambiguities which may arise when only contralateral acoustic reflex is employed are often clarified by the addition of ipsilateral acoustic reflex measurement. The clinician must be aware, however, of the problem of artifact in the measurement of ipsilateral acoustic reflexes.

The ipsilateral acoustic reflex is elicted by presenting an intense reflex-eliciting signal into the same small cavity as the probe-tone. A technical problem arises in separating the acoustic effects due to a muscle contraction from the acoustic effects due to the interaction of the probe tone and the reflex-eliciting signal. Basically, the artifact problem results from the interactions of relatively intense acoustic signals in relatively small ear canal cavities. Although a number of approaches have been developed to overcome this ipsilateral acoustic reflex artifact problem, none has been entirely satisfactory (see Chapter 11). The clinician may avoid interpreting artifact as reflex-activity by carefully observing the direction of the impedance change as recorded by the compliance meter. Actual reflex activity, whether elicited by either ipsilateral or contralateral signal presentation, will be recorded as a *decrease* in compliance (increase in impedance) of the middle-ear system. Ipsilateral artifact, on the other hand, will typically appear as an *increase* in compliance (decrease in impedance). Thus, by simply observing the direction of the impedance change, the clinician can often avoid interpreting artifact as acoustic reflex activity in the measurement of ipsilateral acoustic reflexes. Unfortunately, the artefact is often so large that it masks the actual reflex and the test must be considered ambiguous.

Fig. 29.2 is a schematic representation of the brainstem acoustic reflex arc. The afferent portion also includes the cochlea, eighth cranial nerve, and portions of the brainstem auditory pathways. The efferent portion involves the brainstem pathways, the seventh cranial nerve, and the stapedius muscle. The contralateral reflex pathway crosses the brainstem; the ipsilateral reflex pathway does not (Borg 1973).

A disorder at any portion of the reflex arc will produce a unique effect on the acoustic reflex. A severe cochlear disorder, for example, will result in an 'afferent' effect, or the absence of the acoustic reflex whenever sound is delivered to that ear, regardless of whether the recording situation is ipsilateral or contralateral. A seventh cranial nerve disorder, on the other hand,

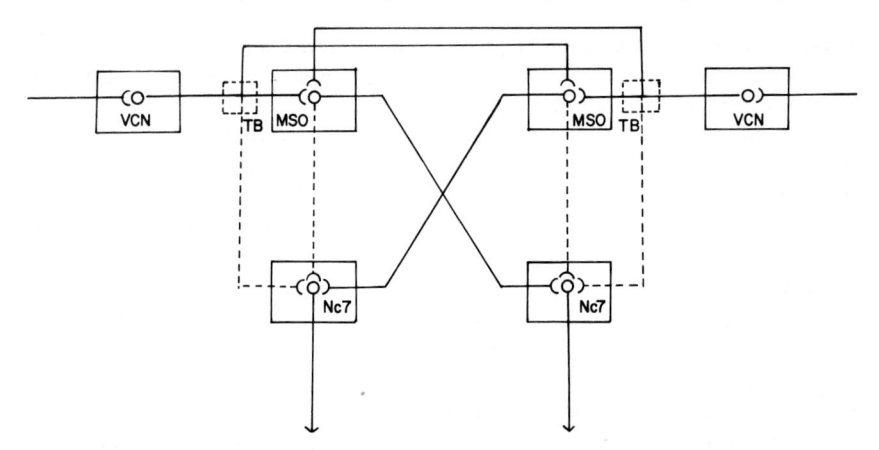

Fig. 29.2. A schematic representation of the acoustic reflex arc (after Borg 1973). The contralateral reflex pathways (solid lines) cross the brainstem; the ipsilateral (dashed lines) does not. (VCN = ventral cochlear nucleus; TB = trapezoid body; MSO = medial superior olive; Nc7 = motor nucleus of the seventh cranial nerve.)

will result in an 'efferent' effect, or the absence of the acoustic reflex whenever the recording probe is in the affected ear no matter which ear receives the reflex-eliciting signal. Finally, a disorder in the brainstem reflex pathways may result in the loss of both the contralateral acoustic reflexes but the preservation of both the ipsilateral acoustic reflexes (Greisen and Rasmussen 1970; Jerger, Neely, and Jerger 1975).

In addition to differentiating disorders in the afferent, efferent and brainstem reflex pathways, the acoustic reflex is also sensitive to middle-ear disorder in two ways. Firstly, when a reflex-eliciting signal is delivered to an ear with a middle-ear disorder and the recording probe is coupled to the opposite, normal ear, the acoustic reflex hearing threshold level (HTL) will be elevated by the amount of conductive hearing loss produced by the middle-ear disorder (Jerger Anthony, Jerger, and Mauldin 1974). Secondly, when the recording probe is coupled to an ear with a middle-ear disorder of even the slightest degree, the acoustic reflex is typically absent. Therefore, the acoustic reflex is sensitive to middle-ear disorders when used in both signal-eliciting and recording (probe) conditions. If reflex HTLs are normal in both ears it is usually safe to conclude that there is no middle-ear disorder in either ear.

The acoustic reflex, therefore, is the most diagnostically significant of the three individual impedance measurements. It is helpful in differentiating afferent (cochlear and eighth cranial nerve), efferent (seventh cranial nerve and middle ear), and brainstem effects. In addition, it is exquisitely sensitive to middle-ear disorder.

Nevertheless, certain ambiguities may arise in interpreting acoustic reflex findings in isolation. Therefore, as in the case of the static compliance test and the tympanogram, the acoustic reflex must be regarded as only one component of the total impedance test battery.

DIAGNOSTIC APPLICATIONS OF IMPEDANCE AUDIOMETRY

Identification of middle-ear disorder

The expected pattern of impedance results in middle-ear disorder is: (i) abnormal static compliance, (ii) abnormal tympanogram (iii) absent or elevated acoustic reflexes.

Results such as a static compliance value of $0.20\,\text{cm}^3$, a type B tympanogram, and absent acoustic reflexes would point decisively to a middle-ear disorder and probable substantial conductive hearing loss.

It is possible, however, for one or two individual impedance measurements to be quite normal even in the presence of a middle-ear disorder. In the case of an ossicular discontinuity, for example, the tympanogram may be a normally-shaped type A. The abnormally large static compliance and absent acoustic reflexes, however, will reveal the presence of the middle-ear disorder in this condition.

In early otosclerosis both the static compliance and the tympanogram may be considered normal. Only an abnormal or absent acoustic reflex reveals the presence of the middle-ear disorder (Terkildsen, Osterhammel, and Bretlau 1973).

The fact that a middle-ear disorder may produce an abnormal impedance result on only one measure of the total impedance test battery suggests a very important point in the diagnostic application of impedance audiometry. That is, if any one impedance measure is abnormal, the presence of a middle-ear disorder must be strongly suspected. In general, we expect all three impedance measures to be abnormal in the presence of a middle-ear disorder. A normal result from any one measurement does not rule out the presence of a middle-ear disorder. Only if results from all three measurements are quite normal is it safe to conclude that middle ear function is normal.

The nature of middle-ear disorder

Impedance audiometry can yield valuable information on the nature of middle-ear disorder. The various pathological conditions resulting in middle-ear disorder frequently form a unique pattern of impedance results. Although this pattern does not diagnose a particular disease process, it is an invaluable adjunct to the total audiological evaluation.

OTOSCLEROSIS

In patients with otosclerosis and related ossicular chain fixation a distinct impedance pattern typically emerges. The tympanogram is a shallow type A, the static compliance is usually in the range from 0.20 to $0.40\,\text{cm}^3$, and the acoustic reflex is usually absent bilaterally. Several variations of this pattern may occur. In some instances, the tympanogram will not be particularly shallow, but relatively normal. In conjunction with this apparently normal tympanogram, the static compliance may also be within the normal range. Finally, in some stages of early stapes fixation, the acoustic reflex may be elicited at relatively normal hearing threshold levels. However, these reflexes will show an abnormal time-course characterized by a negative deflection (decrease in impedance) at both the onset and offset of the eliciting signal (Djupesland 1969).

OTITIS MEDIA

The pattern of impedance results in otitis media is substantially different from otosclerosis. In otitis media, the tympanogram is usually a flat type B, the static compliance falls well below the normal range of 0.30 to 1.60 cm³, and the acoustic reflexes are absent when tested with the probe in the affected ear. In some early or late resolving stages of otitis media, a type C tympanogram may be observed with the point of maximum middle-ear compliance ranging from -100 to -400 mm/H_2O air pressure. If a type C tympanogram is present, acoustic reflexes may or may not be observed. If observed, they typically show a normal time-course, but may show threshold elevation above the normal levels of 75 to 95 dB HTL.

OSSICULAR DISCONTINUITY

Ossicular discontinuity typically results in a deep type A tympanogram, static compliance well above the normal range of 0.30 to 1.60 cm³, and absent acoustic reflexes if tested with the probe in the affected ear. Again there are several possible variations on this pattern. The tympanogram may not be very deep, and the static compliance value may fall within the normal range. Furthermore, the acoustic reflexes may be elicited with the probe tip in the affected ear at relatively normal reflex HTLs. This rather unusual finding arises when there is a functional connection between the stapedius tendon and that portion of the ossicular chain still attached to the tympanic membrane.

A further consideration must be made when interpreting a pattern of results that suggest an ossicular discontinuity. Although a deep type A tympanogram is the typical result of an ossicular discontinuity, any condition that increases the flaccidity of the tympanic membrane will also produce a deep type A tympanogram. Both monomeric and previously scarred tympanic membranes may produce this condition. In differentiating between tympanic membrane disorder and an ossicular discontinuity, the magnitude of the conductive component is an important consideration. The combination of an abnormally deep type A tympanogram and an air–bone gap of 30 to 50 dB suggests an ossicular discontinuity since most of the tympanic membrane conditions resulting in deep type A tympanograms are not associated with substantial conductive hearing loss.

CHOLESTEATOMA

Cholesteatoma may resemble ossicular chain fixation, otitis media, or even ossicular discontinuity, depending on the nature and extent of ossicular chain involvement. If the cholesteatoma produces only slight pressure against the ossicular chain, the impedance pattern of early fixation (type A tympanogram, relatively normal or slightly reduced static compliance, elevated reflex HTLs) will appear. If, however, the 'tumour' occupies much of the middle-ear space, virtually enveloping the vibratory mechanism and substantial mass to the system, then the impedance pattern characteristic of serous otitis (type B tympanogram, low static compliance, absent acoustic reflexes) will usually be seen. Finally, if the cholesteatoma erodes through the lenticular process of the incus, or the incudostapedial articulation, then the impedance pattern characteristic of discontinuity may well appear. In the latter case, it is not unusual to find that the cholesteatoma itself forms a functional link between incus and stapes, leading to a characteristically rounded or flat tympanogram and surprisingly little conductive hearing loss.

PERFORATION OF THE TYMPANIC MEMBRANE

Perforation of the tympanic membrane is the only condition in which the static compliance measurement alone is diagnostically significant. In this condition, the first volume measurement, the volume of air in the external ear canal, may reveal the presence of a perforation not readily visible otoscopically. The typical external ear canal volume measurement is between 0.50 and 1.50 cm^3. A volume in excess of 2.00 cm^3 usually means that the tympanic membrane is perforated. When a perforation is present, neither the tympanogram nor acoustic reflexes can be validly recorded.

In summary, various middle-ear pathologies tend to produce a specific pattern of abnormal impedance results. The resulting impedance patterns, however, should serve only as guidelines in the total audiological evaluation. Impedance measures reflect not the aetiology of the disease, but its effect on the physics of the middle-ear vibratory mechanism. Thus, impedance audiometry is a valuable tool in the diagnosis of middle-ear disorders, but it does not replace the total audiological evaluation.

The nature of sensorineural disorder

Although impedance audiometry was originally advocated primarily for the evaluation of middle-ear disorder, clinical experience has shown that it makes an even more valuable contribution in the evaluation of sensorineural hearing loss. The most dramatic application is the differentiation of cochlear and eighth cranial nerve disorders.

In general, the acoustic reflex is the single most important impedance measurement in evaluation of sensorineural hearing loss. However, the other measurements, the static compliance and the tympanogram, are important in confirming normal middle-ear function.

The acoustic reflex is useful in differentiating cochlear from eighth cranial nerve disorder in two ways. Firstly, the acoustic reflex is characteristically present in ears with cochlear disorder (below a limiting degree of hearing loss) and characteristically absent in ears with an eighth cranial nerve disorder. Secondly, when the acoustic reflex is unexpectedly present in an ear with eighth cranial nerve disorder, it typically exhibits an abnormal time-course in response to sustained signals (reflex decay).

In the ear with a cochlear disorder, the acoustic reflex sensation level (SL) for pure tones in the 500 to 4000 Hz region declines in exact proportion to the degree of hearing loss (Jerger *et al.* 1972; Jerger, Hayes, Anthony, and Mauldin 1978). It is a decibel-for-decibel trade. This relationship is illustrated graphically in Fig. 29.3. Data are based on reflex thresholds (SLs) of 515 patients with varying degrees of cochlear hearing loss. Note that, with no hearing loss, the average reflex SL is 85 dB. However, with a hearing loss of 40 dB, the average reflex SL is only 45 dB. The function decelerates and levels off at an average limiting SL of 25 dB. This sets an upper limit to the degree of cochlear hearing loss that will still show a reflex. If the upper limit of the audiometer producing the reflex-eliciting signal is 110 dB, then the maximum cochlear hearing loss still showing a reflex would be, on the average, 85 dB (110 minus 25). If the upper limit of the audiometer is 125 dB, then the maximum loss will be 100 dB (125 minus 25). This is usually a sufficient range to include most testable sensorineural losses.

The practical implication of this finding is that, if a patient has a sensorineural hearing loss that does not exceed 85 to 100 dB, and if the loss is cochlear, he ought to show a reflex when a sufficiently intense sound is introduced into that ear.

The observation of elevated HTLs associated with a mild hearing loss, or absent acoustic reflexes associated with a mild-to-moderate hearing loss, should always raise the strong suspicion of an eighth cranial nerve disorder.

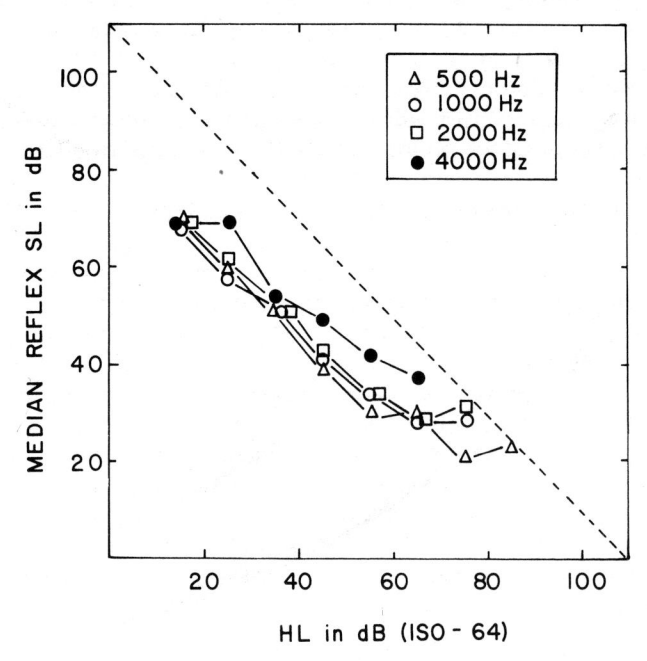

Fig. 29.3. The relationship between the degree of hearing loss (HL) and the acoustic reflex sensation level (SL) in 515 patients with cochlear hearing loss.

Anderson, Barr, and Wedenberg (1969) were the first investigators to describe essentially three abnormal acoustic reflex findings in patients with eighth cranial nerve disorders. These are: (i) elevated acoustic reflex HTLs, (ii) absent acoustic reflexes, (iii) acoustic reflex decay.

The phenomenon of 'elevated' reflex thresholds in eighth cranial nerve disorders refers to the elevation of the reflex HTL in relation to expectation based on normal ears and those with cochlear hearing deficits. In terms of reflex SL, however, the threshold is quite 'normal'. For example, in the normal ear, both reflex HTL and SL might be 85 dB. In the ear with a 30 dB cochlear loss, reflex HTL might also be 85 dB, but reflex SL will be 55 dB (85 minus 30). However, in the ear with a 30 dB loss due to an eighth cranial nerve disorder, reflex HTL will be 115 dB and reflex SL will be 85 dB (115 minus 30).

Since the reflex SL tends to remain 'normal' (i.e. 85 dB) in eighth cranial nerve disorders, increasing hearing loss will eventually drive the reflex HTL beyond the upper limit of the audiometer. If the upper limit of the audiometer producing the reflex eliciting signal is 110 dB, then we would expect the reflex to disappear altogether when hearing loss exceeds 25 dB. It is not surprising, then, that reflexes are the exception rather than the rule in eighth cranial nerve disorder (Jerger, Harford, Clemis, and Alford 1974; Olsen, Noffsinger, and Kurdziel 1975; Sheehy and Inzer 1976; Johnson 1977). Unless the audiometric loss is very slight, the acoustic reflex is usually not elicited at all in eighth cranial nerve disorders.

Fig. 29.4 shows the effects of cochlear and eighth cranial nerve disorder on acoustic reflex HTLs as analysed by Jerger et al. (1974). When the hearing level is within normal limits, the likelihood of the absence of the reflex in eighth cranial nerve disorder is 30 per cent. There is a disproportionate increase in likelihood of the absence of the reflex with increasing hearing loss. For example a sensitivity loss of only 30 dB produced by an eighth cranial nerve disorder, results in a 70 per cent likelihood of absent acoustic reflexes.

A second reflex abnormality associated with eighth cranial nerve disorder is the remarkable phenomenon, reflex decay. When the reflex-eliciting signal is first turned on, the reflex appears normally. However, as the signal is sustained, the amplitude of the reflex gradually decreases and may eventually disappear altogether. Reflex decay may be observed when the signal is presented both ipsilaterally and contralaterally.

Reflex decay has pathological significance only if it is present for signal frequencies of 1000 Hz or less. It is relatively common in normal ears at 2000 and 4000 Hz (Alberti 1974). However, its appearance at either 500 or 1000 Hz is a strong sign of eighth cranial nerve disorder.

The combination of the acoustic reflex threshold test and the reflex decay test is quite sensitive to eighth cranial nerve disorders. Reports by Jerger *et al.* (1974), Olsen *et al.* (1975), Sheehy and Inzer (1976), and Johnson (1977) indicate that the identification rate of eighth cranial nerve disorders by both these acoustic reflex tests ranges from 77 per cent to 86 per cent.

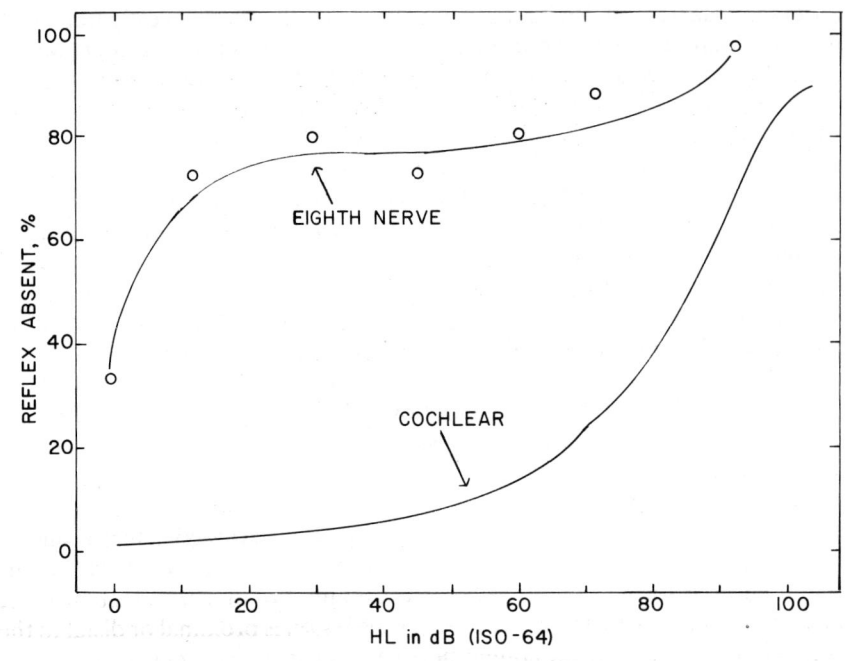

Fig. 29.4. The relationship between the degree of hearing loss (HL) and the likelihood of the absence of the acoustic reflex in cochlear and eighth cranial nerve disorders.

Although acoustic reflex tests cannot replace the total 'test battery' approach to the evaluation of sensorineural hearing loss, these tests are among the most powerful for differentiating cochlear from eighth cranial nerve disorders. However, it is essential to remember, that acoustic reflex tests results, in common with those from conductive hearing loss, cannot be analysed in isolation, but only in relation to results from the pure-tone audiogram.

Site localization of brainstem auditory disorders

One of the most recent diagnostic applications of impedance audiometry is the localization of the site of brainstem auditory pathway disorders. This important application was made possible largely by the addition of ipsilateral acoustic reflex testing to the impedance test battery.

Several acoustic reflex patterns may emerge depending on the site of a brainstem auditory disorder. For example, the finding of totally normal acoustic reflexes in the presence of a brainstem auditory disorder suggests that the lesion is above the level of the central reflex arc in the pons. The presence of normal ipsilateral reflexes, but absent contralateral reflexes, suggests an interruption of the central reflex arc between the ipsilateral cochlear nucleus and contralateral facial (motor nucleus of seven) nucleus (Greisen and Rasmussen 1970). Similarly, the absence of both contralateral reflexes and one ipsilateral reflex suggests an intra-axial brainstem lesion eccentric to the side of the absent ipsilateral reflex (Jergers 1980). A fourth, and very unusual, reflex pattern associated with a brainstem auditory disorder has been reported recently by Jerger, Jerger, and Hall (1979). In this disorder, acoustic reflexes are abnormal with sound to the affected ear on contralateral stimulation only. Both of the ipsilateral reflexes and the other contralateral reflex are normal. This reflex result was observed in a patient with an extra-axial acoustic Schannoma that was found, on surgery, to displace and distort adjacent brainstem structures. It has also been noted in patients with degenerative disease, hydrocephalus, and viral neuritis.

Acoustic reflex testing, then, can provide helpful information in the site localization of brainstem auditory disorders. In combination with other tests of brainstem function, in particular brainstem evoked response (BER) audiometry, the audiological evaluation of brainstem disorders promises to become even more exact.

Seventh cranial nerve disorder

The acoustic reflex test has also become a valuable adjunctive technique for localizing the site of seventh cranial (facial) nerve disorders (Alford, Jerger, Coats, Peterson, and Weber 1973; Citron and Adour 1978). The acoustic reflex is helpful in determining whether the lesion is proximal or distal to the branching of the seventh cranial nerve to the stapedius muscle.

In general, three reflex patterns may emerge depending on the site of a seventh cranial nerve disorder. The first pattern is absence of the acoustic reflex whenever the probe is in the ear on the affected side. No contraction of the stapedius muscle is observed when the reflex-eliciting signal is delivered to either the ipsilateral or the contralateral ear. This pattern may be seen when the seventh cranial nerve disorder is proximal to the branching to the stapedius muscle.

A disorder in this same, proximal site may also show a second pattern of present, but elevated acoustic reflexes. In this case, sound elicits the reflex contraction, but only to abnormally intense signal levels (greater than 100 dB). This pattern may be observed in patients with recovering seventh cranial nerve function.

A third reflex pattern associated with seventh cranial nerve disorder is normal acoustic reflexes. In this pattern, all four reflexes (both contralateral and ipsilateral) are present at normal reflex HTLs. This pattern is typically seen in patients with seventh cranial nerve disorders distal to the branching of the nerve to the stapedius muscle.

Acoustic reflex measurements are helpful not only in localizing the site of a seventh cranial nerve disorder, but also in charting seventh cranial nerve recovery (Citron and Adour 1978). For example, in a patient with idiopathic facial nerve palsy, reflex testing over a period of several days or weeks may show initially absent acoustic reflexes, then present but elevated reflexes, and finally normal reflexes as the disorder resolves from its initial, acute phase to complete recovery.

OTHER APPLICATIONS OF IMPEDANCE AUDIOMETRY

Impedance audiometry has proved to be an invaluable cross-check in the evaluation of hearing in infants and young children (Jerger and Hayes 1976). It is not only sensitive to middle-ear disorders, but, in the case of normal middle-ear function permits quantification of sensorineural hearing level (Jerger, Burney, Mauldin, and Crump 1974). This very important diagnostic application has substantially improved the audiometric evaluation of infants, young children, and the difficult-to-test patient.

The prediction of hearing level from the acoustic reflex is based on the relationship of the acoustic reflex HTL for broad-band noise (BBN) and for pure-tone signals. In normal ears, broad-band noise elicits the acoustic reflex at intensity levels 15 to 20 dB lower than for pure-tone signals. In ears with sensorineural hearing loss, however, the reflex level for noise is elevated while the reflex level for pure tone remains relatively unchanged. Essentially, the broad-band noise signal loses its 'advantage' over narrower band signals. By comparing reflex levels for noise and for pure-tone signals it is possible to make a rough prediction of sensorineural hearing level.

A number of investigations have shown that while the predictive accuracy of this technique is limited in adults it works quite well in children (Jerger, Burney, Mauldin, and Crump 1974, 1978; Jerger, Hayes, and Anthony 1978). For example, Jerger *et al.* (1978) found that in a series of 130 children aged two to twelve years, hearing level was accurately predicted 85 per cent of the time. Furthermore, prediction was 100 per cent accurate for normal hearing and 85 per cent accurate for severe hearing loss. In other words, all children predicted to have normal hearing indeed yielded normal behavioural audiograms, and 85 per cent of the children predicted to have severe hearing loss showed this by behavioural testing.

These findings are among the most exciting in pediatric audiology. Impedance audiometry is not only helpful in confirming the presence of middle-ear disorder when behavioural results suggest a conductive hearing loss, but also allows estimation of sensorineural level when middle-ear function is normal.

SUMMARY AND DISCUSSION

There can be little doubt that impedance audiometry is one of the most important and powerful tools in audiological evaluation. It has proven useful in the evaluation of middle-ear disorder, sensorineural hearing loss, and brainstem, auditory pathway disorders. In addition to all this, impedance audiometry is particularly helpful in the audiological evaluation of infants, young children, and the difficult-to-test patient.

The prudent clinician must constantly bear in mind, however, that impedance audiometry is not a series of three discrete and equally important measures. Rather, impedance audiometry is a total test battery that can be interpreted only in its proper relation to other measures of auditory function. Although it has augmented audiological evaluation, impedance audiometry does not replace the total audiometric test battery. Only when the results of the impedance test battery have been interpreted in relation to other basic audiometric data, has impedance audiometry been effectively carried out.

REFERENCES

ALBERTI, P. (1974). The stapedius reflex and otoneurological diagnosis. Paper presented at the VIth Ibero-American Symposium of Otoneurology, Sao Paulo, Brazil.
—— and JERGER, J. (1974). Probe-tone frequency and the diagnostic value of tympanometry. *Archs Otolar.* **99**, 206–10.
ALFORD, B., JERGER, J., COATS, A., PETERSON, C., and WEBER, S. (1973). Neurophysiology of facial nerve testing. *Archs Otolar.* **97**, 214–19.
ANDERSON, H., BARR, B., and WEDENBERG, E. (1969). Intra-aural reflexes in retrocochlear lesions. In *Nobel Symposium 10: Disorders of the skull base region* (ed. C. Hamburger and J. Wersall) pp. 49–55. Almquist and Wiskell, Stockholm.
BORG, E. (1973). On the neuronal organization of the acoustic middle ear reflex. A physiological and anatomical study. *Brain Res.* **49**, 101–23.
CITRON, D., and ADOUR, K. (1978). Acoustic reflex and loudness discomfort in acute facial paralysis. *Archs Otolar.* **104**, 303–6.
DEMPSEY, C. (1975). Static compliance. In *Handbook of clinical impedance audiometry* (ed. J. Jerger) pp. 71–84. American Electromedics Corp., Dobbs Ferry, New York.
DJUPESLAND, G. (1969). Use of impedance indicator in diagnosis of middle ear pathology. *Int. Audiol.* **8**, 570–9.
GREISEN, O. and RASMUSSEN, P. (1970). Stapedius muscle reflexes and otoneurological examinations in brain-stem tumors. *Acta oto-lar.* **70**, 366–70.
JERGER, J. (1970). Clinical experience with impedance audiometry. *Archs Otolar.* **92**, 311–24.
—— and HAYES, D. (1976). The cross-check principle in pediatric audiometry. *Archs Otolar.* **102**, 614–20.
—— and ANTHONY, L. (1978). Effect of age on prediction of sensori-neural hearing level from the acoustic reflex. *Archs Otolar.* **104**, 393–4.
—— JERGER, S., and MAULDIN, L. (1972). Studies in impedance audiometry: I. Normal and sensori-neural ears. *Archs Otolar.* **96**, 513–23.
—— ANTHONY, L., JERGER, S., and MAULDIN, L. (1974). Studies in impedance audiometry: III. Middle ear disorders. *Archs Otolar.* **99**, 165–71.
—— BURNEY, P., MAULDIN, L., and CRUMP, B. (1974). Predicting hearing loss from the acoustic reflex. *J. Speech Hear. Dis.* **39**, 11–22.
—— HARFORD, E., CLEMIS, J., and ALFORD, B. (1974). The acoustic reflex in eighth nerve disorders. *Archs Otolar.* **99**, 409–13.
—— HAYES, D., ANTHONY, L., and MAULDIN, L. (1978). Factors influencing prediction of hearing level from the acoustic reflex. In *Monographs in contemporary audiology*, Vol. I, pp. 1–20. Maico.
JERGER, S. (1980). Diagnostic application of impedance audiometry in central auditory disorders. In *Handbook of clinical impedance audiometry* (eds. J. Jerger and J. Northern) 2nd edn. American Electromedics Corp., Dobbs Ferry, New York.

—— JERGER, J., and HALL, J. (1979). A new acoustic reflex pattern. *Archs Otolar.* **105**, 24–8.
—— NEELY, J., and JERGER, J. (1975). Recovery of crossed acoustic reflexes in brain stem auditory disorder. *Archs Otolar.* **101**, 329–32.
JOHNSON, E. (1977). Auditory test results in 500 cases of acoustic neuroma. *Archs Otolar.* **103**, 152–8.
METZ, O. (1946). The acoustic impedance measured on normal and pathological ears. *Acta oto-lar.* Suppl. **63**, 1–254.
OLSEN, W., NOFFSINGER, D., and KURDZIEL, S. (1975). Acoustic reflex and reflex decay. Occurrence in patients with cochlear and eighth nerve lesions. *Archs Otolar.* **101**, 622–5.
SHEEHY, J. and INZER, B. (1976). Acoustic reflex test in neuro-otologic diagnosis: A review of 24 cases of acoustic tumors. *Archs Otolar.* **102**, 647–53.
TERKILDSEN, K., OSTERHAMMEL, P., and BRETLAU, P. (1973). Acoustic middle ear muscle reflexes in patients with otosclerosis. *Archs Otolar.* **98**, 152–5.

30 Physiology and pathophysiology of the middle ear—Eustachian tube system

SVEN INGELSTEDT

THE AIR-FILLED EAR SPACES—A SEMI-RIGID GAS POCKET

The various pathophysiological Eustachian tube problems can only be adequately dealt with through an extensive understanding of the normal physiology of the middle ear—Eustachian tube system. The gas exchange in different types of gas pockets within the human body has been studied by Rahn and Canfield (1955). Various mechanisms, viz. ventilation, diffusion, and blood flow through the enclosing structures, are involved. According to Rahn's classification, the gas exchange in the air-filled ear spaces resembles that occurring in a non-ventilated gas pocket. This means that oxygen and nitrogen are continuously absorbed from the gases in the ear, while carbon dioxide remains in equilibrium with that in the lining tissues.

As long as there is no pressure difference across the tympanic membrane the sum of the partial pressures of the gases enclosed always exceeds that in the capillary venous blood in the tissues lining the cavities. This pressure difference is about 6.25 kPa and explains the continuous absorption. If the tube is closed for one hour, the continuous absorption of oxygen and nitrogen will create an underpressure of about 0.3 to 0.5 kPa in the normal middle ear. The rate of this absorption has been determined with different techniques, and extrapolated 24-hour values have invariably proved to be about 1 ml (Van Dishoeck 1941; Riu, Flottes, Bouche, and Le Den 1966; Ingelstedt and Jonson 1967; Elner 1972, 1976, 1977).

TECHNIQUE FOR DETERMINING THE GAS ABSORPTION FROM THE MIDDLE EAR (Ingelstedt and Jonson 1967; Elner 1970, 1972, 1977)

It is possible to determine indirectly the rate of gas absorption from the middle ear (Fig. 30.1), but only in persons in whom equilibration by deglutition is perfect. The subject is instructed to swallow every 5–10 minutes. During the intervals between swallowing the gas absorbed is not replaced. The volume of the gas absorbed is ΔV_{diff} (Fig. 30.1(a)). This results in the gradual creation of a negative pressure $(-P_m)$, which sucks the ear drum inwards. This cupping of the drum causes an inward flow through the flowmeter $\dot{V}_{\text{tm}}$, but the flow is too small to be recorded. However, every 5–10 minutes, when the subject is instructed to swallow, the drum instantaneously resumes its neutral position (V_{tm} in Fig. 30.1(b)). This flow ($\dot{V}_{\text{tm}}$) can be recorded and integrated. The negative pressure created in the ear by the absorption of gas can be measured. The volume of gas passing through the tube every time the subject swallows (ΔV_t) can be calculated if we know the

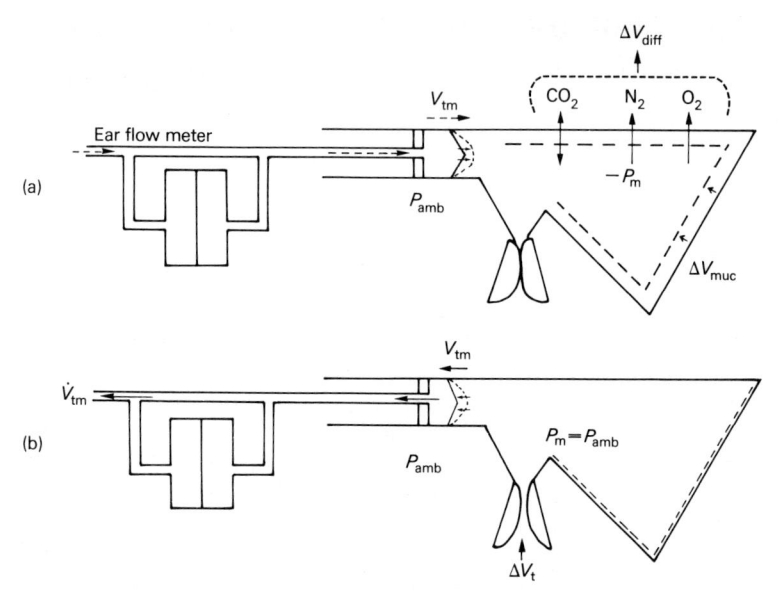

Fig. 30.1. Quantitative study of the rate of gas absorption from the middle ear. P_{amb} = ambient pressure; P_m = middle-ear pressure relative to P_{amb}; V_{tm} = volume displacement of the ear drum in relation to its neutral position, i.e. at which $P_m = P_{amb}$; ΔV_{diff} = the rate of gas absorption from the middle ear; ΔV_t = the rate of air passing through the tube into the middle ear during the act of swallowing; ΔV_{muc} = the pressure-dependent change in volume of the middle ear mucosa. For further explanation, see text and Fig. 30.4.

volume of the air-filled ear spaces and the change in pressure in the middle ear (ΔP_m), and correct for the pressure-dependent change in volume of the middle-ear mucosa (ΔV_{muc}). By adding the gas volumes passing through the tube during the experiment (Fig. 30.2) we can estimate the volume of gas absorbed per 24 hours. Readers interested in such determinations and calculations are referred to Ingelstedt and Jonson (1967) and Elner (1976, 1977). Fig. 30.2 gives the results of two separate recordings made at an interval of one week in the same subject. The precision of the method described above is obvious from the virtual coincidence of the curves.

We have found the mean volume of the closed air-filled ear spaces in 19 normal adults to be 6.6 ml, with SD = 2.4. Even if we were to assume the volume of the gases entering the ear via the tube to be as large as 1 µl per minute, it would still be difficult to imagine that such a relatively small admixture could appreciably change the composition of gas in an ear volume of 6 ml. Further, no gas exchange occurs through the intact tympanic membrane (Elner 1970). Thus the middle ear cavity is not ventilated like a pulmonary alveolus or even like a normal maxillary sinus (Aust 1974).

The composition of gases is an important factor in the milieu of the ear mucosa. There is evidence that the composition of these gases in a non-

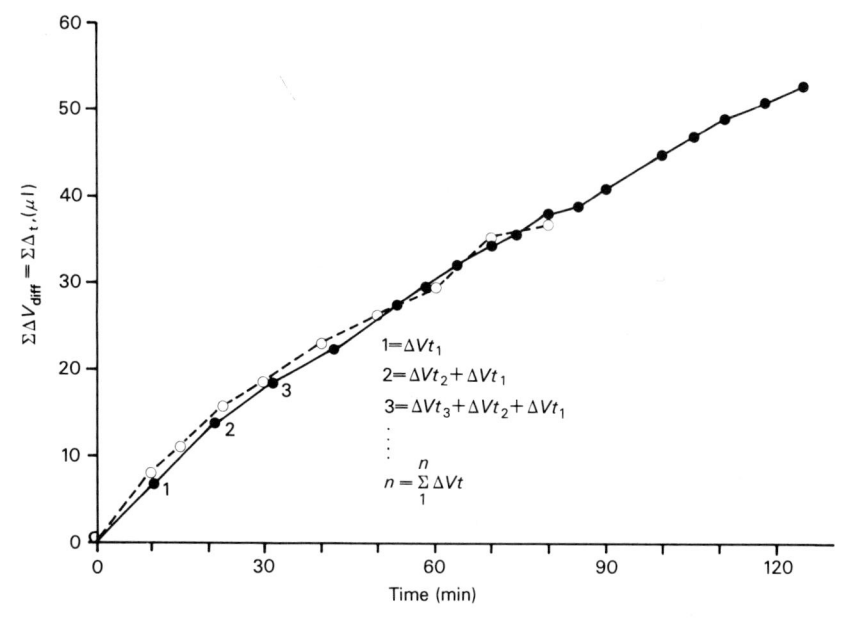

Fig. 30.2. Illustrative example of recording. The blank and filled circles denote the volumes of gas passing into the middle ear during an act of swallowing (ΔV_t). The continuous and interrupted curves denote the cumulative gas volumes passing through the tube and recorded on two different occasions in one subject. $\Sigma \Delta Vt$ equals the gas volume absorbed ($\Sigma \Delta V_{\text{diff}}$). The rate of gas absorption on both occasions was about 30 μl per hour.

ventilated or a closed gas pocket is relatively stable during the period of absorption as long as the pressure in the pocket is close to that of the atmosphere (Rahn and Canfield 1955—elastic subcutaneous pockets in rats; Melville Jones 1961; Riu et al. 1966—normal and dysfunction tube cases; Ingelstedt, Jonson, and Rundcrantz 1975—non-bacterial serous middle ear effusions). The ranges of the values on record for the components of the ear gas are: N_2 84–8 per cent, O_2 5.5–9 per cent, CO_2 5.5–88 per cent.

It should be observed that the methods with which these values have been obtained have inherent sources of error. However, carbon dioxide normally diffuses about 20 times as readily as oxygen, and a state of equilibrium between carbon dioxide in the pocket and that in the surrounding tissues is very soon reached in any non-ventilated or closed gas pocket in the body. There thus seems to be good reason to assume that the pressure of carbon dioxide in the gas in normal ears should be about 5.3–6.0 kPa.

The epithelium of the mucosa between the gas in the ear and the capillaries may be oxygenated from both sides. One might, therefore, assume that in a non-ventilated gas pocket the metabolic activity and oxygenation of the epithelium are chiefly dependent on the diffusion from the capillaries, i.e. the oxygen uptake of the epithelium is virtually dependent on the blood flow through the mucosal lining of the pocket. Observations made *in vivo* in the maxillary sinus of rabbits lend support to this assumption (Reimer, Huberman, Klementsson, and Toremalm 1980).

In tubal dysfunction the pressure to which the lining membrane of the ear spaces is normally exposed may be reduced, and this may in turn affect the diffusion across the membranes and blood flow through the membranes. Oedema of the membranes might increase the average distance of diffusion between the capillaries and the epithelium and possibly also reduce the blood flow through the membranes. Our gas experiments (Ingelstedt et al. 1975) with non-bacterial middle ear effusions containing very few cells indicate that in these cases the blood flow is reduced. In general, however, the P_{O_2} was not so low and the P_{CO_2} not so high as to affect the viability of the mucosa.

EUSTACHIAN TUBE FUNCTION

Inspired mainly by the work of Zöllner (1942), Perlman (1939, 1943, 1951, 1960), Thomsen (1958), and Terkildsen (1957) the 'middle ear research group' was set up at the University of Lund, Sweden, in 1960. Today our main source of inspiration is the Bluestone group in Pittsburgh, who have made invaluable contributions in this field.

Nomenclature of the equilibratory function of the Eustachian tube

The Eustachian tube is a compliant, mucosa-lined conduit connecting the air-filled ear spaces with the nasopharynx. In the normal resting state this airway is collapsed and is intermittently opened on deglutition, for example, by contractions of the tensor veli muscles. There is no convincing evidence that the tube can be closed by muscular contraction.

Normal pressure equilibration in the middle ear and drainage of secretion requires that the Eustachian tube be *patent*, but the tube must also function normally when *collapsed* to prevent respiratory pressure changes and sounds arising in the nasopharynx from being transmitted to the middle ear.

The tube is opened when muscular forces acting on the tube exceed the sum of the closing forces keeping the tube closed. These excess forces separate the lateral wall from the cartilage-supported medial wall of the tube. A second mechanism for tubal opening involves the pressure gradient between the middle ear and nasopharynx. When this pressure difference exceeds the closing forces of the tube, the tube will be forced open without any contraction of the tube-opening muscles. Sometimes both mechanisms may be involved such as during an incomplete muscular opening when a small difference in pressure between the two ends of the tube is often necessary to separate the adherent mucosal walls. But sometimes the tube can be opened by the act of swallowing without any such pressure difference.

The nomenclature used to describe the transport of gas to and from the middle ear is still far from standardized. This hampers complete and uniform discussion of the Eustachian tubal function. The basis for nomenclature used here is: (i) whether the tube is opened by the action of muscles or not, and (ii) on the direction of the transport of gas in relation to the middle ear. The direction of this flow may thus be decided by *any event or procedure* that creates a pressure difference between the middle ear and the nasopharynx.

MUSCULAR OPENING OF THE TUBE
In this case the collapsed tube is opened by contraction of the muscles, e.g. during the act of swallowing or yawning. During inhalation* the flow of gas occurs *from the nasopharynx to the middle ear*, at a relative underpressure in the middle ear. During exhalation the flow of gas occurs *from the middle ear to the nasopharynx*, at a relative overpressure in the middle ear.

PRESSURE OPENING OF THE TUBE
In this case the collapsed tube is opened solely through distension by pressure without any muscular activity. During inflation the flow of gas occurs *from the nasopharynx to the middle ear*, e.g. owing to a relative overpressure in the nasopharynx or Valsalva's manoeuvre. During deflation the flow of gas occurs *from the middle ear to the nasopharynx*, e.g. owing to relative overpressure in the middle ear, during ascent in an aeroplane, or by a relative underpressure in the nasopharynx during a reversed Valsalva manoeuvre.

This distinction between the two mechanisms involved in the opening of the tube, i.e. by muscular opening and by pressure opening, is necessary because only one of the mechanisms may function well in an individual, e.g. there may be no correlation between the results of the Valsalva test and of the inhalation/exhalation tests. In patients with patulous tubes inflation/deflation is good while muscular opening function often is poor, and in alternobaric vertigo (Tjernström 1974) deflation function is reduced, while muscular opening functioning is generally normal.

The closing forces acting on the tube

Proper understanding of the physiology and pathophysiology of the Eustachian tube requires knowledge of the complex mechanisms keeping the compliant tube collapsed. It might therefore be convenient to try to distinguish between the luminal and extraluminal factors involved.

LUMINAL (MUCOSAL) FACTORS
These are qualitatively different variables. There are essentially three factors, viz. the viscosity of secretion, the surface tension of the mucus, and the blood content and elasticity of the mucosal vessels.
The viscosity of secretion. It is obvious that the forces necessary to open the tube vary with the viscosity of secretion. Cantekin (personal communication)

---

* In this chapter the terms *inhalation* and *exhalation* refer not to the act of breathing but to the *ingress* and *egress* respectively of air into and out of the middle-ear cavity from the nasopharynx by way of the Eustachian tube.

has shown with a tubal model, a modified and reinforced Penrose drain, that variations in the viscosity of the 'secretion' favour a pressure-opening of the tube far more than variation in the surface tension of the 'secretion'.

The surface tension of the mucus. Surface tension is a force which is active at any interface between air and liquid. The role of the surface tension of the mucus in opening the Eustachian tube was suggested by Flisberg, Ingelstedt, and Örtegren (1963), and has been studied by Brookler and Birken (1971), Birken and Brookler (1972), and Hagan (1977). Using histochemical and electron microscopic techniques Rapport, Lin, and Weiss (1975) have isolated the mucoplysacharides and glycoproteins active in causing surface tension in the mucus of animals.

The blood content of the mucosal vessels. The pressure-dependent volumetric changes of the mucosa have proved to play an important role in the patency of the Eustachian tube. These are:

1. Postural, hydrostatic venous pressure changes (Perlman 1939; Ingelstedt, Ivarsson, and Jonson 1967; Jonson and Rundcrantz 1969). Even normally the mucosa within the nose and the Eustachian tube is congested in recumbency and the lumina of the airways is therefore reduced. This postural congestion is reflected in the pressure changes in the internal jugular vein measured at the level of the base of the skull. The pressure in the sitting position is about 0.05 kPa and increases to about 1 KPa in the recumbent position (Fig. 30.3). In the semi-recumbent position (20°) the mean volume of air passing the tube is reduced by one-third, and in the horizontal position (0°) by two-thirds, of that in the sitting position (90°).
2. The pressure-dependent volume changes of the middle-ear mucosa were identical whether the pressure was changed directly in the middle ear (traumatic ear-drum perforation) or indirectly (constant air pressure in the middle ear) by alternately increasing and decreasing the ambient pressure (Andréasson, Ingelstedt, Ivarsson, Jonson, and Tjernström 1976).
3. The rate and magnitude of the change in the volume of the mucosa in the closed middle ear is highly dependent on the rate of the ambient pressure change. The slower the given increase in the relative middle-ear pressure the lower the positive pressure in the middle ear necessary for deflation will be, owing to a more effective reduction in the volume of the mucosa. For details see Andréasson *et al.* (1976).
4. Physical activity increases sympathetic tonus and thereby has a decongestive effect on the mucosa.

Luminal factors are discussed further on page 736.

EXTRALUMINAL FACTORS

Elasticity of tubal cartilage and peritubal tissues (muscles, fasciae, ligaments, and vessels). Owing to the elasticity of these extraluminal factors, especially the cartilage, the tube spontaneously resumes its normal collapsed shape after distension. Our experiments in adults have not clearly indicated any

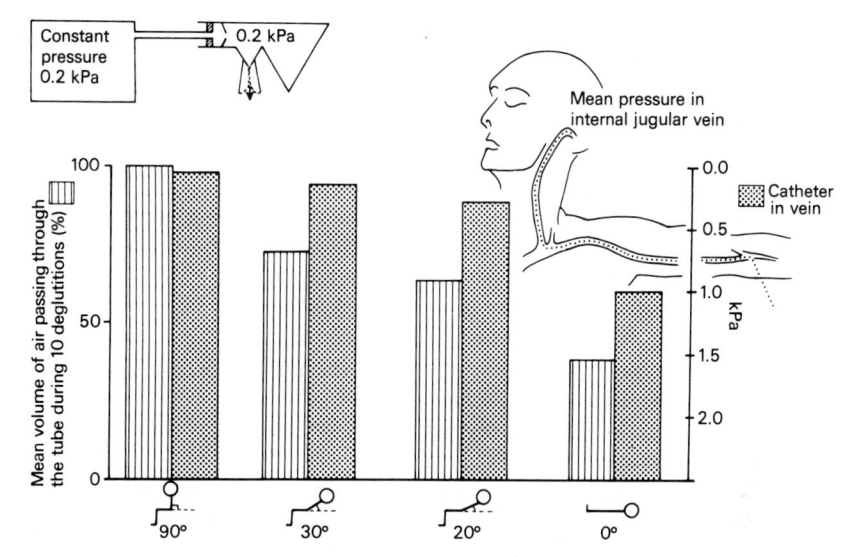

Fig. 30.3. Variation of the venous pressure in the internal jugular vein in different positions of the body. Venous pressure is expressed as a mean value (shaded columns) found in five healthy volunteers. The hatched columns illustrate the mean volume of gases passing through the tube in relation to posture. These mean values were obtained in 16 patients with dry central perforations of the ear drum, all with perfect tubal function and without signs of upper respiratory infection. Constant intratympanic overpressure was applied, while the patient swallowed once a minute for ten minutes. The mean volume of air passing through the tube was determined during this period and in the sitting position (90°). This mean value is expressed as 100 per cent.

fatigue of the tissues operating the closure of the Eustachian tube. The cartilage is mainly a hyaline structure, and the amount of elastic components is considerably greater in adults than in children (Aschan 1954). The tubal compliance seems to be too low ('stiff') in cases with alternobaric vertigo, and to be too high ('floppy') in some children, especially those with chronic middle-ear effusions.

The hydrostatic peritubal tissue pressure. Owing to the high vascularity of the tissues, the peritubal pressure is similarly influenced by variation of the venous pressures with posture.

How does a pressure difference arise between the ends of the tube at ground level when the drum is intact?

1. Atmospheric pressure variations. We generally have to consider small pressure changes of up to about 0.3 kPa in 24 hours in Sweden. More important is the variation of the atmospheric pressure with altitude, i.e. 0.136 kPa per 11 metres at ground level.
2. Pressure changes generated in the closed middle ear.
   (i) The gas absorption.
   (ii) Volumetric changes created by movement of the ear drum, most

commonly by contractions of the tensor tympanic muscle (Ingelstedt and Jonson 1967).
   (iii) Air volume changes in the locked tube at its aural end during attempted opening by deglutition ('negative pressure spikes'—Flisberg, Ingelstedt, and Örtegren 1963c).
   (iv) Changes in the volume of the middle ear mucosa. Thus hydrostatic venous congestion of the ear mucosa brings about an increase in pressure in the middle ear of 0.1 kPa on changing of posture from sitting to recumbent position provided the tube remains closed (Casselbrant, Ingelstedt, and Ivarsson 1978).
3. Pressure changes generated in the nasopharynx.
   (i) Normal pressure changes in the nasopharynx during respiration: approximately ±0.1–0.2 kPa.
   (ii) Toynbee test—swallowing with nostrils occluded.
   (iii) Valsalva test.
   (iv) Reverse Valsalva test—inspiration with occluded nostrils.
   (v) Blowing the nose.
   (vi) 'Sniff'—negative pressure in the nasopharynx at forced nasal inspiration (Ekvall and Magnusson 1977).

BY SPECIAL PRESSURE PROCEDURES
1. Politzer test.
2. Negative and positive square wave pressures applied to otherwise occluded nose during swallowing (Flisberg, Ingelstedt, and Örtegren 1963a).
3. Pressure chamber tests (Ingelstedt *et al.* 1967; Elner, Ingelstedt, and Ivarsson 1971).
   (i) When the subject is instructed not to swallow, the chamber pressure is changed to constant positive or negative pressure levels; thereafter the subject tries to equilibrate by deglutition. It is particularly important to study inhalation, i.e. the gas transport towards the middle ear on deglutition, since it mimics the basic tubal function, i.e. to replace the volume of gases absorbed.
   (ii) During a defined constant lowering rate of the chamber pressure (ascent) the deflation function is measured, i.e. the rate of outflow from the middle ear without any muscular action on the tube. This is the only procedure available to estimate the tube-closing forces and their variables, i.e. the luminal and extraluminal components in subjects with intact ear drums.
4. Gases used for anaesthesia, including pure oxygen (Thomsen and Terkildsen 1965).

Methods indicating tubal openings in subjects with intact ear drums

Only some of the current methods used in clinical or research work will be described.

INSTANTANEOUS VALUE METHODS

The techniques give indications simultaneously with the opening period of the tube.

Integrating microflow method (Ingelstedt et al. 1967; Elner, Ingelstedt, and Ivarsson 1971d). This method permits continuous recording of the volume deviation of the ear drum with respect to its neutral position both by changes of ambient pressure and by pressure within the middle ear. The drum is in communication with the ambient air during these studies. Quantitative studies of the middle ear mechanics are possible by this method (Fig. 30.4).

A pressure chamber is used in which the ambient pressure can be changed to constant positive and negative pressure levels. The ear of the subject is fitted with a catheter running through a rubber disc which is placed against the walls of the inner bony part of the external ear canal so as to be airtight. The other end of the catheter is in connection with the ambient air via the

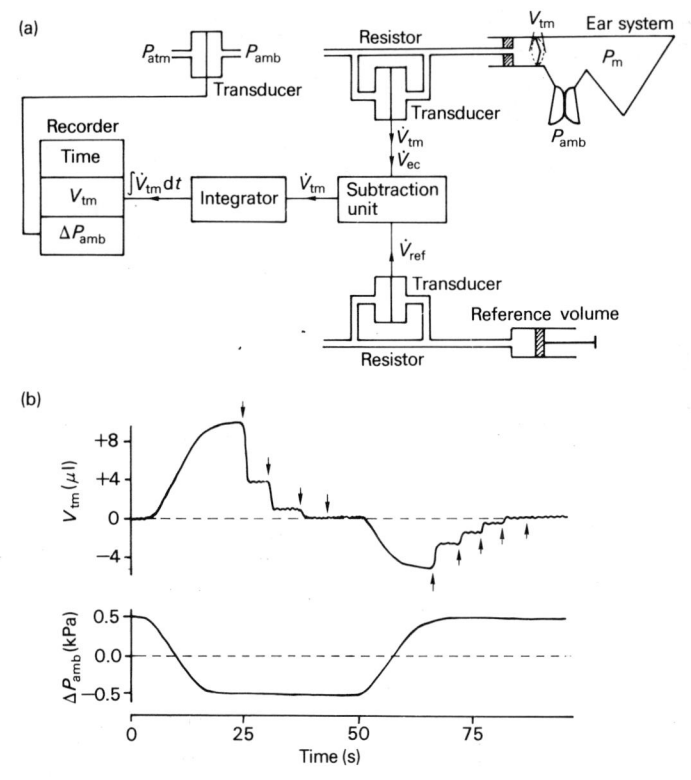

Fig. 30.4 (a). Equipment used for the recording of the ear drum volume displacement (V_{tm}) by changing ambient pressure (ΔP_{amb}) in a pressure chamber. (b) A recorded example: the subject has to equilibrate the static relative overpressure and underpressure in the middle ear by deglutition (arrows). P_{atm} = atmospheric pressure at ground level (in the laboratory); ΔP_{amb} = pressure change in the pressure chamber relative to P_{atm} outside the chamber; P_m = pressure in the middle ear relative to P_{amb}. For details see text.

flowmeter (resistor–transducer). This arrangement makes it possible to record airflows ($\dot{V}_{tm}$, Fig. 30.1) caused by volume displacement of the ear drum owing to changes in middle-ear pressure (P_m). On the other hand, when the ambient pressure (P_{amb}) is changed, the airflow through the flowmeter consists of two components, one caused by the displacement of the ear drum ($\dot{V}_{tm}$) and the other by compression or expansion of the air in the system ($\dot{V}_{ec}$). $\dot{V}_{ec}$ was corrected for by creating a compression and expansion flow ($\dot{V}_{ref}$) within an adjustable reference volume operating a separate identical flowmeter. The flow signal $\dot{V}_{tm}$ was then integrated to allow recording of V_{tm}. In Fig. 30.4 subject has initially equilibrated the middle-ear pressure to ambient pressure, $P_{amb} = P_m$ at 0.5 kPa. The drum is in the neutral position (V_{tm} at 0). The ambient pressure (ΔP_{amb}) is now changed over 25 seconds to a constant level of -0.5 kPa with the subject being instructed not to swallow. The drum bulges outwards ($+$, V_{tm}). Thereafter the subject is instructed to swallow (arrows) and the subject equilibrates completely ($V_{tm} = 0$). This is the exhalation test. The ambient pressure is afterwards increased and the subject has to equilibrate a relative underpressure in the middle ear, i.e. the inhalation test.

Modified acoustic impedance technique (Münker 1972). Changes in pressure across the drum in association with opening of the tube are recorded simultaneously as changes in impedance.

Sonotubometry (Virtanen 1977). This is an interesting and promising method based on conduction of sound at 6, 7, and 8 kHz.

MEAN VALUE METHODS
1. Audiograms.
2. Tympanographic techniques: impedance method and integrating microflow method.

What are the requirements for an adequate analysis of the physiological equilibrating capacity of the Eustachian tube?

An analysis requires investigation of the various mechanisms at work in the middle ear–Eustachian tube system and contributing to the continuous variation in the pressure in the middle ear. The variables involved are: the elastic properties of the ear-drum system (ear drum, ossicles with ligaments, and intra-aural muscles), the volume of the closed air-filled ear spaces, the volumes of gas transported through the tube at different pressure gradients between the ends of the tube, the rate of gas absorption from the gases enclosed within the middle ear, and the pressure-dependent volume changes in the middle-ear mucosa. All these variables have been quantified in experiments behind an intact ear drum except the last, which cannot be measured without incision of the drum (Ingelstedt et al. 1967; Elner et al. 1971; Andréasson et al. 1976).

To be defined as 'normal' a subject must satisfy the following criteria: no history of airway or ear diseases; no noteworthy experience of flying or diving; no subjective or objective signs of catarrhal infections during the last month before the study; no demonstrable otomicroscopic abnormalities including Siegle's test; and a normal audiogram (within 20 dB ISO).

Some concepts of the classification range of physiological variation of the pressure equilibrating capacity of the Eustachian tube

Owing to the lack of pertinent data in the literature, the following concepts are based on our own study of 102 normal adults (Elner *et al.* 1971d). All the tests were performed with the subject seated in a pressure chamber and the measurements were made by the integrating microflow method (Fig. 30.4).

EQUILIBRATION BY MUSCULAR OPENING OF THE TUBE, I.E. INHALATION/EXHALATION DURING THE ACT OF SWALLOWING

Test conditions: with the subject instructed not to swallow the chamber pressure was changed to constant positive or negative pressure levels of 1 kPa, after which he was requested to try to equilibrate by swallowing ten times within 3 minutes. Two such test series were performed (Fig. 30.4). According to their ability to equalize the relative underpressure and overpressure in the middle ear during such tests the subjects were distributed amongst four groups (I–IV) (Fig. 30.5).

By creating a certain amount of ambient pressure increase or decrease in the pressure chamber (P_{amb}) while the tube is closed we have approximated the amount of relative underpressure or overpressure simultaneously built up in the middle ear (P_m) to the same amount as the actual ambient pressure change, i.e. when P_{amb} is reduced by 1 kPa P_m is approximated to 1 kPa

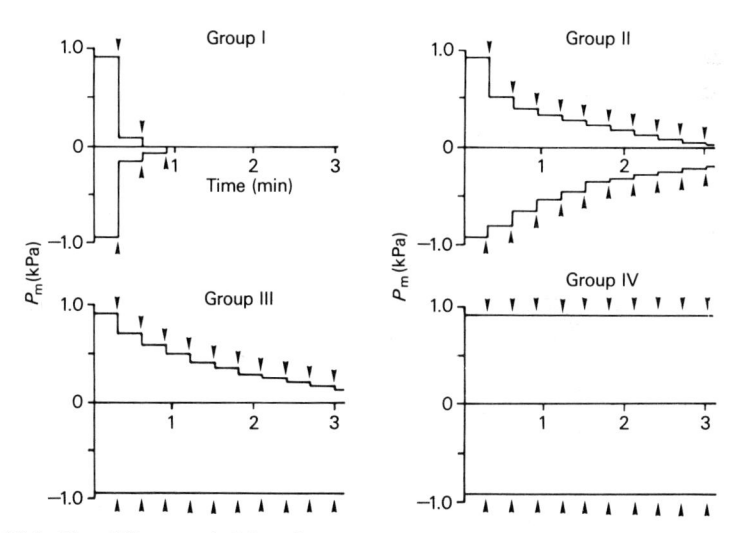

Fig. 30.5. The different tubal function groups. P_m = the middle-ear pressure relative to ambient pressure (P_{amb}) in the pressure chamber. When the negative P_m is reduced by deglutition (arrows) an inhalation test is performed; reduction of a positive P_m, i.e. exhalation test. When P_m reaches zero the ear drum is in its neutral position, i.e. at $P_m = P_{amb}$. For details see text.

relative to P_{amb}. The middle-ear pressure is, however, affected by the outward or inward movement of the ear drum and by the change in volume of the mucosal lining of the cavity and the mastoid cells during the intratympanic pressure change. In adults with normal ears containing relatively large volumes of gas, these factors seem to be of less importance. Thus, for example, if the change in ambient pressure (ΔP_{amb}) is 1 kPa, P_m should be about 0.9 kPa relative to P_{amb} when these ear drum and mucosal factors are corrected for. For detailed information, see Ingelstedt *et al.* (1967).

Characteristics of the tubal function groups based on inhalation/exhalation tests (Fig. 30.5; Table 30.1)

Group I: *perfect equilibration* of relative over- and underpressure in the middle ear during the test period. The residual relative middle-ear pressure after the test does not exceed 5 per cent of the original test pressure just before equilibration.

Group II: *good equilibration* in both directions of flow in the tube.
   II++ : residual relative middle-ear pressure from 6 to 50 per cent.
   II+   : residual relative middle-ear pressure from 51 to 94 per cent.

Group III: *poor equilibration*. No inhalation, i.e. the residual relative middle-ear pressure remains at ⩾ 95 per cent of the original test pressure. Exhalation present, but with a wide range of variation of the residual relative middle-ear pressure from 5 to 94 per cent of the original test pressure.

Group IV: No equilibration either direction of flow, i.e. the residual relative middle-ear pressure is always at least 95 per cent of the original test pressure.

TABLE 30.1. *The distribution in different tubal function groups of residual middle-ear pressure and results of Toynbee's tests*

Classification in 102 subjects	Percentage of inhalation/exhalation function		Residual middle-ear pressure as percentage of original middle-ear pressure at beginning of the tests (kPa)	Percentage in which the Toynbee test opens the tube
Group I, perfect	inhalation exhalation	68	⩽ 5	97
Group II, good	inhalation exhalation	9++ 12+	6–50 51–94	62 50
Group III, poor	inhalation exhalation	2	⩾ 95 5.94	0
Group IV, none	inhalation exhalation	5	⩾ 95	0
Patulous tube	inhalation exhalation	4		100
		100		

It is important for the clinician to understand the results given above in Table 30.1. Observe that in 7 per cent of the material equilibration was poor or non-existent when tested by swallowing as well as in later re-tests. However, hearing was normal in all subjects because these people unconsciously use other techniques, mainly based on inflation, e.g. Valsalva's manoeuvre or blowing the nose. It is clear from the Table 30.1 that the better the muscular equilibratory function in inhalation/exhalation tests the more often the Toynbee tests will be positive (Zöllner 1942; Thomsen 1958).

Criteria used in the classification groups I–IV and the reliability of the inhalation/exhalation tests

1. The initial middle-ear pressure is determined by the integrating microflow method immediately before the first set of tubal function tests (Table 30.2). In cases belonging to group I the pressure in the middle ear is found to be close to that of the ambient pressure. In subjects with 'reduced' function (groups II–IV) the pressure in the middle ear varies (for details see Elner, Ingelstedt, and Ivarsson 1971b).

TABLE 30.2. *Initial middle-ear pressure in different tubal function groups*

Tubal function groups given in Fig. 30.5 and Table 30.1.	Initial middle-ear pressure, i.e. before the pressure chamber test	
	Mean (kPa)	SD (kPa)
I	−0.004	±0.137
II	0.083	±0.115
III, IV	0.15	±0.389

2. The mobility of the ear drum. Total volume displacement of the ear drum when ambient pressure is changed from 1.5 kPa to −1.5 kPa (Fig. 30.6; Table 30.3). These experiments show that the mobility of the ear drum increases significantly with 'reduction' of the tubal function (Elner *et al.* 1971c). The findings argue strongly for the correctness of the classification given in Fig. 30.5 and Table 30.1 and the theory that the inhalation/exhalation results reflect the true mean function. With 'reduced' function the mobility of the ear drum increases, probably due to increased chronic pressure loading of the drum.

TABLE 30.3. *Volume displacement of the ear drum in different tubal function groups*

Tubal function groups given in Fig. 30.5 and Table 30.1	Total volume displacement of the ear drum in μl when ambient pressure is changed from 1.5 to −1.5 kPa while the tube is closed	
	Mean	SD
I	23.2	±5.1
II	31.6	±9.7
III–IV	35.3	±8.9

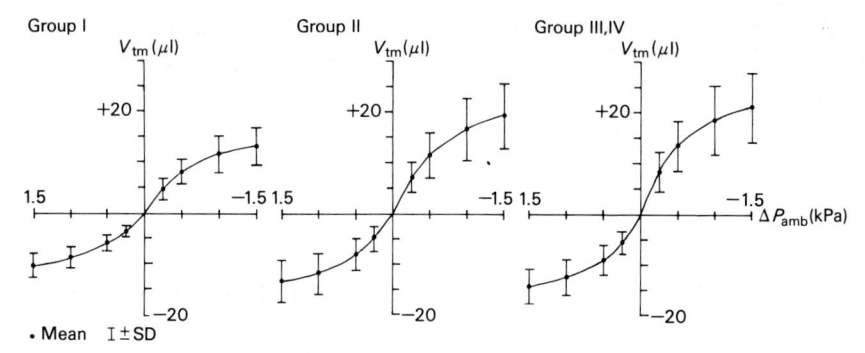

Fig. 30.6. Comparison of the ear-drum mobility between subjects belonging to the different tubal function groups given in Fig. 30.5. The pressure–volume diagrams are obtained by recording the volume displacement (V_{tm} in μl) by changing the ambient pressure (ΔP_{amb}) stepwise from 1.5 kPa to −1.5 kPa in subjects instructed not to swallow. Origo: neutral position, i.e. no pressure difference across the ear drum ($P_m = P_{amb}$). In the upper right quadrant the ear drum has moved outward from its neutral position.

3. Six subjects belonging to group I and six out of seven belonging to groups III and IV were re-examined one month later. Good agreement was found between the results of the first and second inhalation/exhalation tests. On re-examination all subjects in group I had about the same initial middle-ear pressure close to ambient pressure. In subjects belonging to groups III and IV the agreement was less good. But in these groups the pressures were very seldom negative. This supports the assumption that some people use other manoeuvres, mainly based on inflation, for maintaining the middle-ear pressure, e.g. Valsalva, blowing the nose.

PRESSURE OPENING EQUILIBRATION, I.E. INFLATION/DEFLATION
The distensibility of the Eustachian tube is important in any evaluation or attempt to define its elastic properties and structural variation. Complex reaction patterns may be manifestations of the effects of various and hitherto obscure factors. Thus, the length of the collapsed segment of the tube, the properties of the mucosa and the secretion, the elasticity of tubal cartilage and peritubal tissues, and finally the hydrostatic pressure exerted by the vessels in the peritubal tissues are involved.

It is possible today, in subjects with intact drums, to assess the total tubal closing forces by measuring the relative overpressure in the middle ear necessary to open the tube. We can also estimate the magnitude and to some extent distinguish the luminal from the extraluminal components. It should, however, be observed that comparative examination requires a well-defined standard rate of ambient pressure change.

The relative overpressure in the middle ear necessary to open the tube in humans (Andréasson et al. 1976; Cantekin, Saez, Bluestone, and Bern 1979) and in normal rhesus monkeys (Cantekin, Bluestone, Saez, Doyle, and Phillips 1977) depends on the rate at which the middle-ear pressure is increased. The relationship between the magnitude of the opening pressure and the rate at which the middle-ear pressure is increased suggests that the rate of decongestion of the tubal mucosa is of importance in the opening of the tube (Andréasson et al. 1976). According to Cantekin et al. (1977, 1978) the opening of the tube is controlled to a greater extent by luminal viscous and elastic forces than by surface tension forces.

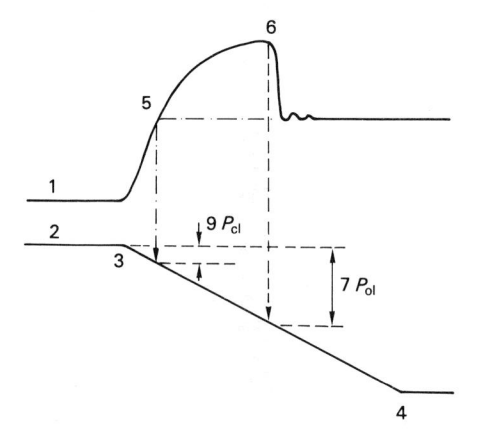

Fig. 30.7. Upper curve—position of the ear drum. Lower curve—ambient pressure in the pressure chamber. Analysis of the pressure opening (P_{ol}) and closing forces (P_{cl}) of the Eustachian tube from the recorded volume displacement of the ear drum. See text for explanation.

The procedure illustrated in Fig. 30.7 has been described by Ingelstedt et al. (1967) and Elner et al. (1971a). The subject is instructed not to swallow and the ear drum is in its neutral position 1, at the ambient pressure 2. If the pressure in the pressure chamber is lowered at a constant rate, 3 towards 4, the ear drum bulges outwards 5. At 6 the relative overpressure built up in the middle ear overcomes the total closing forces of the tube, and the tube is suddenly forced open, i.e. pressure opening. We express this opening pressure as the amount of ambient pressure change necessary to open up the tube (P_{ol}), at the defined change rate in kPa per second. If the lowering of the ambient pressure is continued the tube remains patent, air continues to leak from the ear, i.e. deflation continues, while the ear drum remains in a constant outward position at 5 and will continue to do so even if the ambient pressure change suddenly stops (after 4). This means that 9 expresses the closing pressure (P_{cl}). Thus, we can estimate the total closing forces (7) and the luminal closing forces (9) expressed as the ambient pressure change required at a defined rate of pressure change in kPa per second. (For more details see Fig. 30.10.)

Results of the deflation tests
(i) Pressure opening by an increasing intratympanic overpressure built up

during a constant 'ascent' corresponding to 0.4 kPa per second with the subject refraining from swallowing (Table 30.4).

TABLE 30.4. *Opening and closing pressures in the different tubal function groups*

Tubal function groups given in Figure 30.5 and Table 30.1	Opening pressure (P_{ol} in Fig. 30.7) Mean (kPa)	SD (kPa)	Closing pressure (P_{cl} in Fig. 30.7) Mean (kPa)	SD (kPa)
I	4.58	±1.75	1.89	±1.20
II+	3.90	±1.08	1.67	±0.80
II++	3.46	±1.20	1.84	±0.88
III, IV	3.62	±0.92	1.84	±0.73

(ii) Results of inflation test, i.e. Valsalva. Of the whole sample, 86 per cent were able to inflate the middle ear. The rate of nasopharyngeal pressure change was not recorded during these tests but only the magnitude of pressure required to open the tube. We have, however, found that the nasopharyngeal pressure needed for inflation of the middle ear increases with the rate of the nasopharyngeal pressure change (Ivarsson *et al*. 1979).†

Comparison of the equilibrating capacity in children and adults with normal ears

Such a comparison can be made only if the children and the adults are examined in exactly the same way and *preferably* by the same examiner. Studies in children are limited by the difficulties in obtaining suitable otologically healthy and co-operative test subjects, as well as in finding reliable nontraumatic methods (Bylander 1980).

A modified technique described by Thomsen (1958) with 50 adults and 50 children aged from 4–12 years (mean 7 years) is as follows. The initial middle-ear pressure was measured by tympanometry (conventional impedance bridge). The subject was seated in a pressure chamber. The ambient pressure and that in the external ear canal was adjusted in such a way that the relative middle-ear pressure was ±1 kPa, after which equilibration, if any, was recorded by tympanometry. Equilibration techniques were

† It should be observed that there was *no correlation* between the results of muscular and non-muscular equilibration tests, i.e. muscular versus pressure opening of the tube. This is true for both the Valsalva test and the opening and closing pressures in deflation tests (Table 30.4). It is obvious that the forces closing the tube have not received the attention they deserve. Failure of the tube to close, i.e. a patulous tube or closing forces being 'too weak' may be a contributory cause of middle-ear disease (e.g. chronic adhesive otitis media and retraction pocket cholesteatoma). The negative nasopharyngeal pressure during frequent daily 'sniffing' may evacuate gases from the middle ear by repeated deflation and thereby create a high negative middle-ear pressure which damages the middle ear structures (Ekvall and Magnusson 1977).

standardized as follows: Sequence 1: swallowing ten times during three minutes. Those who could not inhale, i.e. no gas transport into the middle ear, on deglutition, were then examined with sequence 2. Sequence 2: opening the mouth, lateral mandibular movements, yawning, chewing, etc. for up to 20 minutes (Table 30.5).†

TABLE 30.5. *Results of equilibration tests by means of different techniques. The table gives the percentage of subjects who were unable to equilibrate*

	No equilibration, i.e. the residual middle-ear pressure after test sequences was ≥95% of the original middle-ear test pressure. Percentages of subjects with negative results	
	Adults (%)	Children (%)
After sequence 1	12	56
After sequence 2	6	36

Thus a deficient equilibration found in inhalation tests during short test periods and/or variation in the original middle-ear pressure before the pressure chamber tests within the range of ±1 kPa does not necessarily indicate absence of a physiological tubal function, especially in children.

Procedures creating pressure differences between the ends of the tube in cases with perforated ear drums

1. Application of pressure directly to the middle-ear cavity.
   (i) Static negative and positive pressure levels which then are reduced by equilibration, i.e. closed ear canal manometry (Flisberg et al 1963b).
   (ii) Constant middle-ear pressure independent of the rate of equilibratory function, i.e. the flow volume methods (Flisberg 1966; Rundcrantz 1969a, b).
   (iii) Forced-response test by positive pressure (Bluestone, Cantekin, and Beery 1977; Cantekin et al. 1979).
2. Events and procedures changing the nasopharyngeal pressure—see subjects with intact ear drums page 730.

Methods indicating tubal opening in patients with perforated ear drums

Some current instantaneous value methods used in clinical and research work are as follow:
1. Closed ear canal manometry (Flisberg *et al.* 1963) by which the passage of air on inhalation/exhalation, inflation/deflation is recorded by the change in pressure.
2. Flow-volume method by which the passage of air through the tube is

† From the preliminary experiments presented in Table 30.5 it would seem, as expected, that the inhalation, tested over a 20 minute period, is more reduced in children. This could explain why the range of the initial middle-ear pressure in children was wider than in adults.

recorded both in inhalation/exhalation, and inflation/deflation tests (Flisberg 1966; Rundcrantz 1969a, b).
3. Sonotubometry (Virtanen 1977). Useful for inhalation/exhalation and inflation/deflation tests.
4. Forced-response test (Bluestone *et al.* 1977; Cantekin *et al.* 1977, 1979), a combined deflation/exhalation test. The method is so arranged that it is possible to test also inhalation/exhalation. A somewhat similar technique has been described by Flisberg (1966).

Present concepts of a rational approach to differentiation of the causes of tubal dysfunction

It is obvious that new approaches are necessary to elucidate the various hitherto obscure mechanisms which underlie the dysfunction. Such an analysis can *only* be based on test results obtained by *both* inhalation/exhalation *and* inflation/deflation sequences.

In the following a part of the clinical classification according to Bluestone, Beery, and Andrus (1974) is used, i.e. functional and mechanical obstruction. It has to be realized, however, that in most cases there is a combination of the two types. This makes the analysis for classification very complex.

FUNCTIONAL OBSTRUCTION

The 'pure' functional obstruction is extraluminal—insufficient effect of the tube-opening muscles. Tubal function tests show little or no inhalation and exhalation; the pressure opening and closing levels (P_{ol} and P_{cl} in Fig. 30.7) are normal or low, indicating a normal or increased distensibility of the membraneous tube wall.

Such investigations have hitherto been performed only in patients with perforated ear drum (Bluestone *et al.* 1977; Cantekin *et al.* 1977, 1979). An overpressure is created in the middle ear by connecting a constant-speed syringe pump airtight to the external ear canal. The tube is opened by a certain pressure, which is recorded, after which the tube can be kept open during a continuous constant outflow of gases from the middle ear, i.e. the deflation phase.
1. Temporary functional obstruction. Example: children with chronic middle-ear effusions. In many of these cases the distensibility of the wall is increased owing to a malacia of the tubal cartilage (Bluestone *et al.* 1974). In such a condition, a pressure occlusion of the tube might easily occur; this condition should be compared to dynamic compression of extrathoracic airways (Ingelstedt and Jonson 1967). Insufficient muscular effect alone may also cause temporary functional obstruction (Holborow 1975). Both of the above mentioned conditions are often combined and may gradually improve with age.
2. Permanent functional obstruction. Example: cleft palate.

MECHANICAL OBSTRUCTION

Mechanical obstruction is of luminal and/or extraluminal origin. For luminal obstruction see 'Luminal factors' on page 727. For extraluminal obstruction, factors operating the closure of the tube as well as factors exerting compression or restriction of the membraneous tube must be considered. Tubal function tests show little or no inhalation or exhalation; pressure opening and closing levels (P_{ol} and P_{cl} in Fig. 30.7) may be normal, but are more often increased.

Temporary mechanical obstruction. These are due mainly to luminal factors. Examples are mucosal oedema in upper respiratory infections, allergies, and adenoidal hypertrophy. In ear-drum perforation (chronic otitis media and ventilatory tube) the normal mucosal haemodynamics within the tube are completely changed because there is no normal pressure difference between the ends of the tube, as in the nose after tracheotomy. Further it is easy to introduce infections by blowing the nose. Other causes are increased gland formation and increased secretion from the mucosa of the middle ear and the Eustachian tube (Tos and Bak-Pedersen 1977), and a change in the rheologic properties of the effusion, 'poor mucociliary transportation function' (Sadé 1966b, 1974; Sadé, Halevy, and Hadas 1976).

Permanent mechanical obstruction. This is most often due to extraluminal factors, e.g. solid structures such as bone formation, scar tissues, or tumours. (Complete stenosis is extremely rare.)

If the inhalation/exhalation function is little or non-existent, the only possibility left for differentiation between functional and mechanical obstruction is to try to reduce and separate any mucosal factors involved in the dysfunction.

We have to administer drugs exerting a specific influence on the viscosity and surface tension of the mucus or try to decongest the tubal mucosa and then measure the effect from $P_{ol} - P_{cl}$ (Fig. 30.7). Caution must be exercised

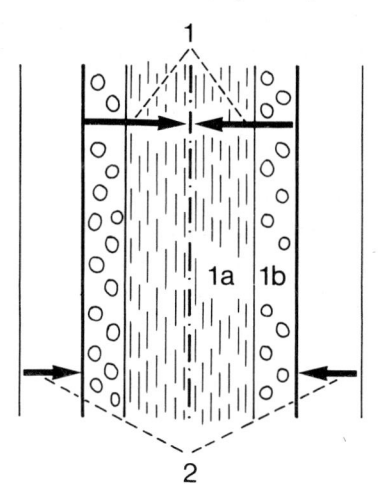

Fig. 30.8. Closing forces acting on the collapsed tube.
1: Luminal closing forces; 1a: viscosity and surface tension of mucus; 1b: blood content and elasticity of mucosal vessels; 2: extraluminal closing forces.

742 Physiology and pathophysiology of the middle ear

in the interpretation of the results of such experiments for differentiation because, for example, a vasoconstrictive drug might increase the viscosity of the mucus and thereby counteract tubal opening. Note that favourable results of experiments on the nasal mucosa cannot be applied directly to the collapsed tube.

Clinical approaches in assessment of the equilibrating capacity

PERFORATED EAR DRUM
1. Politzer test
    (i) If positive, measure the closing pressure immediately after the manoeuvre (Section 1, page 739).
    (ii) Measure the residual pressure after exhalation test (Section 1, page 739).
2. Valsalva's test. If positive, measure the nasopharyngeal pressure necessary for inflation. Try to vary the speed of the increase in nasopharyngeal pressure (kPa per second). Measure as in point 1(i) and (ii) (above).
3. Reverse Valsalva test and sniff. Try to change the speed of the pressure change in the nasopharynx (kPa per second). If positive, measure according to 1(i) and (ii) (above) after inhalation test.
4. Toynbee test. If positive, the inhalation/exhalation function is normal. If negative, proceed with point 5.
5. Inhalation/exhalation tests after direct application of pressure to the middle ear (as presented at 1(i), page 739). Try to equilibrate by a repeated deglutition. If the middle-ear pressure applied is reduced by less than 50 per cent proceed with point 6.
6. In cases of chronic otitis media with central perforation, try to eliminate the temporary mechanical obstruction, which is very often present, i.e. the mucosal congestion within the tube. Instil some drops of 1 per cent ephedrine sulphate in physiological saline into the middle ear. Produce pressure changes in the middle ear by Siegle's technique during deglutition. After ten minutes, re-test points 1–5.

Remaining cases with poor or no function. All of these have a positive Politzer test, some have a negative Valsalva test, and their inhalation/exhalation function is poor or non-existent. In chronic middle-ear effusions, mainly in children, the use of grommets makes expectant treatment possible. The function can be expected to improve with time.

Any further information about the actual dysfunction may require the forced-response test according to Bluestone *et al.* (1977) and Cantekin *et al.* (1977, 1978). This means a deflation/exhalation test by application of positive pressure into the middle ear by a syringe pump. The opening and closing pressures can be determined at a defined rate of pressure change, and after the tube has been forced open it will be kept patent by a constant deflation flow and the pressure–flow relation can be recorded. During this phase any muscular forces tending to dilate the tube can be estimated by a reduction of the positive middle-ear pressure during deglutition and by an increased outflow when the muscular contraction dilates the tube further. In this way we may obtain further information about the degree of functional and/or mechanical obstruction present in a given case.

CASES WITH INTACT EAR DRUMS

Tympanometric determination of the middle-ear pressure is a physiological technique. Serial determinations must be performed to assess tubal function (Brooks 1976). Some information about the dysfunction in cases containing air in the middle ear can be obtained by using investigations according to points 1–4 (see perforated ear drum). If these test results are poor or absent the most atraumatic and physiological method we can recommend is the use of a pressure chamber combined with tympanometry. In this way we can study the inhalation/exhalation function even in small children. Furthermore, we can easily estimate the tube-closing forces and the luminal and extraluminal components, i.e. the inflation/deflation function.

Fig. 30.9 illustrates our new pressure mini-chamber, which can be used both for application of pressure in the investigation of the physiology and dysfunction of the middle and inner ear. It can also be used as a body plethysmograph for studying pulmonary mechanics.

Experiences with preoperative testing of Eustachian tube function in cases of chronic otitis media

Opinions differ on the value of preoperative testing of tubal function. Some investigators (Miller and Bilodeau 1967; Holmquist 1968, 1969b; Siedentop 1968; MacKinnon 1970; Niwa 1972) have found the results of myringoplasty to be better if tubal function is normal before the operation. On the other hand, Ekvall (1970) and Sharp (1970) feel that preoperative testing yields no valuable information, and Smyth Kerr, and Goody (1971) claim that it can safely be excluded. Most investigations are performed only with inhalation/exhalation tests first described by Flisberg *et al.* (1963b) and the Politzer, Valsalva, and Toynbee test.

Andréasson and Ivarsson (1976) made a careful investigation of a large, well-defined collection of cases of chronic otitis media. They found 'perfect' and 'good' tubal function according to the classification presented in Table 30.1 in 70 per cent of the cases based on inhalation/exhalation tests, they also found 4 per cent of cases had patulous tubes. Further, Anndréasson (1976) described a connection between impaired tubal function and a small airspace volume of the ear. In 100 patients subjected to tympanoplasty because of chronic otitis media, Andréasson and Harris (1979) tested tubal function preoperatively by inhalation/exhalation tests. In a review one to three years later, they found no clear correlation between healing and hearing and tubal function on one hand and results of the preoperative inhalation/exhalation tests on the other. Thus, in healed ears there was often an improvement of preoperatively impaired tubal function.

These findings argue strongly at least for the existence of a temporary mechanical obstruction of the tube preoperatively when the function is

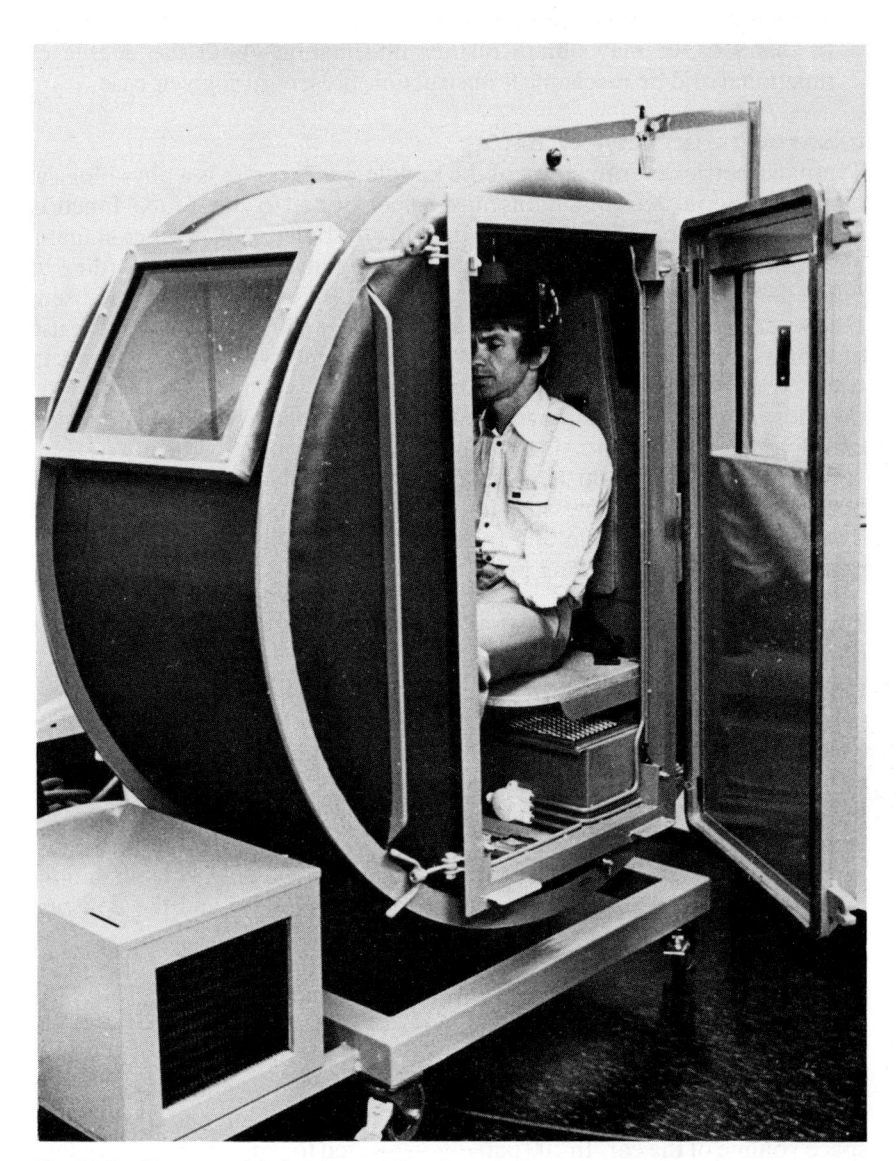

Fig. 30.9. Pressure mini-chamber to allow investigation with the subject in different positions.

impaired, and that the obstruction ceases with the healing of the drum. *Thus, a lack of tubal function tested only by inhalation/exhalation procedure in association with deglutition does not necessarily indicate impairment or absence of tubal function.* Further investigation requires reliable data which in turn require new approaches to the study of tubal function.

Function of Eustachian tube during diving and flying

During flying, and especially during diving, the subject is exposed to rapid and substantial changes in ambient pressure. Consequently equilibration difficulties are a common problem and may even be a disqualifying factor. Normal tubal function is always requested. However, what do we regard as normal? (See Armstrong and Heim (1937) and King (1966).)

An adequate equilibration implies the ability to make the tube patent during sudden pressure changes and the frequency with which the subject is capable of opening the tube. The amount of air allowed to pass through the tube, when kept open, will depend on the time during which it remains open as well as on the rate of the change in the ambient pressure. This complex function can obviously be assessed only during simulated flight and diving in a pressure chamber and the use of a quantitative method (Ingelstedt et al. 1967; Elner et al. 1971d).

Recording of equilibration function (Fig. 30.10)

These recordings were made in 89 of the subjects presented in Table 30.1 (Elner et al. 1971d). From the P_{amb} curve it is possible to calculate the ΔP_{amb} required to induce the pressure necessary to open the tube (pressure opening level—P_{ol}). The ΔP_{amb} required to induce the V_{tm} position (10 μl) is taken as the pressure closing level (P_{cl}). By means of deglutition (indicated in curve as d) the middle-ear pressure is equilibrated ($V_{tm} = 0$), i.e. exhalation. The capacity of the subject for equilibrating by inhalation by means of deglutition is determined as follows; it is checked that the ear drum is in its neutral position ($V_{tm} = 0$). The volume deviation of the ear drum is then recorded during the period of increase of ambient pressure while the subject swallows as frequently as possible (e and arrows in figure). The mean deviation of the ear drum ($V_{tm\ mean}$), from its neutral position during the linear period of the ambient pressure increase (80 per cent), is then calculated by planimetry from the V_{tm} curve. The ΔP_{amb} required to induce this mean deviation ($V_{tm\ mean}$) is regarded as a quantitative measure of the inhalation equilibratory function during the simulated descent (Table 30.6).*

These results strongly support the reliability of the earlier classification into tubal function groups obtained under static pressure conditions

---

* Equilibration, by deglutition, of dynamic pressure changes during descent is thus the most difficult test. It can hardly be performed in subjects other than those belonging to group I. But even among these there is a highly significant difference in the relative 'middle-ear pressure' during the descent period between subjects with a perfect equilibration by swallowing 1–3 times and 4–10 times.

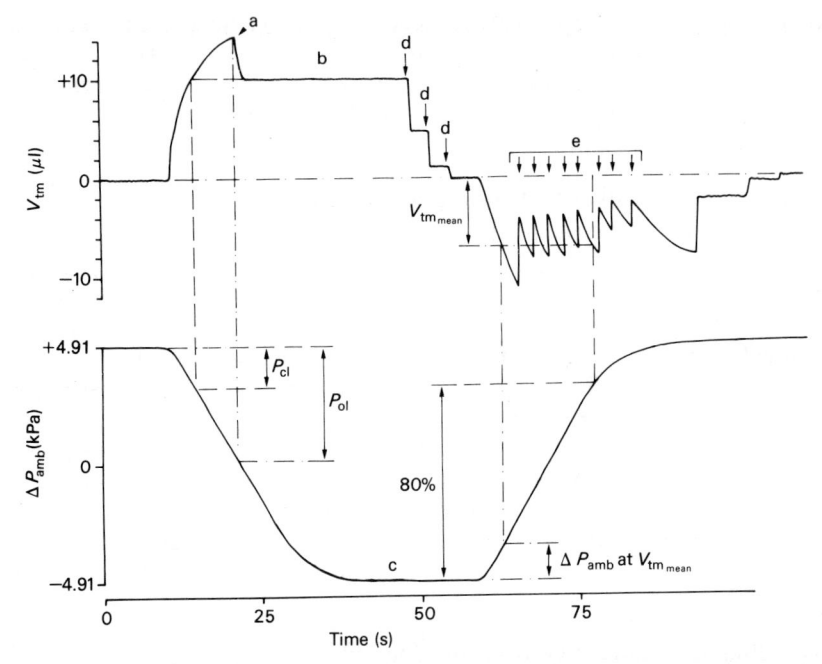

Fig. 30.10. Recording of ear drum displacement (V_{tm} in μl) induced by changes in ambient pressures (ΔP_{amb}, 0.4 kPa/s) in a pressure chamber. Ear drum displacement outwards (+) and inwards (−). The examination starts with an ambient pressure increase of 4.91 kPa, after which it is checked that the middle-ear pressure is equilibrated with the ambient pressure ($V_{tm} = 0$). When the ambient pressure is decreasing the subject is instructed not to swallow, a relative overpressure in the middle ear develops and the sudden drop in the recording (a in figure) indicates the pressure opening of the tube, which occurs when the V_{tm} recording has reached 12 μl. On continued decrease in the ambient pressure (ΔP_{amb}) after the moment the tube has opened the ear drum remains in a constant position, b, i.e. V_{tm} at 10 μl. This means that the relative overpressure in the middle ear is constant, indicating that the gas is continuously leaking from the middle ear. Position c indicates that the ambient pressure has reached a constant level of −4.91 kPa but that the relative overpressure in the middle ear remains at the same level as during the leaking period though the tube is now closed, i.e. V_{tm} persists at 10 μl in the recording.

(Table 29.1). The investigation also illustrates the importance of the fact that a more detailed evaluation of the tubal function under dynamic ambient pressure condtions is necessary for reliable selection of subjects suitable for occupations or sports involving diving or flying.

Furthermore, a relation has been demonstrated between a high-pressure opening level (P_{ol}) and vertigo, i.e. when the relative overpressure in the middle ear exceeds 5.89 kPa expressed as ΔP_{amb} (Ingelstedt, Ivarsson, and Tjernström 1974; Tjernström 1974). This means that the inner ear is stimulated by pressure, i.e. alternobaric vertigo, which appears in about 7 per cent of normal subjects despite usually perfect or good equilibration by deglutition. This transmission of overpressure from the middle to the inner

TABLE 30.6. *The equilibration capacity as evaluated by inhalation/exhalation tests under static pressure conditions in 89 subjects (Table 30.1) is compared with the results obtained in tests performed under dynamic pressure conditions (Fig. 30.9)*

Tubal function groups based on results of inhalation/exhalation tests in Table 30.1		Recorded air passage into the middle ear on deglutition during descent period				'Mean middle-ear pressure' expressed as $\Delta P_{\text{amb mean}}$ according to Fig. 30.9 during descent period on the cases with air passage	
			Absent No. %		Present No. %	Mean kPa	SD kPa
I	Perfect equilibration by 1–3 deglutitions	$n=28$	0	0	28	100	0.98	±0.24
II	Perfect equilibration by 4–10 deglutitions	$n=34$	8	23	26	77	1.37	±0.53
II		$n=20$	18	90	2	10	3.14	±0.41
II, IV		$n=7$	7	100	0	0		

ear has also been used on patients to decompress the endolymphatic hydrops during acute attacks of Ménière's disease (Densert, Ingelstedt, Ivarsson, and Pedersen 1975; Ingelstedt, Ivarsson, and Tjernström 1976).

Obviously, when selecting personnel suitable for flying the inhalation/exhalation equilibratory function must be excellent during dynamic test pressure changes and the pressure opening level of deflation should never exceed 5.89 kPa in one of the middle ears when tested in a pressure chamber at the rate of 0.4 kPa per second.

During diving, the immersion is known to induce a central venous pressure increase of about 2.36 kPa during head-out immersion (Arborelius, Balldin, Lilja, and Lundgren 1972). Ivarsson, Lundgren, Tjernström, Uddman, and Örnhagen (1977) have shown, however, that the head-out immersion (sitting position) has only a minor effect on the diver's ability to equilibrate middle-ear pressures during descent, compared with simulated diving in the recumbent position in a pressure chamber.

The most important point in the selection of suitable divers is inflation/deflation when tested in recumbency. This must be perfect in both tubal flow directions. In general, divers are unable to equilibrate a relative underpressure in the middle ear by deglutitions while diving. This inability is due to the rapidity of the ambient pressure changes which create an intense pressure on the middle-ear–Eustachian tube mucosal vessels.

REFERENCES

ANDRÉASSON, L. (1976). Correlation of tubal function and volume of mastoid and middle ear space as related to otitis media. *Ann. Otol. Rhinol. Lar.* **85**, 198.
—— and HARRIS, S. (1979). Middle ear mechanics and Eustachian tube function in tympanoplasty. *Acta oto-lar.* Suppl. 360, 141.

—— and IVARSSON, A. (1976). On tubal function in presence of central perforation of drum in chronic otitis media. *Acta oto-lar.* **82**, 1.
—— INGELSTEDT, S., IVARSSON, A., JONSON, B., and TJERNSTRÖM Ö. (1976). Pressure-dependent variations in volume of mucosal lining of the middle ear. *Acta oto-lar.* **81**, 442.
ARBORELIUS, M. Jr, BALLDIN U. I., LILJA B., and LUNDGREN, C. (1972). Hemodyanic changes in man during immersion with the head above water. *Aerospace Med.* **43**, 592.
ASCHAN, G. (1954). The Eustachian tube; histological findings under normal conditions and in otosalpingitis. *Acta oto-lar.* **44**, 295.
ARMSTRONG, H. G. and HEIM, J. W. (1937). The effect of flight on the middle ear. *J. Am. med. Ass.* **109**, 417.
AUST, R. Oxygen exchange through the maxillary ostium in man. *Rhinology* **12**, 25.
BIRKEN, E. A. and BROOKLER, K. H. (1972). Surface tension lowering substance of the canine Eustachian tube. *Ann. Otol. Rhinol. Lar.* **81**, 268.
BLUESTONE, C. D. Eustachian tube obstruction in the infant with cleft palate. *Ann. Otol. Rhinol. Lar.* **80**, Suppl 2, 1.
—— and SHURIN, P. A. (1974). Middle ear disease in children. Pathogenesis and management. *Pediat. Clin. N. Am.* **21**, 379.
—— BEERY, Q. C., and ANDRUS, W. S. (1974). Mechanics of the Eustachian tube as it influences susceptibility to and persistence of middle ear effusions in children. *Ann. Otol. Rhinol. Lar.* **83**, Suppl. 11, 27.
—— CANTEKIN, E., and BEERY, Q. C. (1975). Certain effects of adenoidectomy on Eustachian tube ventilatory function. *Laryngoscope, St. Louis* **85**, 113.
—— and —— (1977). Effect of inflammation of the ventilatory function of the Eustachian tube. *Laryngoscope, St. Louis* **87**, 493.
—— PARADISE, J. L., and BEERY, Q. C. (1972). Physiology of the Eustachian tube in the pathogeneses and management of middle ear effusions. *Laryngoscope, St. Louis* **82**, 1654.
BROOKLER, K. H. and BIRKEN, E. A. (1971). Surface tension lowering substance of the Eustachian tube. *Laryngoscope, St. Louis* **81**, 1671.
BROOKS, D. N. (1976). Middle ear effusion in children. *J. Otolar.* **5**, 453.
BYLANDER, A. (1980). A comparison of the Eustachian tube function in fifty children and fifty adults with normal ears. In *Proc. Symp. Physiol. Pathophysiol. Eustachian Tube and Middle Ear.* Thieme, Stuttgart.
CANTEKIN, E. I., BLUESTONE, C. D., and PARKIN, L. P. (1976). Eustachian tube ventilatory function in children. *Ann. Otol. Rhinol. Lar.* **85**, Suppl. 25, 171.
—— SAEZ, C. A., BLUESTONE, C. D., and BERN, S. A. (1979). Airflow through the Eustachian tube. *Ann. Otol.* **88**, 603.
—— BLUESTONE, C. D., SAEZ, C. A., DOYLE, W. J., and PHILLIPS, D. C. (1977). Normal and abnormal middle ear ventilation. *Ann. Otol. Rhinol. Lar.* **86**, Suppl. 41, 1.
CASSELBRANT, M., INGELSTEDT, S., and IVARSSON, A. (1978). Volume displacement of the tympanic membrane at stapedius reflex activity in different postures. *Acta oto-lar.* **85**, 1.
DENSERT, O., INGELSTEDT, S., IVARSSON, A., and PEDERSEN, K. (1975). Immediate restoration of basal sensorineural hearing (Mb Ménière) using a pressure chamber. *Acta oto-lar.* **80**, 93.
EKVALL, L. (1970) Eustachian tube function in tympanoplasty. *Acta oto-lar.* Suppl. 263, 33.
—— and MAGNUSSON, B. (1977). Reverse aspiratory middle ear disease—a

neglected pathogenetic principle. In *11th World Cong. Oto-Rhino-Lar.* Buenos Aires, p. 68.
ELNER, Å. (1970). Gas diffusion through the tympanic membrane. *Acta oto-lar.* **69**, 185.
—— (1972). Indirect determination of gas absorption from the middle ear. *Acta oto-lar.* **74**, 191.
—— (1976). Normal gas exchange in the human middle ear. *Ann. Otol. Rhinol. Lar.* **85**, Suppl. 25, 161.
—— (1977). Quantitative studies of gas absorption from the normal middle ear. *Acta oto-lar.* **83**, 25.
—— INGELSTEDT, S., and IVARSSON, A. (1971a). A method for studies of the middle ear mechanics. *Acta oto-lar.* **72**, 191.
—— —— and —— (1971b). Indirect determination of the middle ear pressure. *Acta oto-lar.* **72**, 255.
—— —— and —— (1971c). The elastic properties of the tympanic membrane system. *Acta oto-lar.* **72**, 397.
—— —— and —— (1971d). The normal function of the Eustachian tube. A study of 102 cases. *Acta oto-lar.* **72**, 320.
FLISBERG, K. (1966). Ventilatory studies on the Eustachian tube. *Acta oto-lar.* Suppl. 219.
—— INGELSTEDT, S., and ÖRTEGREN, U. (1963a). On the function of middle ear and Eustachian tube. *Acta oto-lar.* Suppl. 182.
—— —— and —— (1963b). A 'physiological' test of tubal function. *Acta oto-lar.* Suppl. **182**, 35.
—— —— and —— (1963c). The valve and 'locking' mechanisms of the Eustachian tube. *Acta oto-lar.* Suppl. **182**, 57.
HAGAN, W. E. (1977). Surface tension lowering substance in Eustachian tube function. *Laryngoscope, St. Louis* **87**, 1033.
HOLBOROW, C. (1969). The assessment of Eustachian function. *J. otolar. Soc. Aust.* **2**, 18.
—— (1970). Eustachian tubal function. Changes in anatomy and function with age and the relationship of these changes to aural pathology. *Archs Otolar.* **92**, 624.
—— (1975). Eustachian tubal function: changes throughout childhood and neuromuscular control. *J. Lar. Otol.* **89**, 47.
HOLBOROW, C. A. (1962). Deafness associated with cleft palate. *J. Lar. Otol.* **76**, 762.
HOLMQUIST, J. (1968). The role of the Eustachian tube in myringoplasty. *Acta oto-lar.* **66**, 289.
—— (1969a). Eustachian tube function assessed with tympanometry. A new testing procedure in ears with intact tympanic membrane. *Acta oto-lar.* **68**, 501.
—— (1969b). Eustachian tube function in patients with ear drum perforations following chronic otitis media. *Acta oto-lar.* **68**, 391.
—— (1970). Middle ear ventilation in chronic otitis media. *Archs Otolar.* **92**, 617.
INGELSTEDT, S. (1976). Physiology of the Eustachian tube. *Ann. Otol Rhinol. Lar.* **85**, Suppl. 25, 156.
—— and JONSON, B. (1967a). Mechanisms of the gas exchange in the normal human middle ear. *Acta oto-lar.* Suppl. **224**, 452.
—— and —— (1967b). On the mechanics of the extrathoracic airways: a preliminary report. *Acta oto-lar.* Suppl. **224**, 518.
—— and ÖRTEGREN, U. (1963). Qualitative testing of the Eustachian tube function. *Acta oto-lar.* Suppl. **182**, 7.
—— IVARSSON, A., and JONSON, B. (1967). Mechanics of the human middle

ear. Pressure regulation in aviation and diving. A non-traumatic method. *Acta oto-lar.* Suppl. 228.

IVARSSON, A. and TJERNSTRÖM, Ö. (1974). Vertigo due to relative overpressure in the middle ear. An experimental study in man. *Acta oto-lar.* **78**, 1.

—— and —— (1976). Immediate relief of symptoms during attacks of Ménière's disease, using a pressure chamber. *Acta oto-lar.* **82**, 368.

—— JONSON, B., and RUNDCRANTZ, H. (1975). Gas tension and pH in middle ear effusion. *Ann. Otol. Rhinol. Lar.* **84**, 198.

—— TJERNSTRÖM, Ö., and UDDMAN, R. (1979). Patency of the eustachian tube in different body positions. *ORL* **41**, 329.

—— LUNDGREN, C., TJERNSTRÖM, Ö., UDDMAN, R., and ÖRNHAGEN, H. (1977). Eustachian tubal function during immersion. *Undersea biomed. Res.* **4**, 9.

JONSON, B. and RUNDCRANTZ, H. (1969). Posture and pressure within the internal jugular vein. *Acta oto-lar.* **68**, 271.

KING, P. F. (1966). Otitic barotrauma. *Proc. R. Soc. Med.* **59**, 543.

MACKINNON, D. M. (1970). Relationship of preoperative Eustachian tube function to myringoplasty. *Acta oto-lar.* **69**, 100.

MELVILL JONES, G. (1961). Pressure changes in the middle ear after altering the composition of contained gas. *Acta oto-lar.* **53**, 1.

MILLER, G. F. Jr (1965). Eustachian tubal function in normal and diseased ears. *Archs Otolar.* **81**, 41.

—— and BILODEAU R. (1967). Preoperative evaluation of Eustachian tubal function in tympanoplasty. *S. med. J, Nashville* **60**, 868.

MÜNKER, G. (1972). *Funktionsanalyse der Tuba Eustachii.* Medizinische Habilitationsschrift, Freiburg.

NIWA, H. (1972). The study on the measurement of the Eustachian tubal function. *J. Otolar. Jap.* (Abstracts) **6**, 2.

PALVA, A. and KÄRJÄ, J. (1970). Eustachian-tube patency in chronic ears. Preoperative evaluation correlated to postoperative results. *Acta oto-lar.* Suppl. **263**, 25.

PERLMAN, H. B. (1939). The Eustachian tube; abnormal patency and normal physiologic state. *Archs Otolar.* **30**, 212.

—— (1951). Observations on the Eustachian tube. *Archs Otolar.* **53**, 370.

—— (1960). Physiological basis for tubal function tests. *Archs Otolar.* **71**, 384.

—— (1967). Normal tubal function. *Archs Otolar.* **86**, 632.

RAHN, H. and CANFIELD, R. (1955a). Volume and gas composition changes of subcutaneous gas pockets immediately following the injection of various gas mixtures. In *Studies in respiration physiology* (eds. H. Rahn and W. O. Fenn) p. 409. WADC Technical Report 55–357. Wright Air Development Center, Dayton, Ohio.

—— —— (1955b). Volume changes and the steady state behaviour of gas pockets within body cavities. In *Studies in respiration physiology* (ed. H. Rahn and W. O. Fenn) p. 395. WADC Technical Report 55–357. Wright Air Development Center, Dayton, Ohio.

RAPPORT, P. N., LIM, D. J., and WEISS, H. S. (1975). Surface-active agent in Eustachian tube function. *Archs Otol.* **101**, 305.

REIMER, Å., HUBERMAN, D., KLEMENTSSON, K., and TOREMALM, N. G. (1981). The mucociliary activity of respiratory tract. Experiments on the effect of changing pO_2 and pCO_2 in ambient atmosphere and arterial blood. *Acta oto-lar.* **91**, 139–48.

RIU, R., FLOTTES, L., BOUCHE, J., and LE DEN, R. (1966). *La physiologie de la trompe d'Eustache.* Librairie Arnette, Paris.

RUNDCRANTZ, H. (1969a). Posture and Eustachian tube function. *Acta oto-lar.* **68**, 279.
—— (1969b). Posture and Eustachian tube function. *Acta oto-lar.* Suppl. **263**, 15.
—— (1970). The effects of position change on Eustachian tube function. *Otolar. Clin. N. Am.* **3**, 103.
SADÉ, J. (1966a). Middle ear mucosa. *Archs Otolar.* **84**, 137.
—— (1966b). Pathology and pathogenesis of serous otitis media. *Archs Otolar.* **84**, 297.
—— (1974). The biophathology of secretory otitis media. *Ann. Otol. Rhinol. Lar.* **83**, Suppl. 11, 59.
—— and BERCO, E. (1976). Atelectasis and secretory otitis media. *Ann. Otol. Rhinol. Lar.* **85**, Suppl. 25, 66.
—— HALEVY, A., and HADAS, E. (1976). Clearance of middle ear pressures. *Ann. Otol. Rhinol. Lar.* **85**, Suppl. 25, 58.
SIEDENTOP, K. H. (1968). Eustachian tube dynamics, size of the mastoid air cell system and results with tympanoplasty. *Otolar. Clin. N. Am.* **5**, 33.
—— TARDY, M. E., and HAMILTON, L. R. (1968). Eustachian tube function. *Archs Otolar.* **88**, 386.
SHARP, M. (1970). The manometric investigation of tubal function with reference to myringoplasty results. *J. Lar. Otol.* **84**, 545.
SMYTH, G. D., KERR, A. G., and GOODY, R. J. (1971). Current thoughts on combined approach tympanoplasty. I. Indications and preoperative assessment. *J. Lar. Otol.* **85**, 205.
TERKILDSEN, K. (1957). Movements of the ear-drum following intra-aural muscle reflexes. *Archs Otolar.* **66**, 484.
THOMSEN, K. A. (1958). Investigations on the tubal function and measurement of the middle ear pressure in pressure chamber. *Acta oto-lar.* Suppl. **140**, 269.
—— and TERKILDSEN, K. (1965). Middle ear pressure variations during anesthesia. *Archs Otolar.* **82**, 609.
TJERNSTRÖM, Ö. (1974a). Function of the Eustachian tubes in divers with a history of alternobaric vertigo. *Undersea biomed. Res.* **1**, 343.
—— (1974b). Further studies on alternobaric vertigo. Posture and passive equilibration of middle ear pressure. *Acta oto-lar.* **78**, 221.
— (1974c). Middle ear mechanics and alternobaric vertigo. *Acta oto-lar.* **78**, 376.
TOS, M. and BAK-PEDERSEN, K. (1977). Goblet cell population in the pathological middle ear and Eustachian tube of children and adults. *Ann. Otol. Rhinol. Lar.* **86**, 209.
VAN DISHOECK, H. A. E. (1941). Negative pressure and loss of hearing in tubal catarrh. *Acta oto-lar.* **29**, 303.
VIRTANEN, H. (1977). Eustachian tube sound conduction. Sonotubometry: an acoustical method for objective measurement of auditory tubal opening. Thesis, Helsinki, Finland.
ZÖLLNER, F. (1942) *Anatomie, Physiologie, Pathologie and Klinik der Ohrtrompete.* Springer, Berlin.

Section 7
Electrophysiological tests of hearing

31 Bio-electric potentials available for electric response audiometry: indications and contra-indications

H. A. BEAGLEY and L. FISCH

Of recent years there has been much interest in various bio-electric potentials of the central nervous system which can be utilized as neurophysiological indicators of auditory function and their applications to clinical audiometry. The potentials of principal interest to audiometry will now be described briefly, and the indications and contra-indications for their use in clinical practice reviewed.

Starting at the periphery (the cochlea) and progressing along the auditory pathways to the cortex we have:
1. Endocochlear potentials and compound auditory nerve action potential.
2. Brainstem evoked potentials.
3. Middle latency responses.
4. Cortical evoked potential (V-potential).
5. Cortical d.c. potentials.

The endocochlear potentials of clinical significance are those which are elicited in the course of electrocochleography (ECochG), the details of which are outlined in Chapter 33. There are at least three potentials mixed together and how these are separated is indicated in the section on ECochG.

ENDOCOCHLEAR POTENTIALS

(i) The compound auditory nerve action potential

This is generated by the fibres of the auditory nerve with a latency of about 2 ms when the cochlea is stimulated by sound especially if the onset of the sound is fairly abrupt. It has been established by Teas, Eldredge, and Davis (1962) that the individual action potential in each auditory nerve fibre is a diphasic spike potential. But when the response of the whole auditory nerve is recorded the compound action potential has the typical shape with a prominent negative peak, N_1, generally followed by a second negative peak N_2, and occasionally a third, N_3, (Fig. 31.1). The reason for this is that the Békésy travelling wave activates a series of nerve fibres as it passes along the basilar membrane (see Chapter 4) and the slightly out-of-phase individual action potentials become convoluted together to produce the typical compound action potential. As the auditory nerve fibres originating in the basal turn are to a large extent synchronized by the sound stimulus (but not completely so) the typical compound action potential has its main origin here. More apically the travelling wave has slowed down to some extent and

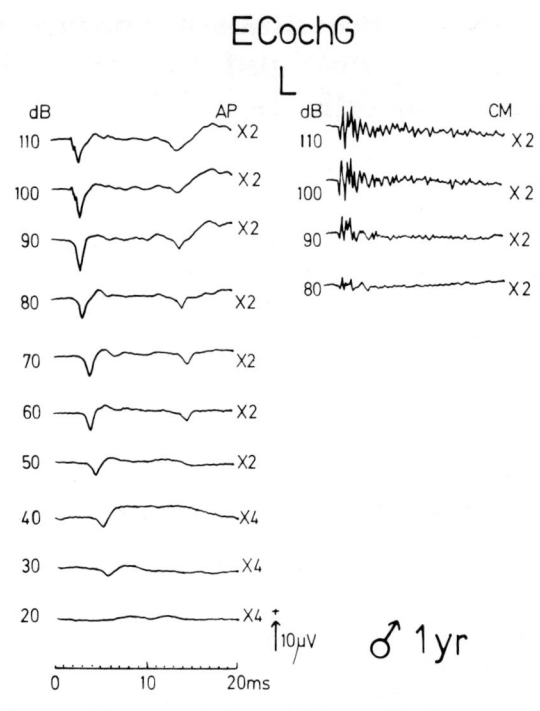

Fig. 31.1. The electrocochleogram of a boy aged 1 year. Hearing was normal by this test.

the individual action potential are essentially out of phase with one another and a clear compound action potential is extremely difficult to record from the apical region. Thus the action potential recorded during ECochG gives information mainly from the basal turn of the cochlea, and to a lesser extent, from the middle turn.

(ii) The cochlear microphonic

This is generated by the hair cells of the organ of Corti. It has no perceptible latency and can be regarded as a receptor potential and it gives a reasonably faithful reproduction of the incident sound stimulus, e.g. a pure tone, which is an acoustic sine wave, produces a sinusoidal microphonic in the cochlea. This is the reason for the term 'cochlear microphonic'. Destruction of the cochlear hair cells will abolish the cochlear microphonic. The CM has limited value in ECochG because it is virtually impossible to quantify. It has no physiological threshold as does the action potential and cannot therefore be used for hearing evaluation, but it does have some limited value in differential diagnosis as will be seen later.

(iii) The summating potential

This is regarded as a receptor potential and like the cochlear microphonic has no perceptible latency. Its origin, however, is complex. It can be regarded simplistically as being the response of the cochlear end-organ to the envelope of the second stimulus and can be thought of as biasing the basilar membrane in one direction thus causing a d.c. off-set potential, usually negative, at high sound intensities. It is of value in differential diagnosis, e.g. of Ménière's disease and acoustic neuroma.

(iv) The endolymphatic potential

The steady-state potential of about 80 mV located within the endolymph of the scala medial of the organ of Corti, was first described by Békésy (1950). Although useful in investigations on experimental animals it currently has no application in clinical audiology and is not recorded by the usual techniques of electrocochleography.

BRAINSTEM EVOKED POTENTIALS

These very small potentials whose amplitude rarely attains one microvolt were described by Sohmer and Feinmesser (1967) and Jewett and Williston (1971). Unlike the endocochlear potentials which are recorded by a 'near field' technique, i.e. with the recording electrode close to the site of generation of the potential (as in ECochG), the brainstem potentials, often called the 'brainstem electric responses' (BSER), are recorded using a 'far-field' technique where the recording electrodes are at a considerable distance, in this case generally on the vertex (or high frontal region) and the earlobe (or mastoid). Typically there are five peaks separated by about 1 ms. Of these the first, Wave I, is the auditory nerve action potential and is very clear in children but less definite in adults. The remaining peaks II to V are generated by the passage of synchronized neural responses passing along the auditory pathways of the brainstem by way of the cochlear nucleus, the superior olivary complex, the nucleus of the lateral lemniscus and finally the inferior corpus quadrigeminum (Fig. 31.2(a) and (b)). Despite their very small amplitudes these potentials are of value both in audiological diagnosis and even more so for neurological investigations in such cases as early disseminated sclerosis or other discrete lesions of the brainstem.

MIDDLE LATENCY RESPONSES

The responses are so called because their latency lies between that of the *early* responses, the endocochlear and brainstem potentials, on the one hand and the *late* cortical potentials on the other; the latencies of the various peaks of the middle responses range from 10–50 ms. The discovery and investigation of the middle responses are associated with the work of Goldstein and Rodman (1967) and of Mendel and Goldstein (1969) *inter alia*. The site of generation of the middle responses has not been defined precisely, but almost certainly it is situated in the auditory radiations in the thalamic region, and in the primary auditory cortex in the temporal lobe. Although potentially useful as indicators of auditory function, with the advantage over

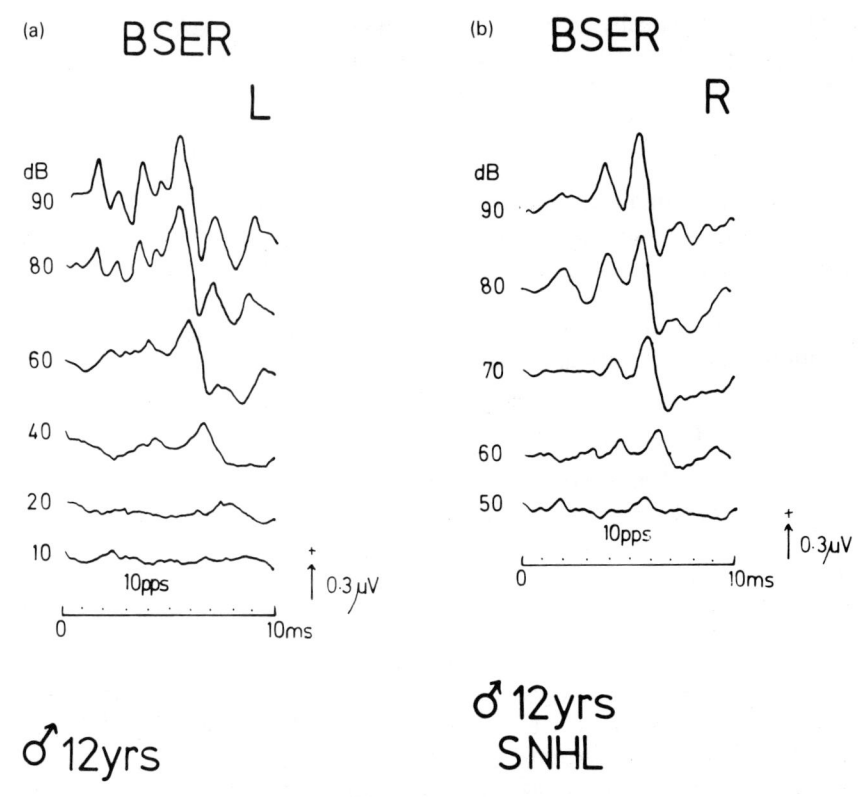

758 *Bio-electric potentials available for audiometry*

Fig. 31.2. (a). Brainstem evoked responses (BSER) from a boy of 12 years; Left ear, normal hearing. (b). BSER from the right ear which showed a sensorineural loss of 45 dB.

the action potential and brainstem responses that they are frequency sensitive they have proved to be somewhat labile in the hands of many investigators and have not so far achieved clinical acceptance outside one or two centres (Fig. 31.3). More will probably be heard of them in the future. In this respect the 40 Hz Event Related Potential (ERP40) described by Galambos and his collaborators (1980) is of particular interest (personal communication).

CORTICAL EVOKED POTENTIAL (V-POTENTIAL)

The auditory evoked cortical potential was the first potential to be developed for audiometric purposes. This potential, often called the 'vertex potential' or 'V-potential', was extracted from the background EEG as the definitive physiological indicator in electric response audiometry (ERA), although the latter term is today a generic one covering all the potentials used in the so-called objective testing of hearing. The V-potential is a late cortical response consisting of three main peaks, P_1 at about 60 ms, N_1 at about 100 ms, P_2 at about 175 ms, and sometimes an N_2 at 200–250 ms

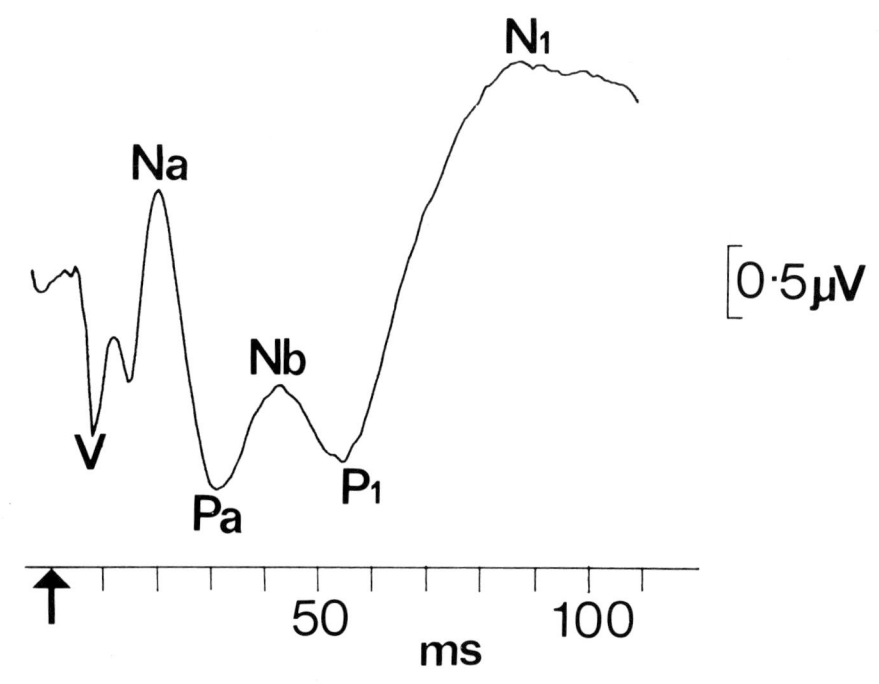

Fig. 31.3. An example of middle latency responses. This is the average of the responses from 35 normal subjects, using binaural click stimulation at approximately 90 dB above threshold. (Dr P. Rudge, courtesy of the Editor, *Brain*.)

(Fig. 31.4). It is probably not the primary response of the auditory cortex to sound in view of its latency, but the auditory cortex and the adjacent cortical areas are undoubtedly involved. It is probably related in some way to auditory perception and it is certainly useful as a test of auditory function as it can be elicited by means of tone bursts within the typical audiometric frequency range. How it is extracted from the EEG for audiometric purposes is described in Chapter 33.

CORTICAL d.c. POTENTIALS

There are two d.c. potentials of cortical origin which may have some application to audiometry in the future. These are (i) the contingent negative variation (CNV) described by Walter (1964) and (ii) the perstimulatory d.c. responses recorded by Keidel (1971) and Finkenzeller (1979). The difference between the two responses is that perstimulatory response is coterminous, in time, with the auditory stimulus and can be elicited, of course, only if d.c. amplifiers are employed; the CNV, on the other hand, is recorded during operant conditioning, also by d.c. amplification. Both potentials are of interest to psychologists studying perception but have not so far been embodied into current clinical audiological tests, although a

ERA (V-potential)

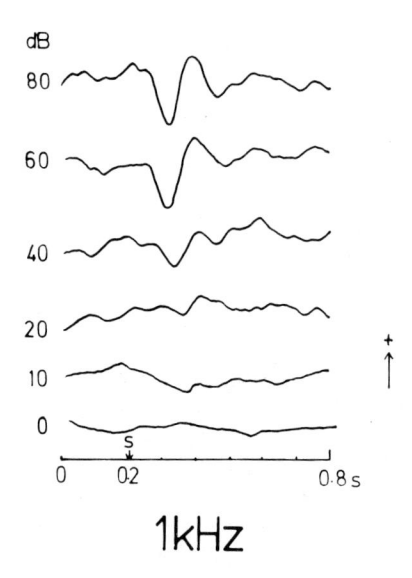

[Figure: Cortical ERA traces at 1 kHz, recorded at 80, 60, 40, 20, 10, and 0 dB; time axis 0 to 0.8 s with stimulus marker at 0.2 s]

1kHz

♀ 19yrs

Fig. 31.4. Cortical ERA from a young woman of 19 years with normal hearing. The cortical evoked potential can be traced down to 10 dB HL, indicating a hearing threshold of 5 dB at 1 kHz.

promising method of objective speech audiometry based on the CNV has been proposed by Burian, Gestring, Gloning, and Haider (1972).

INDICATIONS AND CONTRA-INDICATIONS FOR ELECTROPHYSIOLOGICAL TESTS

Audiometry carried out with the help of electrophysiological techniques which record involuntary changes in some parts of the hearing system is not a substitute for pure-tone threshold audiometry based on the conscious co-operation of the subject. Electrophysiological tests should be considered instead as useful adjuncts to be used in those not particularly numerous cases where co-operation is not possible so that behavioural responses to sound stimulation fail to provide the diagnostic answers that we seek.

It is important to be aware of the indications and contra-indications of the various electrophysiological hearing tests which are discussed in greater detail in Chapter 33. The tests based on reflex responses such as the acoustic stapedial reflex or the post-auricular myogenic response will not be considered in this context although these reflexes can of course be produced without the active voluntary co-operation of the subject. Only those tests which are based on the recording of a bio-electric potential will be reviewed and they will be discussed from peripheral to central starting with the endocochlear potentials and ending with those of cortical origin. As the needs of adults and children are somewhat different in this respect, it is better to consider them separately.

IN ADULTS

(i) **Electro-cochleography**

In adults this test is rarely ever required as a test of hearing as such; instead it is used more in neuro-otological practice in cases of suspected retrocochlear disorder especially acoustic neuroma or similar lesions, cerebellopontine angle tumours, angiomata, or vascular anomalies in these regions. It is also useful in investigating endocochlear disorders such as endolymphatic hydrops, or Ménière's disorder, and in the differential diagnosis of unilateral Ménière's from suspected acoustic neuroma which is always an important and sometimes difficult clinical distinction to make.

It is often used in the investigation of sudden, unexplained total deafness especially if it is unilateral as this may, not infrequently, be a manifestation of acoustic neuroma. In one series of such cases followed up in the Royal National Hospital, London there were no less than 9 per cent which had this underlying etiology (Graham, personal communication).

(ii) **Brainstem electric responses (BSER)**

These tests are today attracting much attention in the field of audiology and neurology. In the case of adults the neurological aspect predominates. Examination of these responses, and especially of their latencies, which are often prolonged in disease processes affecting the brainstem, are often carried out to clarify the neurological diagnosis. Examples are cerebellopontine angle space occupying lesions which may cause pressure on the brainstem, as well as small discrete lesions within the substance of the brainstem proper, such as plaques of multiple sclerosis or other demyelinating process, punctuate haemorrhages or small intramedullary tumours, and tumours of the cerebello-pontine angle.

(iii) **Cortical evoked potentials**

The principal audiological test based on the cortical response (sometimes known as the vertex-potential or V-potential) is often simply called 'ERA', from the old name 'evoked response' audiometry which is now replaced by the more precise name *electric* response audiometry. It is more akin to conventional audiometry than either of the two preceding tests, in that a true audiogram can be constructed from it. This is comparable in all ways with an ordinary pure-tone audiogram. In adults this test is reserved essentially for those whose pure-tone audiometry results are suspect, or frankly unreliable. Such patients must give at least passive co-operation, permitting the surface electrodes to be affixed and thereafter sitting still in a comfortable chair for up to one hour. Those who flagrantly refuse to co-operate to this extent are included in that very rare group where ECochG must be contemplated—the others in this category are patients with severe epilepsy which completely obscures the ERA traces. Having said this, it becomes clear that ERA is virtually restricted to the investigation of non-organic hearing loss (including malingering) and medicolegal cases, to confirm other audiograms and give some idea of their validity. Another fairly rare indication is to clarify the diagnosis of central deafness. A tumour in the midbrain, for example, may show normal peripheral auditory activity as shown by ECochG and even by BSER, yet subjective hearing may be lacking. A negative result based on the V-potential will help clinch the diagnosis.

IN CHILDREN

There is no single hearing test which can provide all the answers for the full diagnosis of hearing impairment. There are single tests which can undoubtedly confirm that there is no hearing loss. For example, in a co-operative child pure-tone threshold audiometry can tell us that hearing is normal, or, in an infant and very young children below the age of $2\frac{1}{2}$ years a properly carried out free-field test based on behavioural observation can safely exclude hearing impairment of serious consequence or significance, although this should be confirmed by full audiometry as soon as possible.

However, once a hearing impairment is confirmed, by any method, several tests will be necessary to obtain the answers to the following questions:
  (i) What is the frequency distribution of the loss?
  (ii) What is its extent?
  (iii) What type is it—conductive, sensorineural, or mixed?
  (iv) To what degree is hearing of speech sounds affected?
  (v) Are there, apart from loss of sensitivity, other hearing disorders such as abnormality of loudness perception (hypersensitivity or loudness recruitment)?

Obviously in small children not only can we not obtain all the answers by any single test, but we cannot in many cases obtain them in a reasonably short time by applying the necessary tests in quick succession. When asked to examine a child we must first decide which test will give us a reliable answer to the crucial question of whether the child has a hearing impairment or not. One cannot and should not make a decision before a general examination of the child, including behavioural observation, is carried out by an audiological physician. The need to decide what should be the appropriate test to obtain an answer as soon as possible, by the most informative and economical procedure, so that any rehabilitation procedure that may be necessary can commence almost at once, is the very essence of the first examination.

In a well established audiology centre the techniques of play audiometry will be well known and the audiology team skilled in applying them. Co-operation for play audiometry is possible from the age of $2\frac{1}{2}$ years in otherwise physically and mentally healthy children and, therefore, all efforts should be made to accomplish this test. Naturally it is most useful in any case to obtain first of all a general impression of the child's reaction to a variety of test sounds in free-field, including speech sounds which will give a fairly good, yet approximate idea about the child's hearing ability. This will also provide us with much useful information about many aspects that are of importance from the diagnostic point of view. An account of these tests is given in Chapter 25.

When no co-operation is possible (in children below the age of $2\frac{1}{2}$ years or older children who have other difficulties, e.g. mental or physical impairment, behavioural difficulties, psychological disturbances) tests by behavioural observation should be carried out first of all. In a well established audiology clinic facilities for observation and tests based on behavioural reactions exist. It is essential to have a spacious, acoustically insulated and well ventilated room specially devoted to examining children, including those who have various difficulties mentioned earlier. There should be facilities for observation via a one-way viewing window or closed circuit television and facilities to apply test sounds, either by the tester himself or by means of prerecorded sounds delivered through suitably placed loudspeakers. When such facilities and the necessary skill exist, in the great majority of children a direct test by behavioural observation will tell us whether there is a significant hearing impairment or not. Reactions to test sounds should be compared with behavioural reactions to other types of sensory stimulation such as touch, light, puff of air on the skin, and vibration. These can be important in children who are apathetic, or have suffered sensory deprivation.

It is clear that the environment should be structured in such a way that the natural anxiety of the child is reduced to the minimum so that his confidence can be gained. This should enable us to manage and test restless children who cannot keep still (when unnecessary stimulation can be eliminated) as well as apathetic children (who need special stimulation). It would be, for example, futile to try to obtain responses by behavioural change from a child who is very anxious or frightened by an unsuitable room which is ill-equipped for this type of examination. It would be then incorrect to state that it is not possible to test that particular child by behavioural observation and that other methods should be tried. It is not in such a case the child who is difficult or the method inappropriate. The difficulty may lie in a different area, namely an unsuitable environment or possibly a relatively inexperienced examiner.

It can be very difficult to make precise audiological measurements in free-field and to determine exactly in terms of decibel levels the intensity of the test sound heard by the child. Threshold tests are virtually impossible in these clinical situations in free-field. It is advisable not to pretend that precise measurements are being carried out. At this stage one should be deliberately imprecise and should adopt the so-called 'rough sketch method' of assessment (Fisch 1978). Attempts to measure hearing accurately in these situations can be very misleading. The imprecision of the rough sketch does not preclude anyone changing or improving the original assessment on the basis of later observation and testing. However, when testing behavioural observation in free-field in a properly structured environment we can almost invariably assign the hearing ability to one of three broad categories:

1. The child's hearing is not seriously impaired which means that he certainly should hear at least a slightly raised conversational voice.
2. The child's hearing is moderately impaired so that he is bound to have considerable difficulty hearing a mezzo-forte conversational voice.
3. The child's hearing is severely impaired and he will have great difficulty in hearing normal speech or possibly may not hear it at all.

Accordingly, we can then take the necessary remedial measures and arrange further observations which eventually will lead to an accurate assessment, but if we try to be very precise from the beginning we may embark on time consuming procedures which may not be successful with many children, and therefore postpone assessment and commencement of remedial measures. This unhurried approach allows us to draw a rough sketch of what is wrong fairly quickly and in most cases, commence the programme of remedial measures almost at once. We continue then with the design process until a precise picture emerges.

Such a careful and unhurried observation of a child suspected of hearing loss is perfectly in order when the observer is an experienced paedo-audiologist working in a suitable audiological centre, for by such methods the clinical picture can be established and any remedial measures that are required can be instituted without procrastination or undue delay. However, these ideal circumstances do not always prevail. The child with suspected hearing loss, slow speech development or multiple handicaps may be seen initially in a remote area where a paedo-audiology centre does not exist. In such a case the assessment of the hearing status of the child in a busy hospital outpatient department, especially one dealing mainly with adults, may present great difficulties. A firm diagnosis may not be made at an early date and valuable time may be lost. Even if the child is referred subsequently to a paedo-audiology centre the child may still prove difficult to assess. To avoid further undersirable delays in such cases, testing by means of electrocochleography or brainstem responses may offer the best method of resolving the diagnostic dilemma without further loss of time.

Although as stated above, no single test can provide us with the answer concerning all aspects of hearing impairment, pure tone threshold audiometry is still the most informative single test which can be carried out economically in a reasonably short period of time, with relatively simple equipment. It is, therefore, the most important single hearing test which gives us a very good idea about the physiological condition of the hearing system. Every possible effort should be made to obtain a reliable result with this test in all children found to have a hearing loss as a result of either behavioural observation or an electrophysiological procedure. Ultimately, it is pure-tone audiogram which is stable over a reasonable period of time which gives the most valid picture of the child's hearing. Follow-up audiometry should not be omitted just because electrophysiological methods have been used to make the initial diagnosis.

Children who are difficult to assess by reason of hyperactivity, apprehension, retardation and so on, those in whom it is essential to make a firm diagnosis without further delay so that remedial measures can be instituted, and those coming from abroad and available for testing for a fairly brief period of time, may be considered as suitable candidates for electrophysiological testing. But apart from these cases there are certain clinical situations in which electrophysiological testing is much more clearly indicated.

Blind infants, where hearing is suspect, are prime candidates for ECochG or BSER. A child with, for instance, Norrie's disease or other severe visual defect will be almost impossible to diagnose with confidence by behavioural methods and the matter should be clarified by elective ECochG or BSER. The rubella syndrome is a special case which is familiar to all paedoaudiologists. Such children can have numerous disabilities apart from hearing loss including physical and mental retardation, heart anomalies and defective vision. While the hearing loss can usually be confirmed or disproved in most of these cases by behavioural methods, those with serious visual defects may require electrocochleography. The possibility of a hearing defect which is severe in middle frequencies, but rather better in high and the low frequencies should be kept in mind because as has been pointed out earlier, both ECochG and BSER record preferentially from the basal cochlear region and may perhaps underestimate the hearing loss to some extent for this reason. In practice, however, this has not proved much of a difficulty and in many of the severer cases of rubella syndrome the high frequencies may be just as severely affected as the middle frequencies.

Gross hyperkinesia, psychosis and autism may also present the audiologist with severe problems when attempting behavioural assessment and in the end electrophysiological testing, ECochG or BSER, may be called for. The fact that these two tests can be carried out under general anaesthesia is a very great advantage in these cases and in some hyperkinetic children anaesthesia permits the first really adequate otoscopic examination permitting the otologist who conducts the ECochG the opportunity, in some cases, of removing impacted wax or even foreign bodies, and assessing the tympanic membrane for the possibility of middle-ear effusion. Far from being a disadvantage in such cases, general anaesthesia can be a distinct advantage.

Athetoid cerebral palsy in a young child can be a difficult matter when hearing assessment is required. In the hands of a highly skilled paedo-audiologist experienced in testing such cases a careful behavioural examination is often possible and with patience it is often possible to teach such a child to perform an adequate pure-tone audiogram despite his neuromuscular problems. This will allow the hearing to be assessed (including the hearing for high frequencies), and will show whether or not a hearing aid is required. If the difficulties are such that electrophysiological testing is thought necessary, the type of test is dictated in part by his age. As stated in Chapter 34 which deals with anaesthesia, children below 3 years of age are usually given Ketamine without intubation because of resistance in the respiratory circuits that intubation would entail. Ketamine abolishes sensation but some muscular movements may persist in a child with athetosis. This makes it mandatory to use ECochG rather than BSER because the latter would be made more difficult by muscular contractions, but ECochG would be unaffected. But a child of 3 years and over can safely be anaesthetized with Halothane and intubated. This would mean that muscular relaxation would occur during the test and both ECochG and BSER could be carried out, as neither is affected by general anaesthesia. BSER may be quite useful in such cases as the possibility of brain stem lesions in the region of the cochlear nucleus are thought to occur in some cases of cerebral palsy.

Clearly the use of ECochG and BSER in young children is largely restricted to assessment of hearing in those difficult cases, often with multiple handicaps in whom conventional clinical tests are of limited value or are impossible to apply. An exception to this generalization is the distorted AP waveform, widened and monophasic in its configuration, which is seen in some cases with a history of kernicterus. This resembles the distorted waveform seen in some adults with acoustic neuroma. Recently one of us (HAB) was called upon to test a child of 3 years 4 months in whom the mother had noted an apparent unilateral hearing loss. As there was a family history of neurofibromatosis (von Recklinghausen's disease), the mother was concerned that the child may be developing a lesion of this sort. As neurofibromatosis which affects the auditory nerve often produces a striking distortion of the AP, it was decided to carry out ECochG. Ketamine anaesthesia was used despite the fact that he was just over 3 years of age so that he could be carried directly to the Radiology Department for tomography if the AP findings were suspicious.

In fact the AP showed particularly florid example of widened monophasic distortion in the affected ear. Brainstem responses were not attempted as experience has shown that it is not possible to elicit BSER in cases with the type of AP distortion mentioned (probably on account of desynchronization of the nerve impulses). Instead the child was taken directly for hypocycloidal tomography while still asleep under the influence of Ketamine, and the results of this examination were most revealing. The internal auditory meatus on the affected side was grossly widened and eroded, with the erosion appearing to extend to the middle and posterior aspects of the petrous bone. This would appear to confirm the presence of a tumour within the internal auditory meatus. This was apparently a solitary lesion (at least at present) and is the youngest example of this sort of lesion that we can recall. Surgical exploration and removal of the tumour was successfully carried out and histological examination showed it to be a meningoma. Meningiomata, sometimes multiple, are quite often encountered in cases of neurofibromatosis.

ELECTROPHYSIOLOGICAL TESTS IN OLDER CHILDREN

So far we have discussed the indications and contra-indications of these tests in infants and young children. Older children also need such investigation in some cases. In general these children have established speech and are attending school, but are referred to audiologists with bizarre hearing problems. Clinical assessment often indicates non-organic hearing loss (NOHL) see Chapter 27 and electrophysiological tests are sometimes needed to clarify the picture.

The ideal test for a school age child would be ERA based on the V-potential; this permits an audiogram to be obtained at any required audiometric frequency. ERA can often be obtained quite easily in reasonably co-operative school children. For a shorter confirmatory test BSER can be carried out and this will indicate, in general terms, the hearing status, i.e. whether there is normal hearing or a certain degree of hearing loss, but BSER, like ECochG does not give an audiogram as such, as only the frequencies from 2–8000 Hz are easily tested in contradistinction to ERA where all frequencies can be tested. In general, cases of NOHL are quite co-operative and the electrophysiological confirmatory tests can be applied without difficulty. Only in very rare cases is the opposite the case, but where co-operation is not forthcoming it is possible, if necessary, to carry out ECochG under sedation. This is rarely ever required.

We may sum up by saying that the great majority of children can be assessed by behavioural methods if these are applied in the appropriate manner by a patient and skilled examiner in a suitable test environment. It is only when such methods fail to yield at least a reasonable estimate of the child's hearing within a reasonable length of time does electrophysiological testing become necessary. Only in extremely rare cases (e.g. blindness) should it be considered as the first choice and limitations of the results of ECochG and BSER should be borne in mind, namely the fact that the low frequencies are not adequately tested by these methods. And finally, behavioural observation and testing should be continued even after electrophysiological diagnosis so that ultimately a stable pure-tone audiogram is obtained and recorded in the patient's case notes.

REFERENCES

BÉKÉSY, G. VON (1950). D-C potentials and energy balance in the cochlear partition. *J. acoust. Soc. Am.* **22**, 576–82.

Burian, K., Gestring, G. F., Gloning, K., and Haider, M. (1972). Objective examination of verbal discrimination and comprehension in aphasia using CNV. *Audiology* **11**, 310–16.

Finkenzeller, P. (1979). Auditory evoked potentials—late cortical responses. In *Auditory investigations: the scientific and technological basis* (ed. H. A. Beagley) pp. 507–25. Clarendon Press, Oxford.

Goldstein, R. and Rodman, L. B. (1967). Early components of averaged evoked responses to rapidly repeated auditory stimuli. *J. Speech Hear. Res.* **10**, 697–705.

Keidel, W. D. (1971). DC potentials in auditory evoked response in man. *Acta oto-lar.* **71**, 242–8.

Jewett, D. L. and Williston, J. S. (1971). Auditory evoked far fields averaged from the scalp of humans. *Brain* **167**, 1517–18.

Mendel, M. I. and Goldstein, R. (1969). Stability of the early components of the averaged electroencephalographic response. *J. Speech Hear. Res.* **14**, 829–40.

Sohmer, H. and Feinmesser, M. (1967). Cochlear action potentials recorded from the external ear in man. *Ann. Otol. Rhinol. Lar.* **76**, 427–35.

Teas, D. C., Eldredge, D. H., and Davis, H. (1962). Cochlear responses to acoustic transients: an interpretation of whole-nerve action potentials. *J. acoust. Soc. Am.* **34**, 1438–59.

Walter, W. G. (1964). Slow potential waves in the human brain associated with expectancy. *Archs Psychiat.* **206**, 309–22.

32 Auditory myogenic responses

ELLIS DOUEK

It has always been common knowledge that sounds will cause an involuntary response in the muscles of the body. These responses are of two main types: (i) *To loud sounds*—these form part of the startle response. The most well-known, most frequently used aspect of this response is the blink reflex. In small infants this is often accompanied by an out-stretching of the arms and legs (Moro reflex). (ii) *To quiet sounds*—these have been much less clearly understood, but electrical recordings using modern averaging techniqeues have shown that there is a generalized response to quiet sounds in all the muscles of the body. This is not surprising if it is considered that animals treat a quiet sound as a warning of danger or of the presence of prey. Clearly some sort of preparation for sudden muscle activity is required.

One type of response to quiet sounds has been recognized since before records were kept and this is the ability that animals have to prick up their ears when they hear a quiet sound. Because of Preyer's description in 1881 this has generally been known as Preyer's reflex.

It is only when averaging techniques became available that electrical recordings were made in response to sounds. Geisler, Frishkopf, and Rosenblith (1958) recorded responses to clicks which occurred in the scalp although they did not recognize their muscular origin.

In 1963 Bickford, Jacobson, and Galbraith demonstrated that these scalp recordings were myogenic and also showed that similar responses could be obtained from muscles in all parts of the body. The stimuli that they used were loud clicks of 100 dB or more. They noted the difference in latency between a response recorded from the muscles at the inion (8–10 ms) and the startle response (25 ms) as well as the voluntary movement response of 100 ms. Using curarization techniques Bickford *et al.* (1963) and Cody, Jacobsson, Walker, and Bickford (1964) confirmed the myogenic nature of these responses. Among the responses from the various muscles four have received closer attention: those from the inion, the parietal, postauricular region, and the jaw. As of these, only the postauricular reflex has had clinical applications it will be dealt with last, and in more detail.

THE INION RESPONSE

This can be obtained from an electrode placed on the inion. It is difficult to be sure of the origin of this response as many muscles, not to speak of neurogenic elements, are present in that general area. The most massive contribution however must come from the neck muscles. It is indeed complex with a negative peak at 30 ms latency.

The inion response has aroused some interest from the theoretical point of view since Cody and his colleagues (1964) showed that it could be obtained from deaf patients with normal vestibular function.

The association with the vestibule was used by Tabor and his colleagues in 1968 and later by Pignataro (1972) in attempts to use this response in the study of vestibular function.

Problems have arisen, however, as it appears that stimuli, vestibular or cochlear, can give rise to a response. Cody and Bickford (1969) for instance, showed that even visual and tactile stimuli can produce measurable responses even though they may lie at different latencies. It is because of the non-specific nature of the inion response that it has not yet been put to clinical use.

THE PARIETAL RESPONSE

Interest arose here as far back as 1967 when Goldstein and Redman claimed that they could use responses obtained from parietally placed electrodes in the middle latency area as a method of objective audiometry. Clinically, however, this has not been found useful to other workers during the ensuing years.

The nature of these responses is complex as the major component is probably neurogenic although it has not been possible to separate absolutely the myogenic from the neurogenic.

Today it is more common to discuss these middle latency parietal responses under the general title of 'early cortical' rather than of myogenic.

THE ACOUSTIC JAW REFLEX

Meir-Ewert, Gleitsmann, and Reiter (1974) have demonstrated a response to high-intensity sound which can be elicited from the jaw muscles if they are kept under tension. It has not found a clinical use mainly because the response is only to very loud sound whereas the main clinical requirement has been up to recently in the field of objective audiometry.

THE POST-AURICULAR RESPONSE

Among the many recordings made from the surface at the time, Kiang, Crist, French, and Edwards (1963) reported a response obtained from an electrode placed behind the ear with a maximum peak latency of about 15 ms. It appeared to be myogenic in origin and showed signs of fatigue and habituation. On the other hand it was quite clearly a low-threshold response to quiet sound.

In 1969 Cody and Bickford studied this response using tone bursts as stimuli. These had a rise and decay time of 1 ms and were presented at a rate 2 per second. With these stimuli they found that many subjects yielded no response at all and those who did required intensities of around 90 dB.

In the same year, however, Yoshie and Okudaira found that using clicks instead of tone bursts of slower rise-time the response was more consistent and could be obtained to low-intensity sounds.

The main obstacle to its use as a clinical tool remained the inconsistencies resulting from changing muscle tone. Lack of tone would produce a weak response requiring high intensity sound stimulus whereas a moment of increased muscle tension would result in a prominent response.

Douek, Gibson, and Humphries (1973) introduced the post-auricular myogenic response as a clinical tool. The problem of variable muscle tone was mitigated by recording from both sides simultaneously. This meant that in the majority of head movements at least one side retained enough tension to produce an adequate response. In this way it was possible to obtain an objective indication of hearing acuity in the moving child. To stress the fact that the test was based on the crossed, bilateral and consensual nature of this reflex it was discussed under the name of crossed acoustic response (CAR).

Latency measurements could be made and one side compared to the other so that a place for the CAR in the diagnosis of brainstem lesions emerged (Douek, Ashcroft, and Humphries 1976).

THE CHARACTERISTICS OF THE POST-AURICULAR RESPONSE

The largest responses are obtained from an electrode placed immediately behind the pinna with the reference electrode on the ear-lobe, though almost equally good responses can be obtained with the reference below the tip of the mastoid process. An earth electrode may be placed anywhere convenient usually on the wrist or the leg.

The stimulus

The poor responses obtained in 1969 by Cody and Bickford using a relatively slow rise time tone must compare significantly with Yoshie and Okudaira's (1969) excellent responses using clicks. It is the onset of the stimulus which evokes the response (Gibson 1974) although in the case of a pure-tone burst a response can be obtained at the end of the sound suggesting that it is the sudden change in sound intensity which is responsible for the electrical potential. Experiments on normal subjects have shown that the rise time of the stimulus is critical and should be less than 250 µs if responses are to be obtained to low intensity sound.

Recovery time and habituation

Recovery time is quite rapid as Kiang *et al.* (1963) had found that they could still obtain identifiable responses at rates of over 200 per second while Yoshie and Okudaira (1969) showed that there had been a 90 per cent recovery of amplitude after an interstimulus interval of only 100 ms. Complete recovery occurred after 140 ms. A click stimulus rate of 10 per second was found to be entirely adequate for clinical purposes (Douek *et al.* 1973).

Prolonged stimulation, however, posed a different problem. Many workers had found evidence of habituation and fatigue (Kiang *et al.* 1963; Davis, Engelbretson, Lowell, Mast, Sallerfield, and Yoshie 1963; Gibson 1974). In practical terms fatigue does occur particularly if the subject or patient is tired or bored.

Effects of muscle-tone changes

All workers who have studied this response have noted the changes in amplitude which result from different head positions while Cody *et al.* (1964) pointed out that curarization abolished the responses altogether.

Clinically this is reflected in three problems. Firstly that of sleep, tiredness, or boredom and is specially important in the testing of small babies sleeping after a feed (Fig. 32.1).

Variation of amplitude of response with muscle tone

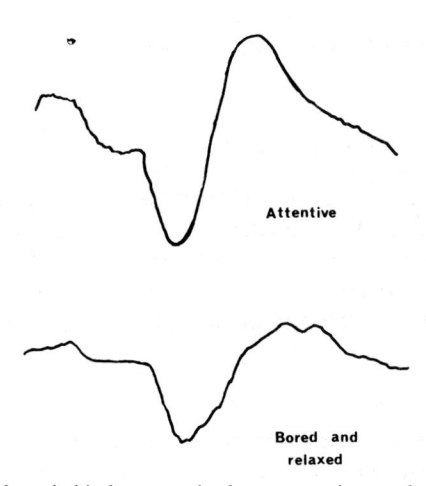

Attentive

Bored and relaxed

Fig. 32.1. Recording from behind one ear in the same patient under different conditions.

Secondly in the matter of head position. The response is largest with the head tilted towards the side where the recording is being made. Voluntary muscle contraction and forced smiling are helpful in increasing the amplitude of the response.

Thirdly drugs such as diazepam or even alcohol will adversely affect the amplitude of the response.

Amplitude of the response

It is clear from the preceding comments that the amplitude of the response is exceedingly variable, dependent on a number of factors including, of course, the technical one of the number of stimuli which have been averaged; apart from the effects of muscle tone the main variation depends on the intensity of stimulus stretching from as little as 2 μV to almost 30 μV if measured from positive to negative peak.

Configuration of the response

There is considerable variation in the shape of the response but the following characteristics have been noted:
  (i) a small positive peak;
  (ii) a negative deflection which is the most sharply defined;
  (iii) a second positive peak.

Variations in the size, sharpness, and slope of these peaks are very wide but it is the peak of the negative deflection (ii) which is used as the latency of the 'crossed acoustic response' and it is the difference between the peaks at (ii) and (iii) which is used as a measure of amplitude.

The latency

The latency of response is best measured at the peak of its negative deflection as this is the sharpest and most consistent. This latency tends to become longer as the amplitude diminishes and falls between 12–18 ms.

Alteration of the band-width recording limits

Thornton (1975) analysed the power spectrum of the post-aural response. He found that the main spectral peak was at 600 Hz, the spectrum extending from 100 to 1600 Hz. By using a wide-band recording system five peaks are found, three positive and two negative. The latencies are in chronological order—$P1:10$ ms; $N1:12$ ms; $P2:15$ ms; $N2:19\cdot5$ ms; $P3:24$ ms.

There are some advantages to setting the low-cut filter at 200 Hz as much of the background activity disappears and $N1$ and $P3$ predominate as much cleaner identifiable responses.

The bilateral nature of the response

The post-auricular electrical response which has been discussed together with its characteristics can be considered a reflex. It is certainly part of the automatic response to quiet sound produced in the body's voluntary musculature and can only be a vestigial equivalent of any animal's ability to prick up its ears when they hear the first suggestion of a sound.

Other reflexes such as the visual contraction of the pupil to light, the tactile corneal reflex and in particular the closely related stapedius reflex are all bilateral and consensual.

The post-auricular muscle response is no different and a sound which is able to produce a reflex electrical change in the muscle behind the ear will automatically produce an equal response with the same latency behind the contralateral ear.

All the evidence associated with the bilateral nature of this response has confirmed that it truly crosses the brainstem in the same manner as all the other brainstem reflexes.

It is to the bilateral aspect of this response and to the fact that the pathways must cross the brainstem that we owe the major part of clinical applications of the reflex in the form of a test and it is for this reason that when used in this way it has been referred to as the 'crossed acoustic response' (Douek et al. 1973; Clifford-Jones, Clarke, and Mayles 1979).

THE CROSSED ACOUSTIC RESPONSE (CAR) (Fig. 32.2)

Studied as a crossed acoustic reflex the bilateral simultaneous recording of the post-auricular myogenic response had been put to clinical case in two ways.
1. As an objective test of hearing.
2. As a tool in neurological diagnosis.

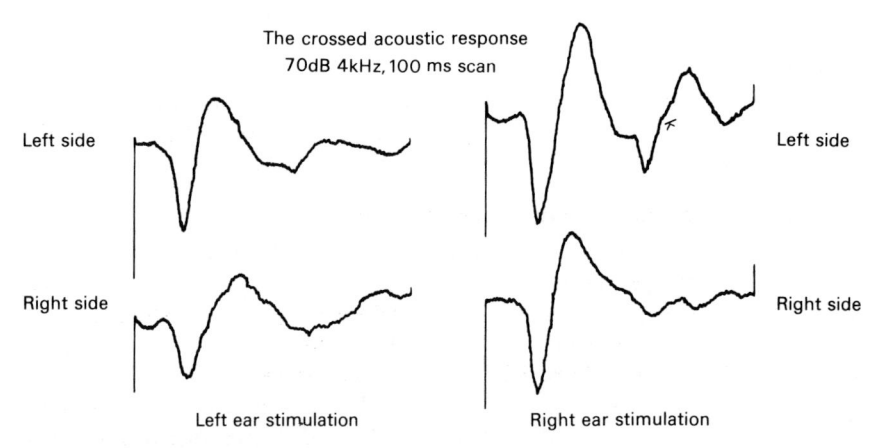

Fig. 32.2. Normal responses obtained from electrodes behind each ear and with stimulation on each side separately.

An objective test of hearing

This was first described in 1973 (Douek *et al.*) and the reliability and place of this system studied over many hundreds of cases in the setting of a standard routine clinic (Douek *et al.* 1974, 1975; Humphries, Gibson and Douek 1976). The system evolved requires a stimulus generator which produces clicks at a rate of 10 per second. A response should be visible by 15 seconds and the stimulus should not be continued for too long as the element of fatigue is introduced after about two minutes.

A high-quality transducer is necessary to maintain the acoustic wave-form of the click and the sound itself can be administered either through earphones in the older child or through an electrostatic loudspeaker. If earphones are used it is possible to test each ear separately provided wide-band masking is applied in the other ear.

For babies, where the test is used principally as a screening technique a loudspeaker stimulating both ears simultaneously is the proper instrument to use.

Standard EEG silver-cup electrodes are used as active and earth electrodes and a light clip on the ear-lobe as the reference electrode. The low-noise biological amplifiers have a high input impedance and a high common-mode rejection ratio. The main amplifier is housed with the averager and a small pre-amplifier can be attached in a harness at the back of the child to allow greater freedom of movement. A filter is set to a narrow bandwidth to eliminate as much background noise as possible.

A two-channel averager receiving responses separately from behind each ear is essential in neurological investigations as latency comparisons are required. In tests of hearing acuity only, it is possible to feed in responses from each ear to be 'mixed' into a common averager (Douek and Clarke 1976) (Fig. 32.3). In this case there is a yes or no answer to whether the child hears.

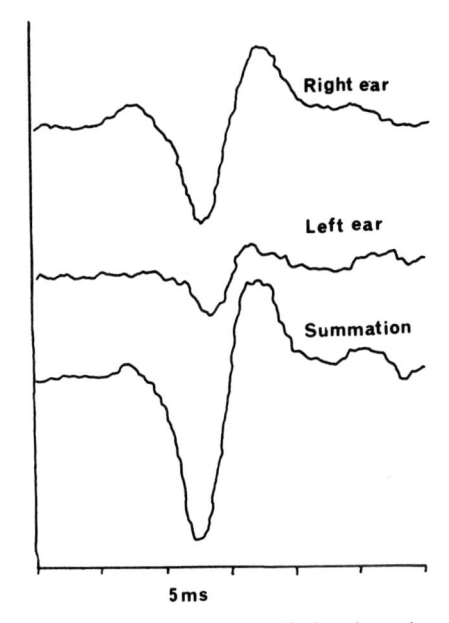

Fig. 32.3. Result of mixing the responses from behind each ear into a single average.

The contribution that this method makes to the testing of hearing is that it is a rapid, painless technique which can be used on the mobile child.

In the Hearing and Language Clinic at Guy's Hospital, London where the CAR test has had its most extensive investigation the following conclusions have been reached:
1. The technique should only be used as an adjunct to clinical methods and not as an answer in itself. This is because the results, although of a yes or no type require interpretation in the light of the child's behaviour as a whole.
2. As the test is actually done during the clinic and the results are available

within a few minutes of the clinical examination it has a major confirmatory importance even in cases where an objective test is not strictly necessary. This is of particular value to the more inexperienced examiners who obtain an immediate confirmation of their own clinical assessment. Although it cannot be quantified this immediate feedback of information appears to be of some advantage in the training of junior staff as well as in more positive diagnosis.
3. It is of special value in the assessment of mentally retarded children who cannot be tested in other ways.
4. It gives negative results in children who are sedated, who suffer from a hypotonic condition or sometimes, who are simply asleep.
5. Children with glue ears give variable results as often the response seems near normal when the child hears higher tones adequately. In other cases, however, the results indicate deafness. It has not been possible to correlate these differences directly with the middle-ear pressure nor with the quality of the secretions.
6. Neonates respond extremely well and the C A R is a good screening test of babies' hearing at birth. The exception is premature babies where the response does not become apparent until chronological maturation has taken place.
7. There are no false positives.
8. High-tone loss responds as deaf.

Recent reports (Hazel, Conway, Fraser, and Keene 1977; Fraser, Conway, Keane, and Hazel 1978) have used a simple form of maching scoring to obtain a completely objective result. They recorded the post-aural response from behind one ear only and in a series of 102 subjects produced no false positive results and only a small percentage of normally hearing adults and children failed to produce a response (Fig. 32.4).

Neurological investigations

The use of the C A R in neuro-otological investigation is based on the concept of fibres crossing over the brainstem from the auditory connections on one side to the motor system both on the same and on the other side.

The anatomy and physiology of this response is not entirely clear.

In a general sense the afferent pathway consists of the auditory nerve and cochlear nucleus. This time taken from generation of the impulse in the cochlea can be calculated from the latency of the second brainstem electrical response and is about 2.4 ms. The efferent pathway is the motor neurones of the facial nerve from its nucleus to its termination in the post-auricular muscle endings. The length of the nerve is not much above 5 cm so that at a nerve conduction velocity of 50 m/s and a neuromuscular transmission velocity of less than 1 m/s so that the time taken for the impulse to travel in the peripheral segment is a little above 5 ms.

The central pathway from the cochlear nucleus on one side to the seventh nucleus on either side remains quite unknown, but if by extrapolation it takes about 3 ms then about four synapses are involved.

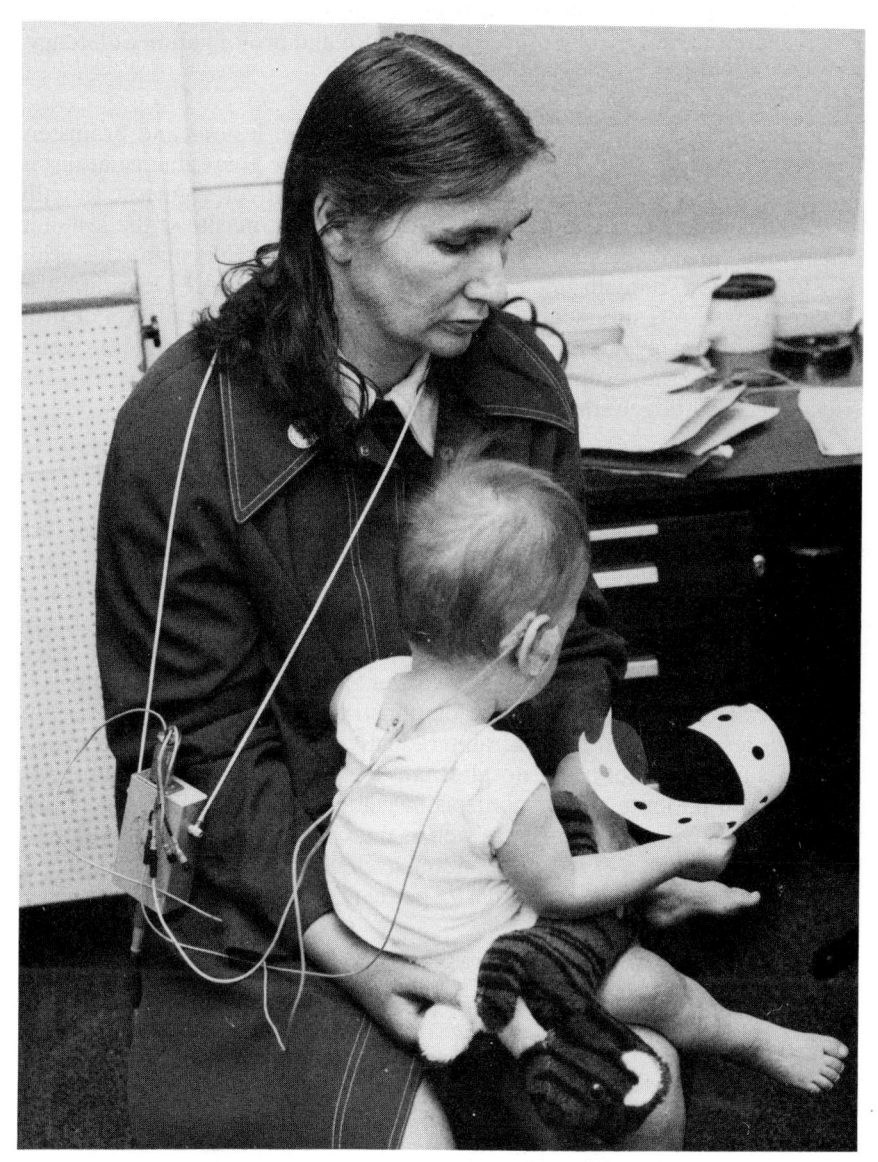

Fig. 32.4. Recording from behind one ear only in a child at University College Hospital. (With permission, P. Martin.)

778 Auditory myogenic responses

The abnormalities which have been studied in relation to neurological disease are of two types. Absence of response and prolongation of latency.

Absence of response

A group of cases including cerebellopontine angle lesions and brainstem tumours were reported (Douek et al. 1976) to show gross abnormalities in the response on one or other side or in the cross-over segment. Initially attempts were made to correlate these findings with the site of the lesion in the brainstem and in some cases this was possible, though in many the lesion was too gross. Today brain-scanning techniques have made localization of tumours by CAR in association with other neuro-otological tests of little importance, however, the distinction can be made between tumours which interfere with the propagation of these electrical responses and other ischaemic and degenerative lesions which do not.

Prolongation of latency (Fig. 32.5)

MULTIPLE SCLEROSIS

It was noticed early (Douek et al. 1973) that a few cases of multiple sclerosis showed a prolonged latency on either one side or in the cross-over. Later (Douek et al. 1976), 18 cases were reported all of which showed an increased latency. Little work was done in assessing the place of the CAR in the diagnosis of multiple sclerosis until the publication of an important series (Clifford-Jones et al. 1979). These workers accepted that the diagnosis of multiple sclerosis depends on the demonstration of objective evidence of *multiple* lesions within the central nervous system white matter of a patient with a suitable history and no alternative explanation. They examined a series of 66 patients and 53 controls in whom they carried out visual and somesthetic-evoked responses as well as the CAR. The aim was to look for subclinical evidence of lesions in systems which did not show clinical signs. Abnormal latencies were found in 73 per cent of the patients' CARs 63 per

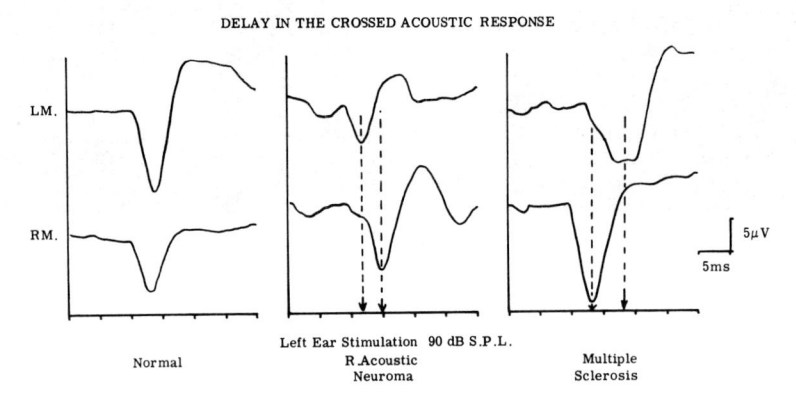

Fig. 32.5. Example of prolonged latency in the cross-over. Note the loud stimulus used as the purpose of the test is to measure the latency and not the threshold.

cent in the visual and 73 per cent somesthetic evoked response. A combination of CAR and VER abnormalities was present in 90 per cent of patients with multiple sclerosis. This suggests that a combination of these two measurements produces a very sensitive test.

CHROMOSOME ABNORMALITIES

Among CAR tests done on children who had normal hearing at Guy's Hospital a small group of 17 were found to have prolonged latency. Of these, 12 turned out to have chromosomal abnormalities with excess chromatin. It was also found that this group fell among those children who had considerable delay in speech despite normal hearing and a lack of global delay of sufficient magnitude to prevent speech development.

OTHER SYNDROMES

Prolonged latencies have been found in conditions which appear to involve a slowing of neuronal conduction. A case of Leigh's syndrome produced this effect.

These examples are given to demonstrate that a prolonged latency is not evidence of a specific disease but rather of malfunction of CNS tissue. The CAR can be used in combinations with other findings, as in the case of multiple sclerosis, to help in coming to a conclusion.

There is no doubt that the CAR, both as a test of hearing acuity and as a measure of brainstem function, requires more study to establish its full potential. What is clear, however, is that, as in the case of other evoked responses, its place remains only a part of the clinical findings which together help to form a diagnosis.

REFERENCES

BICKFORD, R. G., JACOBSON, J. L., and GALBRAITH, R. F. (1963). A new audiomotor system in man. *Electroenceph. clin. Neurophysiol.* **15**, 720.

CLIFFORD-JONES, R. E., CLARKE, G. P., and MAYLES, P. (1979). Crossed acoustic response combined with visual and somatosensory evoked responses in the diagnosis of multiple sclerosis. *J. Neurol. Neurosurg. Psychiat.* **42**, 749–52.

CODY, D. T. R. and BICKFORD, R. G. (1969). Average evoked myogenic responses in normal man. *Laryngoscope, St. Louis* **79**, 400–16.

—— JACOBSON, J. L., WALKER, J. C., and BICKFORD, R. G. (1964). Average evoked myogenic and cortical potentials to sound in man. *Ann. Otol. Rhinol. Lar.* **73**, 763.

DAVIS, H., ENGEBRETSON, M., LOWELL, E. L., MAST, T., SATTERFIELD, J., and YOSHIE, N. (1963). Evoked responses to clicks recorded from the human scalp. *Ann. N.Y. Acad. Sci.* **112**, 224.

DOUEK, E. E. and CLARKE, G. P. (1976). A single average crossed acoustic response. *J. Lar. Otol.* **90**, 1027.

—— ASHCROFT, P. B., and HUMPHRIES, K. N. (1976). The clinical value of the post-auricular myogenic (crossed acoustic) responses in neuro-otology. In *Disorders of auditory function* (ed. S. D. G. Stephens) Vol. II, p. 139. Academic Press, London.

—— Gibson, W. P. R., and Humphries, K. N. (1973). The crossed acoustic response. *J. Lar. Otol.* **87**, 711.

—— —— —— (1974). The crossed acoustic response and objective tests of hearing. *Dev. Med. child Neurol.* **16**, 32.

—— —— —— (1975). The crossed acoustic response. *Revue Lar. Otol. Rhinol.* **96**, 121.

Fraser, J. G., Conway, M. J., Keene, M. H., and Hazell, J. W. P. (1978). The post-auricular myogenic response: a new instrument which simplifies its detection by machine scoring. *J. Lar. Otol.* **92**, 293.

Geisler, C. D., Frishkopf, L. S., and Rosenblith, W. A. (1958). Extracranial responses to acoustic clicks in man. *Science, N.Y.* **128**, 1210.

Gibson, W. P. R. (1974). Investigations of the post-auricular myogenic responses, M.D. Thesis, University of London.

Goldstein, R. and Rodman, L. B. (1967). Early components of averaged evoked responses to rapidly repeated auditory stimuli. *J. Speech Hear. Res.* **10**, 697–705.

Hazell, J. W. P., Conway, M. J., Fraser, J. G., and Keene, M. H. (1977). Audiological screening using the post-auricular myogenic response and a machine scoring system. Paper read at 5th Symposium of International ERA study group. Jerusalem.

Humphries, K. N., Gibson, W. P. R., and Douek, E. E. (1976). Objective methods of hearing assessment and a system for recording the crossed acoustic response. *Med. Biol. Engng*, **42**, 1.

Kiang N. Y.-S., Crist, A. H., French, M. A., and Edwards A. G. (1963). Post-auricular electrical response to acoustic stimuli in humans. Quarterly progress report No. 68, Research Laboratory of Electronics, MIT Cambridge, Massachusetts.

Meir-Ewert, K., Gleitsmann, K., and Reiter, F. (1974). Acoustic jaw reflex in man. *Electroenceph. clin. Neurophysiol.* **36**, 629.

Pignataro, O. (1972). Early evoked potentials by sound stimuli. Paper read at 11th International Congress of Audiology. Budapest.

Preyer, W. (1881). *Die Seele des Kindes.* Leipzig.

Thornton, A. R. D. (1975). Distortion of averaged post-auricular muscle responses due to system bandwidth limits. *Electroenceph. Clin. Neurophysiol.* **39**, 195.

Yoshie, N. and Okudaira, T. (1969). Myogenic evoked potential responses to clicks in man. *Acta oto-lar. Suppl.* **252**, 89.

ECochG is carried out clinically using one of the available commercial systems. An electrode is placed close to the cochlea. Usually this is by means of a transtympanic needle electrode which passes through the tympanic membrane so that its tip rests on the promontory of the middle ear, immediately superficial to the basal cochlear turn. The tip of the needle electrode is thus sited a little anteriorly to the round window niche of the cochlea (see Fig. 33.2). Potentials developed within the cochlea are measured between this needle electrode and a reference electrode on the earlobe or mastoid. Physiological amplifiers with a gain of 10^4 or greater amplify the electrical output and pass the amplified signal to the averager which reduces the noise background rendering the endocochlear potentials readily visible. The bandpass of the amplifier system is fairly wide for ECochG, 3 Hz to 3 kHz being typical. A series of sound stimuli is presented, 128 to 512 being the number commonly used. The sound stimuli have certain essential requirements:

1. They must have an abrupt onset—thus a wideband click produced by using an electrical square pulse to activate a sound transducer (e.g. a loud speaker) is commonly used. This produces an acoustic click with a sudden onset and an 'after ring', the latter being due to the mechanical properties of the transducer activated. The frequency content is very wide—in fact it contains some of all the audible frequencies, hence the name 'wideband click' but inevitably there will be some concentration of energy at certain frequencies and this depends largely upon the transducer. The click used should be checked for its spectral density. Often the maximum concentration of energy is in the 3 kHz region.

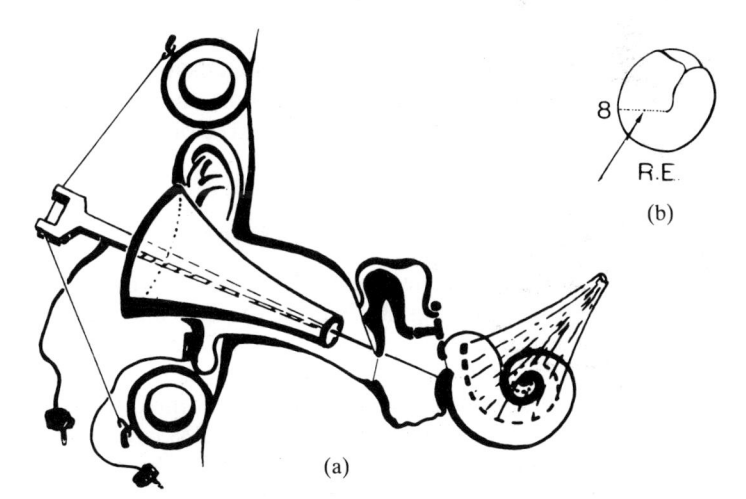

Fig. 33.2. (a). This sketch shows the position of the circumaural retaining ring, the retaining elastic band, the electrode holder and the electrode which penetrates the drum and comes to rest on the promontory anterior to the round-window niche. (b). This shows the site of entry of the electrode halfway between the umbo and the posterior meatal wall, or a little anterior to this. (From Portmann and Aran 1971.)

2. Short high-frequency tone bursts are also useful in ECochG. Such bursts are generated in various ways and again the onset time must be quite fast and the plateau is quite short. Typical values are a rise-time of 1 ms, a decay-time also of 1 ms, and an overall duration of about 6 ms. Such short-tone bursts are very suitable for ECochG. The frequency of such tone bursts can range from 2 to 8 kHz. Lower frequency tone-bursts are less satisfactory as will be explained later.

3. The onset of the click or tone-burst used is of great importance. It is the sharpness of the rise-time which ensures the greatest synchrony of neural output from the cochlear nerve fibres from the basal region of the cochlea. This is why a wideband click is such a good stimulus in this respect but the short-tone bursts described above operate in much the same way. Well synchronized volleys of action potentials generated by such stimuli are readily recorded by the averager. As the frequency is steadily reduced the degree of synchrony due to the onset of tone is steadily lost until a series of small action potentials is generated by each oscillation of the sine wave used. This is the state of affairs at frequencies below 1 kHz. Added to this the rate at which low frequencies are propagated towards the cochlear apex is somewhat variable and this leads to loss of synchrony between the small action potentials generated by each cycle of the sine wave. Such asynchronous action potentials cannot be extracted satisfactorily by averaging and at present it is not possible to record satisfactorily from the apical turn of the cochlea with certainty and such responses as are obtained originate mainly at the basal turn and to some extent in the second cochlear turn whether or not they are produced by tone-bursts of high or low frequency.

4. Polarity of the stimuli is crucial for ECochG. To understand this we have to consider the other endocochlear potentials, the CM and the SP as well as the AP. It is in order to obtain the AP free of CM that the method of polarity reversal is used.

REMOVAL OF CM FROM THE ECochG RECORD

The CM is generated by cochlear hair cells and it tends to follow the acoustic wave-form rather closely. Fig. 33.3 shows the CM and the AP first mixed together and later separated from one another. The method of separation depends upon fundamental differences of AP and the CM. The AP is invariant in its general shape and polarity whereas the CM follows the shape and polarity of the acoustic stimulus. Thus the CM can be annulled by the averager if the polarity of the acoustic wave-form is alternately reversed; the AP is unaffected by this, being produced essentially by the *onset* of the tone burst or click, and it always has the same polarity. Thus a series of action potentials contaminated with CM is obtained free of the CM if the latter occurs in alternate polarity owing to the alternating polarity of the stimulus—but the AP is not so affected and is thus obtained alone and free of CM.

ECochG

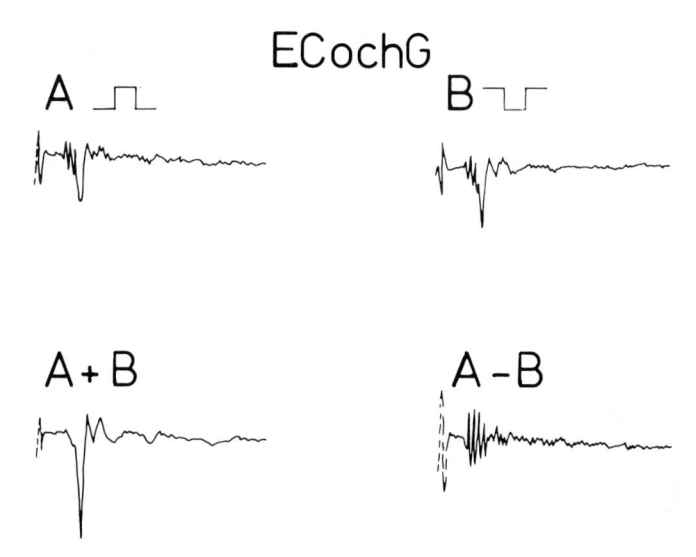

Fig. 33.3. In averaging systems with a split memory (as in most commercial apparatus) the AP and CM from all acoustic stimuli in one polarity go to memory A, whereas AP and CM in response to stimuli in the *opposite* polarity go to memory B. By simply moving a switch to A + B the cochlear microphonic (which is in the same phase as the acoustic stimulus) is cancelled, leaving the AP freed of CM. Turning the switch to A−B, however, will cancel the AP, leaving the CM.

While such a method preserves the AP the CM is lost. However, a refinement in the instrumentation permits the AP or the CM to be obtained at will. To do this the averager must have a split memory, each half of which is designated A or B. An electronic switching manoeuvre directs all the responses from acoustic stimuli of one polarity to enter memory A where they are recorded, and all the responses to stimuli of the *opposite* polarity to go to memory B. It is then a simple matter to separate AP and CM—if memories A and B are added, the action potentials being alike, simply add together, but the cochlear microphonics being in opposite polarity, are cancelled. Thus A plus B gives AP only. On the other hand is memory B *subtracted* from memory A and the action potentials are then cancelled, but the cochlear microphonics, due to the subtraction are not cancelled; instead they are doubled in amplitude. Thus A minus B gives CM only (Fig. 33.3). This device is available on most modern commercial ECochG systems.

CALIBRATION OF SOUND STIMULI FOR ECochG

This is an important aspect of hearing testing using this technique as the usual method of sound measurements used in audiometric calibration is not available owing to the short duration of the stimuli. For details see Knight 1979. The short tones used are measured either biologically so that the levels are stated in decibels Hearing Level (dB HL) or in terms of peak equivalent sound pressure level (p.e.SPL).

SUMMATING POTENTIAL (SP)

Polarity reversal of the stimuli can be used successfully to separate AP from CM as described above, but there is another potential recorded in ECochG called the summating potential (SP) which is not removed by this method. The SP is generally recorded together with the AP and different methods are needed to remove it. The SP is a complex potential which will not be described in detail here. It is essentially a d.c. potential and represents a reaction to the *envelope* of the waveform of the acoustic stimulus. It is generally seen at high intensities and is in large part due to biasing of the basilar membrane in one direction and generally, but not always, results in a negative deflection and is therefore called −SP. The mixture of −SP and AP is visible in Fig. 33.4 and separation of AP and −SP, when necessary, can be achieved by making the AP adapt and finally disappear by speeding up the rate of stimulation. This leaves only the −SP. In practical terms it is achieved as follows:

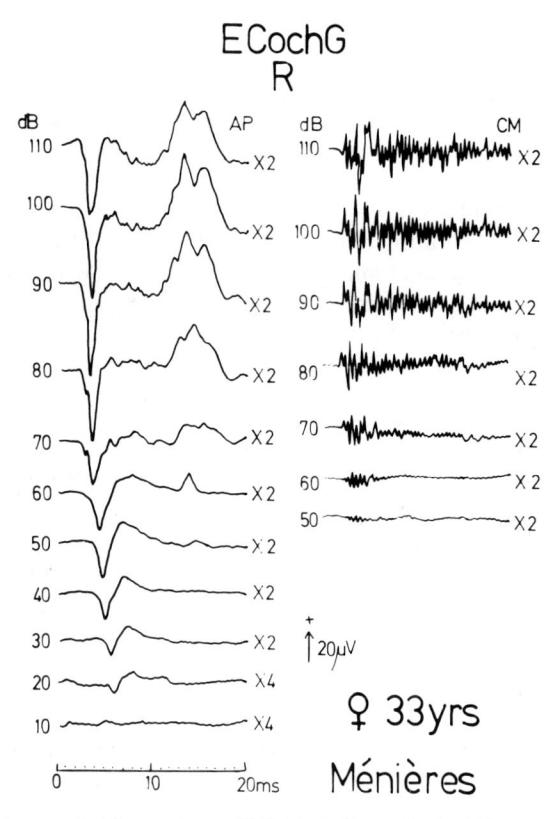

Fig. 33.4. This patient with symptoms of Ménière's disease had a fairly normal AP, but there was quite a prominent −SP which is clearly visible at 100, 90, 80, and 70 dB; see also Fig. 33.5.

1. A fairly high intensity tone-burst (say 80 dB) is delivered at the normal rate, 5/s. This will produce a mixture of AP and −SP. This is stored in memory A.
2. Next, the same series is delivered at a much faster rate, say 100/s. This causes the AP to 'adapt' and disappear, leaving the −SP only. This is stored in memory B.
3. Subtract memory B from memory A, i.e. A−B gives AP only, without the −SP, which is present in each memory and is removed by subtraction. This procedure is shown in Fig. 33.5, but it must be emphasized that the adaptation process is sometimes incomplete; some AP remains in memory B but its latency is increased and subtraction will then give rise to an artefact in the form of a falsely diphasic AP. In spite of this however, the technique as originally developed by Eggermont and Spoor (1973) is useful in identifying the presence of −SP and measuring its magnitude.

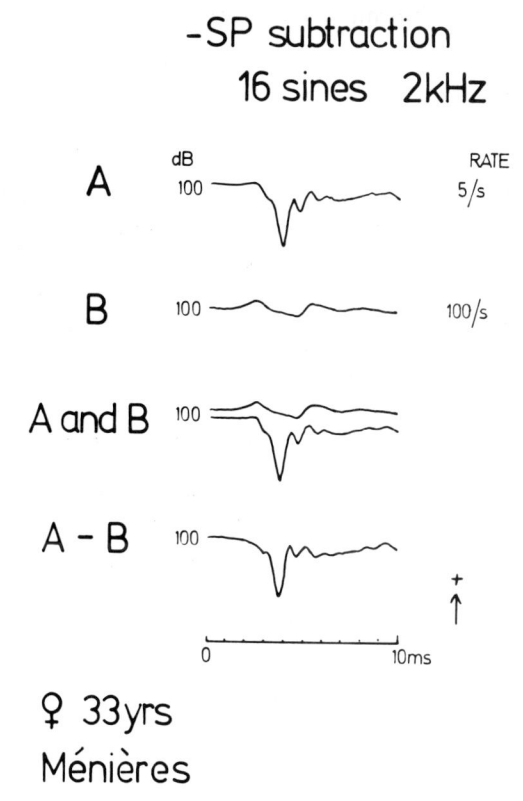

Fig. 33.5. This trace is from the same patient as in Fig. 33.4. (A) AP and −SP produced by stimuli at the rate of 5/s. (B) the same trace modified by a rapid rate, 100/s. (A) and (B) shows the two traces. Note that the AP has virtually disappeared due to adaptation, the result of very rapid stimulation; this leaves only the −SP. (A − B) in this trace B (−SP) has been subtracted from A(AP and −SP). This results in a normal AP without −SP. This result is very revealing if complete adaptation can be achieved.

ALTERNATIVE ELECTRODES FOR ECochG

The transtympanic electrode gives the best means of recording the endocochlear potentials and the AP recorded by this method has a mean amplitude in the region of 10 μV. This is due to the close proximity of the electrode to the subjacent cochlear generators. Alternative electrode placements include:
1. An electrode which penetrates the skin of the deep external auditory meatus (Elberling and Salomon 1971).
2. A ball, wick, or wire electrode placed in contact with the external surface of the drum (Cullen, Ellis, Berlin, and Lousteau 1972) (Khechinashvili and Kevanishvili 1974). These methods give a very much smaller amplitude by a factor of about ten.
3. A vertex electrode as used for brainstem responses also records the AP quite clearly in children but much less clearly in the case of adults.

THE TECHNIQUE OF ECochG

The development of ECochG as a test of hearing is largely the result of the researches of Portmann, Aran, and Le Bert of Bordeaux (1968) and of Yoshie in Japan (1968). The sketch in Fig. 33.2 shows the transtympanic electrode in place against the promontory of the middle ear and secured in position by a fine elastic band which is hooked on to a retaining ring. This ring encircles the ear and is strapped around the head to fix it firmly. In this way the tip of the electrode is held lightly against the promontory in front of the round window. The sketch also shows the position on the drum where the electrode is inserted. This is a very simple procedure for an otologist.

The drum is visualized through a non-conducting plastic ear speculum, using an operating microscope. The speculum is steadied *in situ* by a piece of Sellotape which attaches it to the retaining ring. Occasionally a second piece is required, usually at right angles to the first. Before inserting the electrode any debris or wax is carefully lifted out of the meatus with a probe or crocodile forceps. It is preferable not to syringe the ear or to instil any antiseptic fluids into it prior to or following ECochG.

ANAESTHESIA

For adults a light spray with an anaesthetic, e.g. Cetocaine in an aerosol spray is sufficient.* Some otologists, however, prefer iontophoresis to 'drive' the molecules of local anaesthetic into the drum surface. In practice the author has not been impressed with the advantages of this method because the inner surface of the drum is not anaesthetized, nor is the mucosa of the middle ear. In spite of this, the discomfort of the procedure is

---

* More recently the author has abandoned even local anaesthetic sprays and now uses no topical anaesthesia at all, finding it ineffective, and can vouch from personal experience that insertion of the electrode causes trivial, or indeed no discomfort.

minimal, being similar in magnitude to that of venupuncture which is habitually practised without anaesthesia. The very occasional adult who is excessively nervous can be calmed by appropriate sedation, e.g. intravenous Valium (diazapam—see Chapter 34). Those adults who do feel anything as a result of ECochG usually speak of a sensation in the throat, probably from the innervation of the glossopharyngeal nerve which supplies the middle-ear mucosa. Children, on the other hand, require general anaesthesia and this is one of the chief advantages of ECochG in difficult children. It is the practice in the Royal National Hospital to anaesthetize children of less than three years with Ketamine and those of three years and over by means of Halothane and nitrous oxide using endotracheal intubation. The technique is fully described in Chapter 34. Upon completion of the ECochG the child is allowed to sleep off the anaesthetic in an adjacent recovery area—this takes a couple of hours in the case of Ketamine, but recovery from Halothane is very rapid. Thus, in virtually every case the child can return home after the test and hospital admission is rarely required.

ASEPSIS

Conventional sterilizing procedures are used to sterilize all forceps or probes used. Plastic specula are stored in Hibitane solution and washed in sterile water after use. The transtympanic electrodes are sterilized according to their method of manufacture. Where acrylic varnish is used as an insulating material it is usual to sterilize them in a hot air oven; electrodes coated with Teflon are autoclaved. This electrode, it will be remembered, is the only which penetrates the tissues. The electrode is mounted in an electrode holder (which is stored in formalin vapour)* and care must be taken to see that electrical conductivity is complete when the electrode and its holder are assembled as a unit. This is done by using a small piece of sterile aluminium foil against which the tip of the electrode is touched as shown in Fig. 33.6. Electrical conductivity is shown by the meter going over to short circuit (i.e. zero ohms). If it fails to do so the electrode should be rotated in the holder to improve contact or the tip can be 'brightened' by stroking it across the sterile aluminium. This often results in good conductivity. Prior to attaching the circumaural fixation ring the reference electrode will have been attached to the ear lobe and the earth electrode to the forehead. These electrodes consist of silver–silver chloride discs as used in EEG and are attached to the skin with a double-sided adhesive disc. Electrode jelly is inserted through the perforation of the disc electrode using a syringe with a cut-off venupuncture needle (size 18). This is used to rub the skin gently, by rotating the cut-off end of the needle against it. An electrode impedance of about 2000 ohms should be obtained between the earlobe and forehead electrodes, using an EEG electrode impedance meter for this purpose. Up to 5000 ohms is acceptable, but 2000 ohms is ideal.

At this point the otologist takes up the electrode holder with its transtympanic electrode and under direct vision inserts the tip of the electrode

* Now discontinued.

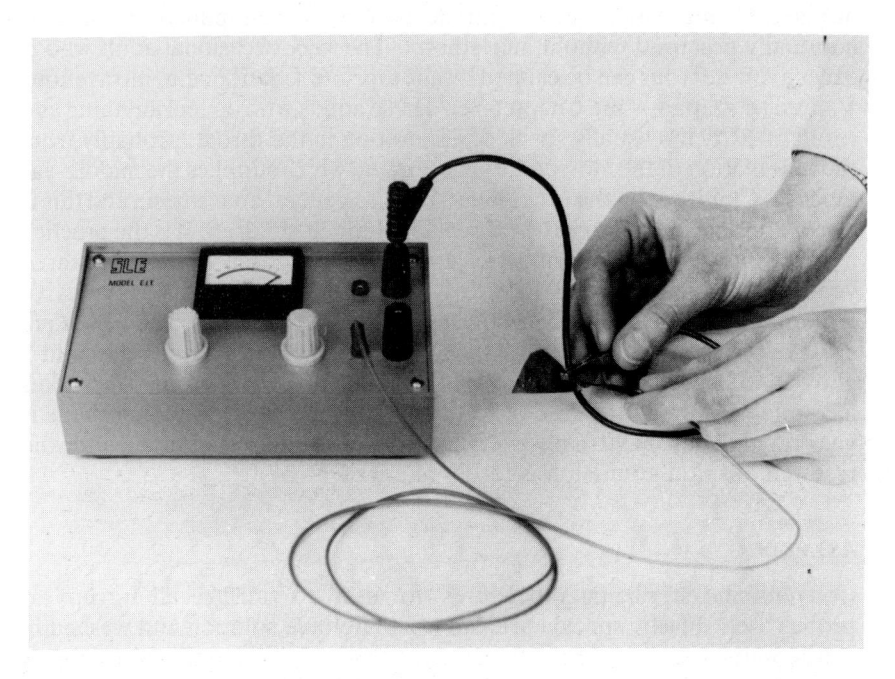

Fig. 33.6. This shows how the transtympanic electrode is tested for electric conductivity. The electrode and a piece of sterile aluminium foil are both attached to a resistance meter (an E E G impedance meter is very suitable). When the tip of the electrode is brought into contact with the aluminium foil a short circuit will result, i.e. zero ohms on the dial. This indicates good electrical conductivity and the electrode can now be used with confidence.

through the drum at the level of the umbo, but behind it as shown in Fig. 33.2 and its tip comes to rest on the underlying promontory. The elastic band is attached so as to retain the electrode gently against the promontory. All three electrodes are now plugged into the pre-amplifiers which are mounted close to the patient's head and the loudspeaker is brought to the standard distance from the patient's ear; at this Hospital it is 50 cm from the front grill, but 66 cm from the cone of the speaker (see Fig. 33.7). This means that a sound will take just 2 ms to travel from the loud-speaker to the patient's ear.

TEST ENVIRONMENT

As with all audiometric tests, a quiet environment is needed. An anechoic chamber would be the ideal for ECochG testing, but this is usually impracticable. In the Royal National Hospital a large I A C booth 4 × 3 metres (internal measurement) is used. This gives adequate room for the patient, tester, anaesthetist, anaesthetic equipment, instruments, and assistants. A smaller enclosed space would make the procedure very trying. The I A C

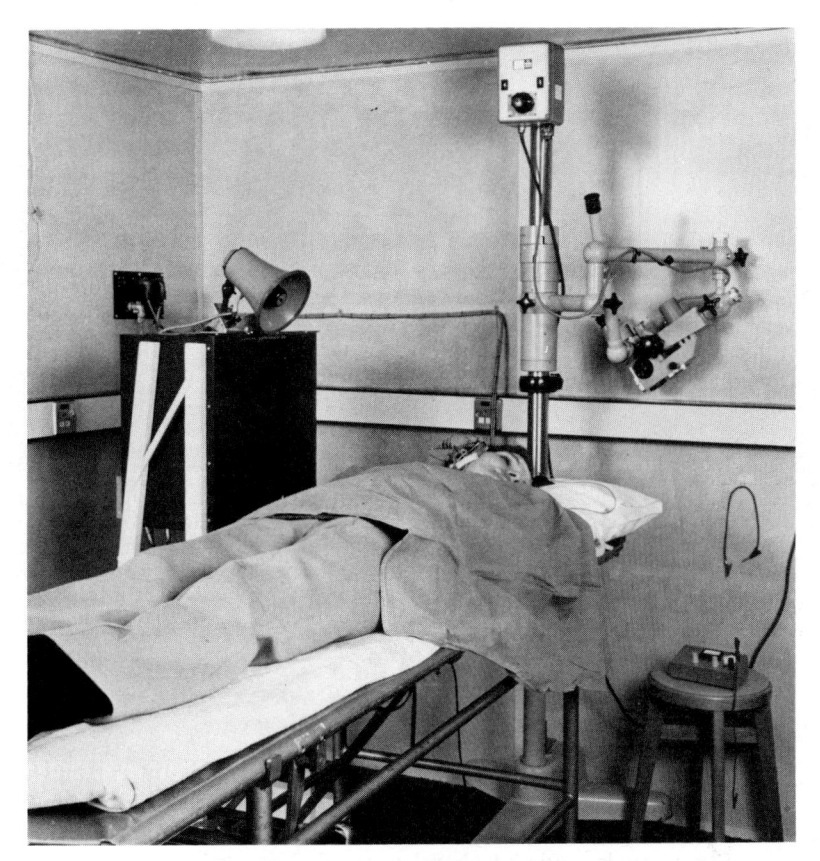

Fig. 33.7. The loudspeaker is brought the standard distance (50 cm in this case) so that sound stimuli are delivered at the correct intensity for electrocochleography.

booth is made with a perforated steel lining and this is earthed with a thick copper earth wire. All mains electric supplies are carried in copper conduits and can be turned off by means of an external isolator switch should electrical interference be a problem. This is only rarely needed, but battery lighting should be available if it is necessary to open the isolator switch. A large I A C booth as used at the Royal National Hospital provides a suitable acoustic and electrical environment for ECochG (see Fig. 33.8(a) and (b)).

In hospitals where a suitable enclosure is not available for ECochG it may be necessary to employ a closed acoustic system instead. For this, a TDH-39 headphone is encased in mu-metal in a special capsule to prevent electromagnetic radiation to the electrode. It is attached by means of a magnetic ring to a special magnetized circumaural retaining ring. Care must be taken to ensure that the top of the electrode holder sits *below* the level of the circumaural ring so that it is not pressed on by the encapsulated headphone. But, in fact, a free-field method is preferable if a suitable test room can be provided.

792 Electrophysiological tests of hearing

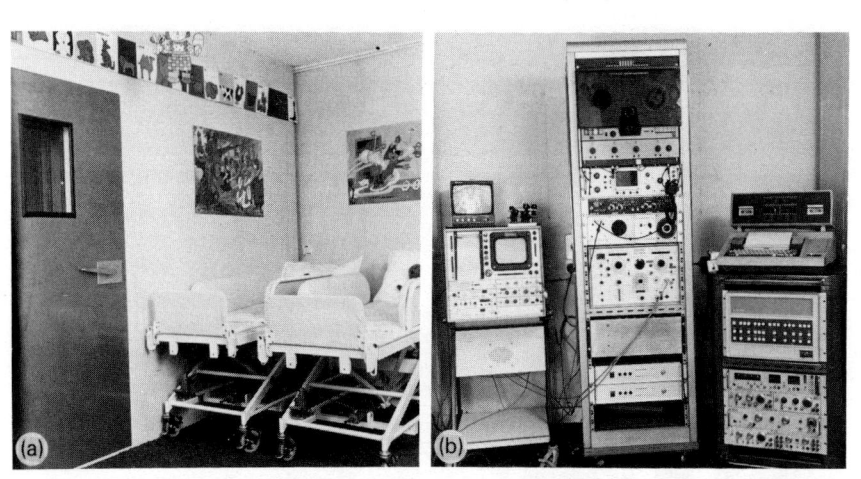

Fig. 33.8. (a). This shows the door (left) to the large IAC (Industrial Acoustic Company) booth used in the Royal National Throat, Nose and Ear Hospital. Outside is the recovery area where anaesthetized children can sleep off the effect of the general anaesthesia before returning home. (b). This view shows the recording equipment situated outside the test booth. All clinical electrophysiological hearing tests can be carried out with the commercial apparatus on the left. The other equipment is mainly for research purposes.

RECORDING TECHNIQUE

With the patient lying quietly on the couch in the test booth, the AP and CM are recorded with the apparatus which is sited outside the booth. Commonly 128 to 512 stimuli are used, 10 per second being a convenient rate. A 10 or 20 ms analysis time is used and a band pass of 3–3000 Hz is selected as a rule. Starting with the selected stimulus (e.g. wide band click) at a high-intensity level (say 100 db HL) AP and CM are recorded and this is repeated at successively lower levels until the threshold of the AP is determined. In the case of normally hearing subjects this is in the region of 20 dB HL (Fig. 33.9) but is correspondingly higher if the hearing is impaired (Fig. 33.10). The CM has no threshold, but there is a pseudo-threshold at about 60–70 dB in most cases. If there is a severe hearing loss no AP at all may be detected; however a CM is sometimes detected in such cases in which case it is inferred that the auditory nerve is not functional but that some cochlear hair cell activity still persists, suggesting a neural hearing loss (Fig. 33.11).

The wide-band click threshold agrees fairly well with the mean threshold values (if available) at 1, 2, 4, and 8 kHz, or with 3 kHZ. High-frequency tone bursts of 2, 4, 6, and 8 kHz can be used to explore the configuration of the audiometric threshold, but reliable threshold information cannot at present be elicited for stimuli of 1000 Hz or less. A deaf child, for example, may give no definite AP response, yet a subsequent audiogram when available, may indicate substantial *low-tone* hearing which the ECochG does not measure. This can happen with a 'ski-slope' hearing loss.

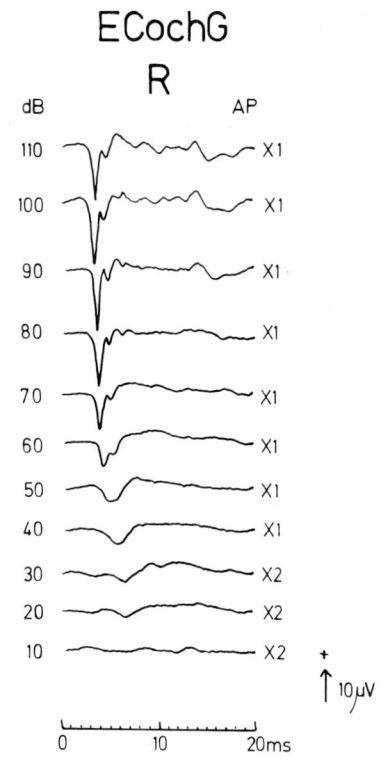

Fig. 33.9. A normal AP from a patient with unimpaired hearing. The AP can be traced down to 20 dB but is not observed at 10 dB.

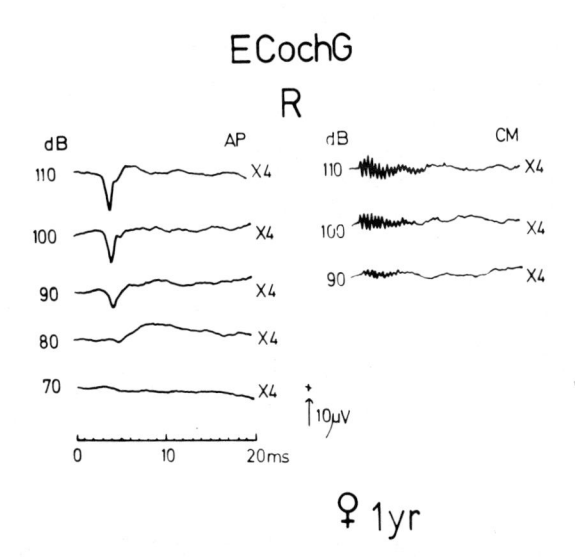

Fig. 33.10. The AP of a child with impaired hearing.

ECochG

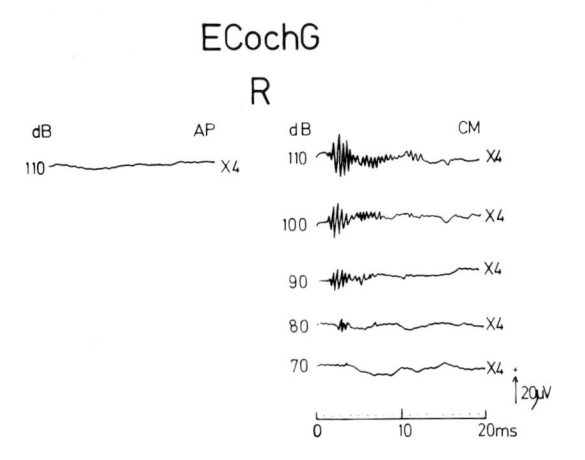

R

```
dB        AP              dB                    CM
110  ————————— X4         110  ~|||~~~~~~~ ——— X4
                          100  ~|||~~~~~~ ——— X4
                           90  ~|||~~~~ ————— X4
                           80  ~~~~~~~~~~~~~ X4
                           70  ~~~~~~~~~~~~ X4
                                              | 20μV
                              └────┴────┘
                              0    10   20ms
```

♀ 47yrs
Acoustic Neuroma

Fig. 33.11. This patient had a right acoustic neuroma with total hearing loss on the affected side. Note that there is no AP at all but that a well-marked CM is observed at various levels of stimulation. This indicates that at least some cochlear hair cells are functioning, but that the auditory nerve is not. It in fact confirms a *neural* hearing loss and was the factor which indicated the presence of the acoustic neuroma.

CASES SUITABLE FOR ECochG TESTING

Children

Difficult children may be tested by ECochG if conventional testing is impracticable. It can be carried out at any age from a few months old until puberty. It is often required for very hyperactive and unco-operative children, multiply handicapped cases (e.g. blind and suspected of deafness), or children with athetosis etc. The indications and contra-indications are set out in Chapter 31.

Fig. 33.10 shows traces from a child who was assessed by ECochG and found to have partial hearing. Fig. 33.12 shows no AP on either side and no definite CM either. Tomography was carried out while the child was still anaesthetized and gross cochlear dysplasia was discovered. Fig. 33.13 shows a distorted AP in a child with a history of hyperbilirubinaemia and Fig. 27.5 (Chapter 27) is from an untestable child with psychiatric symptoms and non-organic hearing loss (NOHL).

Adults

It is rarely necessary to use ECochG to determine the hearing in an adult, But Fig. 33.14 is one such rare case, a young adult suspected of NOHL with

ECochG

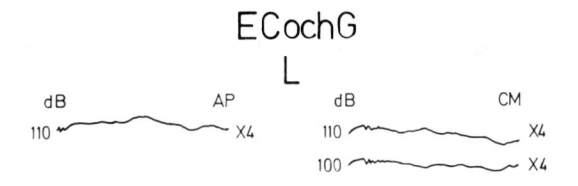

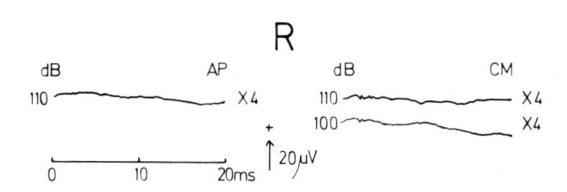

L

R

♀ 2 yrs
Bilateral Cochlear
and Vestibular dysphasia

Fig. 33.12. This extremely deaf in fact showed no AP in either ear and little or no CM. While still anaesthetized hypocycloidal tomography was carried out and this revealed gross cochleovestibular hypoplasia.

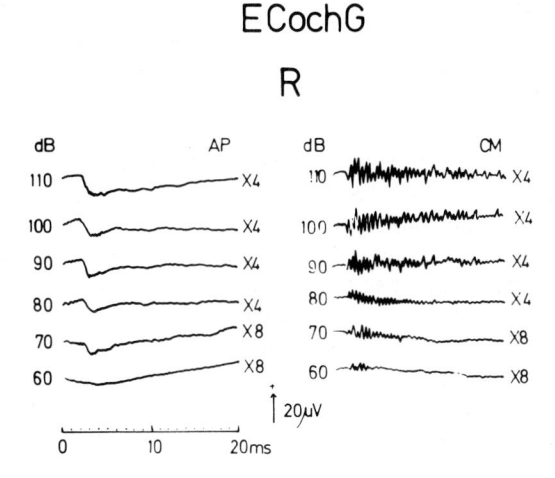

ECochG

R

♂ 5yrs
Kernicterus

Fig. 33.13. AP and CM from a child with a history of kernicterus. Note the widened, monophasic AP which is attributed to a partial block of the auditory nerve. This is also seen in some cases of acoustic neuroma.

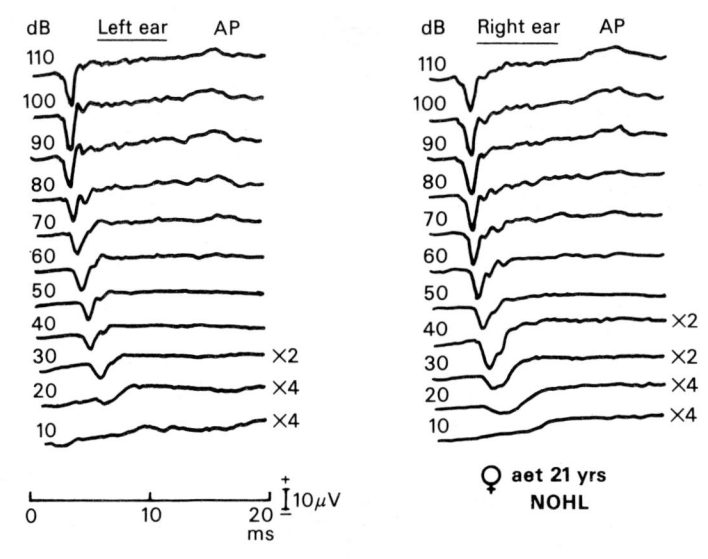

Fig. 33.14. The electrocochleogram of a young adult suspected of non-organic hearing loss, but too unco-operative for ERA. ECochG with sedation showed normal hearing. (Beagley and Gibson (1978). Courtesy Academic Press.)

very variable audiograms and too unco-operative for cortical ERA. ECochG under Valium (diazepam*) sedation (i.v.) confirmed normal hearing in each ear.

More frequently ECochG is used to diagnose the presence of acoustic neuroma in adults with unexplained, progressive sensorineural hearing loss, generally unilateral and sometimes of rapid onset. Such cases must always be suspected as being examples of acoustic neuroma and ECochG prior to Myelodil (iofendylate) cysternography is desirable. Various ECochG changes can be seen in the affected ear in cases of acoustic neuroma.

(i) Widened, distorted, monophasic AP (Fig. 33.15).
(ii) AP threshold better than subjective threshold suggesting a neural block which prevents the nerve impulses reaching the higher centres normally (Fig. 32.15) or not at all, in some cases.
(iii) A well marked CM with an absent or largely suppressed AP, suggesting a neural rather than a cochlear lesion, which would favour the diagnosis of acoustic neuroma (Fig. 33.11).
(iv) Very occasionally the AP is normal in some medially placed acoustic neuromas (Fig. 33.16). In these cases pressure of the tumour on the brainstem can lead to delayed brainstem conduction time (*vide infra*). In testing a case of suspected acoustic neuroma it is wise to test the normal ear first and use the traces as a comparison for the traces from the affected ear. Other space occupying lesions in the posterior fossa may show electrocochleographic changes similar to those caused by acoustic neuroma. Examples are meningioma, congenital cholesteatoma,

* NB Beware of accidental intra-arterial injection with diazepam.

ECochG

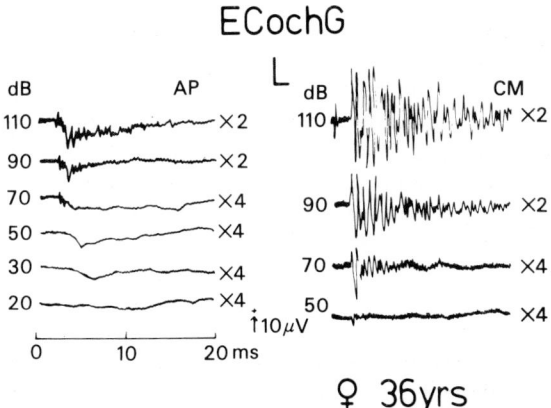

♀ 36yrs
Acoustic Neuroma

Fig. 33.15. This shows the widened monophasic AP from a patient with an acoustic neuroma. The pure-tone audiogram showed a hearing loss of 70 dB, yet the AP in this case could be traced down at least to 30 dB. Both these findings are typical of acoustic neuroma. (Adapted from Beagley and Gibson (1978). Courtesy Academic Press.)

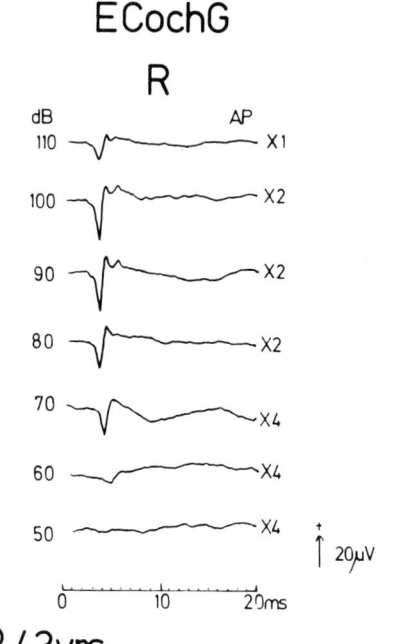

ECochG

♀ 43yrs
Acoustic Neuroma

Fig. 33.16. This patient had a large cystic medially-placed acoustic neuroma. Apart from loss of sensitivity (shown also by the pure-tone audiogram) the AP trace is unremarkable. The BSER showed marked prolongation of brainstem conduction time, a difference of 0.6 ms on the affected side.

798   *Electrophysiological tests of hearing*

secondary tumours, angioma and ectasia of basilar artery (Beagley and Gibson 1976). Disseminated sclerosis in the form of an isolated plaque on the cochlear nerve can also mimic acoustic neuroma.

Ménière's disease, especially when unilateral may present problems of differential diagnosis with respect to acoustic neuroma. ECochG is often helpful. Sometimes no abnormalities at all are noted, but more often a widened notched AP is visible. This is attributed to an enhanced − SP owing to the hydrops (Fig. 33.17). If the adaptation technique described above is used the − SP can be subtracted revealing an essentially normal AP (Fig. 33.5). This favours the diagnosis of Ménière's disease.

Brainstem electric responses Brainstem electric responses (BSER) are creating a great deal of interest in present-day audiology and neurology. The

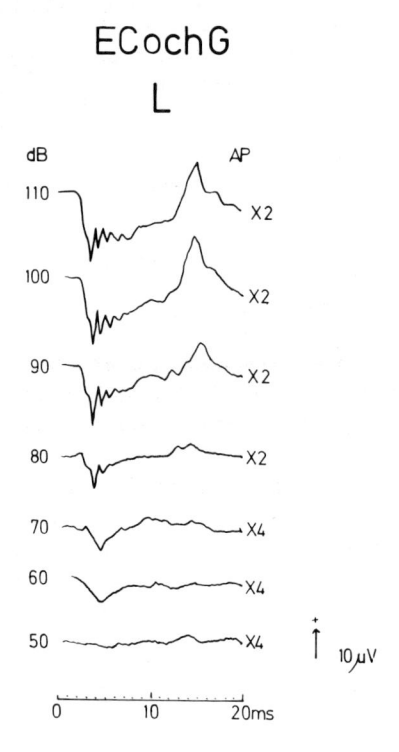

ECochG
L

♂ 52yrs
Ménières

Fig. 33.17. Many, but not all, cases with symptoms of Ménière's disease show this widened and notched AP. It is attributed to a very large −SP which distorts the AP. When the −SP can be demonstrated by *total* adaptation of the AP (see Fig. 33.5) it can be subtracted from the widened AP and what is left is generally a normal looking AP. The −SP in such cases is probably a result of the hydrops. (Note the prominent postauricular myogenic response at 15 ms.)

waves of the BSER as discussed in the preceding chapter are small in amplitude (<1 μV) and are recorded by a 'far-field' technique with the recording electrodes placed at about the same distance from the brainstem generators, generally the vertex and the earlobe, although other placements are possible. It is to be remembered that under these conditions the concept of an *active* electrode and a *reference* electrode is not valid. In BSER recordings both vertex and earlobe electrodes are 'active' and both contribute to the waveform.

Much of the instrumentation for BSER is similar to that used for ECochG, only minor adjustments need to be made. The stimuli, clicks, and high-frequency tone bursts which are suitable for ECochG serve equally well for BSER.* The condition most usually varied is the pass-band of the physiological amplifiers. For ECochG the pass-band is usually quite wide, 3–3000 Hz, but for BSER this is often narrowed by raising the high-pass filter cut-off. Many experts in this field use a pass-band of 250–3000 Hz; this is especially helpful in removing low-frequency artefacts and mains hum at 50 Hz (60 Hz in some countries). This pass-band also removes a large low-frequency potential, however, which is passed by a wider pass-band (e.g. 0.8–3000 Hz) which enhances the amplitude of all the waves, and especially wave V, which 'ride' on the large slow wave and wave V in particular has its amplitude increased as a result (Robinson and Rudge 1977). Individual users will select the pass-band best suited to their requirements. For audiological purposes 250–3000 Hz has many advantages.

The analysis time selected is usually 10 ms which gives plenty of time to see all five waves of the BSER, but in some patients with prolonged latencies (e.g. neonates) at stimulus levels close to threshold it may be desirable to increase the analysis time to avoid truncating the response.

The number of stimuli has to be greater than that used for ECochG. In some cases 500 repetitions may be enough, but usually it is safer to use 1000 stimuli; more than this number is rarely indicated. The repetition rate is typically 20 per second, which means that a series of 1000 stimuli can be delivered in less than one minute, which is not unduly burdensome either for the tester or for the patient who must lie quite still during this period, as muscle artefacts can easily obscure the small brainstem potentials. Repetition rates of 10/s may give a clearer view of some of the earlier waves, but

---

* Interest has recently been aroused by reports by Davis and Hirsh (1979) of a modified form of BSER using low-frequency tone bursts (500 Hz) which permit testing of low frequency hearing in children. To do this the high-pass filter setting is relaxed from 250 Hz to 30 or 40 Hz and this permits a wave described at SN_{10} (slow negative wave at 10 ms) to appear. This is said to be a good indicator of low-frequency hearing. Another interesting technique for testing low-frequency hearing (e.g. 500 Hz) is to use the BSER and record the response to short 500-Hz tone bursts while concurrently masking the test ear with white noise which is 'notched' at 500 Hz by suitable filtering. In this way that part of the basilar membrane not masked is allowed to respond to the tonal stimulus while the other basilar membrane structures, and particularly the basal region, are inhibited. The BSER under these conditions can be presumed to have its provenance in the apical cochlear region. This method has been proposed by Picton, Ouellette, Hamel and Smith (1979) and may well provide the answer to improved frequency specificity in BSER testing.

faster rates, e.g. 50/s, may have the effect of diminishing some of the waves, except wave V which seems the most 'durable' of the response components.

In view of the small amplitude of the BSER steps must be taken to see that electrical artefacts do not obtrude and obscure the brainstem potentials. For this reason a loudspeaker may not be the ideal method of delivery unless extensive antimagnetic shielding is employed. As this involves expensive mu-metal sheathing it is probably better to use a mu-metal sheathed headphone. One commercial system uses a TDH-39 headphone, sheathed in mu-metal and encapsulated in a sound deadening plastic cup which is attached by a magnetized ring to a corresponding headband. Mu-metal sheathing of the headphone effectively eliminates troublesome electromagnetic radiation which could cause artefacts.

The patient is usually tested relaxed in the recumbent position on a bed or couch. A child should have a parent or an assistant with him if he is nervous. A very nervous child can, if necessary, be sedated, or even anaesthetized, as drugs of this sort do not affect the BSER; in fact it is possible to do both an ECochG and a BSER on an anaesthetized child at the same session.

One obvious advantage of BSER over ECochG is the fact that superficial electrodes only are required, unlike ECochG where an electrode is generally passed through the tympanic membrane which means that some otological training is mandatory, whereas BSER can safely be carried out by non-medical personnel.

The audiological uses of the BSER include the hearing assessment of children who cannot be assessed by more conventional techniques. Of course a child tested in this way must lie quite still and this is sometimes a limiting factor. If the child is very nervous, or hyperactive, then sedation is essential if clear recordings are to be obtained. In cases where muscular movements are a problem, e.g. athetoid cerebral palsy, then anaesthesia may be required. If the athetoid child is under three years of age and intubation not desirable, Ketamine anaesthesia would generally be employed but this may not abolish the muscle movements in which case ECochG will give better results than BSER. But apart from these exceptional cases BSER is generally a practicable procedure. In cases of suspected non-organic hearing loss (NOHL—Chapter 27) in school-age children seen in the course of a clinic attendance, it is generally possible to get a BSER during the initial visit and this can give information of crucial significance (Figs. 33.18 and 33.19).

In adults BSER is used more for neurological type investigations. Cerebellopontive angle tumours which compress the brainstem can often be detected from increased latencies of the brainstem waves, especially wave V. Fig. 33.20 shows the latencies of wave V from a group of normal hearing adults with the 95 and 99 percentiles. Prolonged wave V latencies are often seen in early punctate lesions of the brainstem such as multiple sclerosis (Robinson and Rudge 1977). Large medially placed acoustic neuromas sometimes cause no specific changes in the ECochG but prolongation of wave V latency is often seen. A difference between the two sides of 0.3 ms is

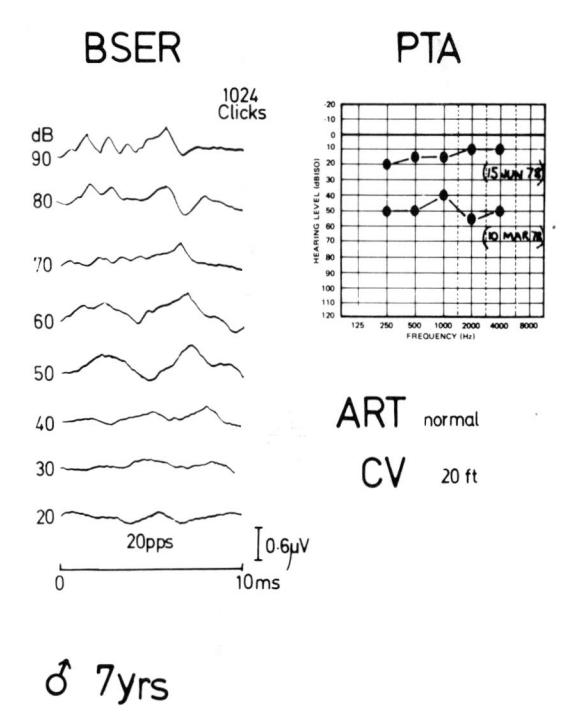

Fig. 33.18. This child was suspected of non-organic hearing loss with an apparent loss of 50 dB shown in the audiogram. The wave V of the BSER can be traced down to at least 30 dB suggesting that the child's hearing was within the normal range. A subsequent pure-tone audiogram three months later confirmed this.

probably significant clinically. The time interval between the crest of wave I and the trough following wave V is often called the 'brainstem conduction time' and is a little over 4 ms normally. In cases of cerebellopontine angle tumour with brainstem compression the affected side may show a significant increase in brainstem conduction time as compared with the normal side. As wave I is sometimes not very clear in the BSER* of some adults, the N_1 of the AP of the ECochG will give a very clear reference point from which to measure the brainstem conduction time.

Cortical evoked potential (V-potential) The vertex (or V-) potential is the cortical response evoked by an auditory stimulus. It has been developed as a method of so-called 'evoked response' audiometry and it represents the first serious attempt to develop an objective test of hearing based on the recognition of an evoked potential from the cortex. It is sometimes called 'Cortical ERA'.

As described in the preceding chapter the V-potential involves the auditory cortex but it is too late (at 50 ms) to represent the *primary* cortical response. It is almost certainly a *secondary* cortical manifestation, in view of its duration of about 200 ms, and is undoubtedly related in some way to

* See note added in proof on page 808.

802 *Electrophysiological tests of hearing*

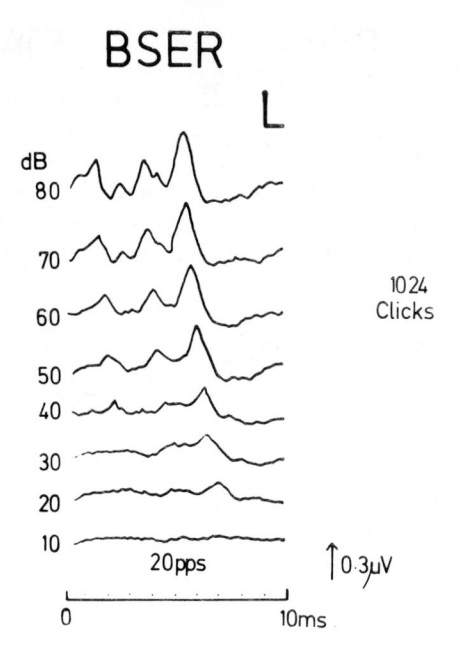

Fig. 33.19. A very clear set of BSER traces from a girl of 12 years.

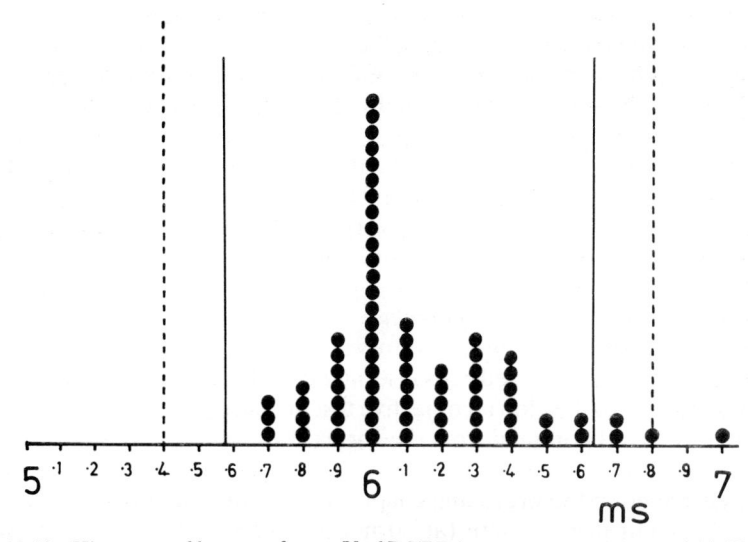

Fig. 32.20 Histogram of latency of wave V of BSER in a sample of adults aged 14–79 years with 95 and 99 percentiles. (Beagley and Sheldrake (1978). Courtesy *British Journal of Audiology*.)

perception. The V-potential produced by sound stimuli is effectively an onset response; an off-set response can be elicited under appropriate conditions, but it is not generally seen in V-potential when it is used as an audiometric procedure. The V-potential can be elicited by any acoustic stimulus used in audiometry and it is frequency specific. Thus clicks or tone-bursts of various frequencies are suitable stimuli. If tone-bursts are used their duration should be in excess of 30 ms (50–100 ms is often selected) and their rise-decay time should be fairly brief, about 10–20 ms being suitable. The response is not affected by the polarity of the pure-tone and phase locking is not required.

The same pre-amplifiers and amplifiers are used as for ECochG and BSER but the pass-band is very much restricted. As the frequency of the V-potential is only 6–10 Hz a pass-band 0.5 to 15 or 30 Hz is satisfactory. In this, the Royal National Throat, Nose and Ear Hospital the pass-band generally selected is 0.8 to 16 Hz which seems quite suitable. The rate of stimulus presentation can vary from 0.5 to 1 stimulus per second and the number of stimuli used is commonly about 50 or 60. In this Hospital 64 stimuli at the rate of 1 per second are generally used.

Superficial silver–silver chloride EEG disc electrodes are attached, the active one on the vertex (attached with Celloidin), the reference electrode on one ear lobe (or mastoid) and on earth (ground) electrode on the forehead; these two latter electrodes are attached to the skin by means of double-adhesive discs. Electrode jelly is injected through the central perforation in the dome of the electrode using a syringe with a cut-off hypodermic needle (18 gauge) and the electrode impedance is reduced to about 2000 ohms by gently rubbing the skin by rotating the needle. The impedance is measured by means of an EEG impedance meter. An impedance of >5000 ohms is unacceptable.

The patient is usually tested seated in a comfortable chair with a high back against which he reclines his head to relax the neck musculature. This obviates many of the muscular artefacts which might otherwise obscure the recordings. The patient has to sit still during the minute or so during which the series of sound stimuli is being delivered. To ensure that the patient remains reasonably still during the test the tester should be able to observe him by means of a mirror strategically placed in the sound-treated booth and visible through a viewing panel, or by means of a small television monitoring camera supplying a television screen outside the booth and easily observed by the tester (see Fig. 33.8(b)).

The sound stimuli can be delivered by a loudspeaker, but more conventionally earphones are used. This permits monaural testing and permits masking to be applied to the non-test ear when necessary. In this respect cortical ERA is exactly comparable to pure-tone audiometry. It is often convenient (but not essential) to have alternative means of generating stimuli, e.g. a stroboscopic flash and a vibrator to test for a visual or vibrotactile evoked potentials respectively, each of which can be recorded with the electrode configuration used in ERA. The purpose of this manoeuvre is to test for a visual, or vibroactile response in those cases in which an auditory evoked potential cannot be elicited. If the alternative stimulus is effective in eliciting a response while the auditory one is not, this will help to confirm the tester's observation that the auditory evoked potential is indeed absent and that the patient presumably has a marked hearing impairment.

The analysis time ('window') is generally 0.5 to 1.0 second in duration. In this Hospital an analysis time of 0.8 s is used and the stimulus is released 0.2 s *after* the averager has commenced its sweep. This gives 0.2 s of averaged EEG record prior to the period in which the V-potential will be seen (Fig. 33.21). The stimuli are presented in descending order of intensity, starting well above the presumed threshold; e.g. if it is thought that the patient has substantial hearing capability it is probably best to start at 70 or 80 dB HL—but if considerable hearing loss is likely it is preferable to start at the maximum output of the audiometer, say 110 dB. Once a well-marked response has been recorded at high intensities, the sequence is repeated 20 dB lower, until the response becomes smaller in amplitude, and its latency slightly prolonged at which point the steps are reduced to 10 dB and the stimulus presented until the V-potential can no longer be discerned. The

ERA (V-potential)

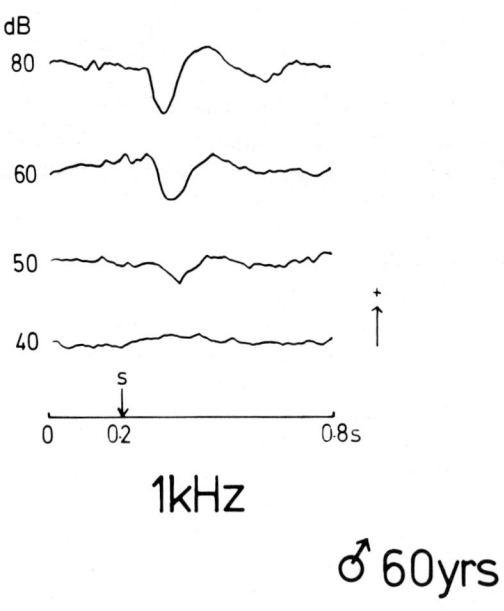

1kHz

♂ 60yrs

Fig. 33.21. An example of an ERA from a patient with impaired hearing (1 kHz only in this trace). Other frequencies also gave evidence of hearing loss, confirming the validity of the pure-tone audiogram. This information was required for medicolegal purposes.

value taken as indicating subjective threshold is half way between that at which the response was last observed and the level 10 dB less intense at which the response was judged to be absent.

It is customary to observe the average building up on the screen of the oscilloscope as the sequence of stimuli is presented. In this way the response can often be noted quite clearly after only 10 or 20 presentations at high intensity levels in which case the series can be curtailed and recommenced at a lower level. But unless time is really pressing it is preferable to complete the series—say 64—and write out the final average on a graphic recorder for later scrutiny.

It is also advisable to keep an eye on the unaveraged EEG from time to time especially if the background is 'noisy' or the traces indistinct. An excess of alpha rhythm may mean that the patient has closed his eyes or even dozed off. He should be told *not* to close his eyes; it is a good idea to provide him with a book to read. It is also desirable to inform him (if he has any hearing) before each series of sound stimuli is released. This helps to keep the patient in a 'neutral' state of attentiveness, i.e. not unduly anticipatory, nor unduly apathetic. Head and body movements, chewing movements, even excessive eye blinks, may contaminate and obscure the record; observation of the patient visually will help the tester as the patient can be cautioned to sit still and if necessary the presentation of tones can be repeated with the aim of obtaining a clearer record.

In interpreting the record the tester should adopt a sceptical state of mind, accepting as positive only those traces which bear a distinct resemblance to the high level trace which serves as a subjective template. As the intensity of stimulation is reduced the amplitude steadily falls away especially below 50 dB HL and the latency of the waves increases, especially below 30 dB HL. At threshold the latency may be increased by 50 to 100 per cent. In no case does the latency shorten as the intensity is reduced. If at low intensities an apparent response is observed which has a *shorter* latency than the preceding trace, then the tester should be very wary about accepting it as a positive response and should repeat the stimuli at the same level to clarify the situation. In judging the V-potential it will be noted from the high-level response that there is a prominent N_1 peak at about 100 ms and a prominent P_2 at 150–200 ms. The $N_1 - P_2$ segment is the most conspicuous feature of the V-potential and is the feature upon which the tester should concentrate his main attention. In no case should the tester accept a response as positive unless he is convinced that it is so, as false positive responses are always possible. A random deflection in the averaged EEG record at very low intensity levels may suggest a response to the tester—but he should be wary of accepting such a fluctuation as a response especially if the latency seems unrealistic without confirming by one or more repetitions at the same stimulus level. In this way the scoring of false positives will be diminished.

Any desired audiometric frequency can be used for ERA* but as the

---

* 'ERA' in this Chapter means cortical ERA, the abbreviation ERA denoting 'evoked response audiometry'.

technique is time consuming it is usual to restrict it to two or three frequencies. For medicolegal purposes 1, 2, and 3 kHz are often used as these frequencies form the basis of assessing hearing handicap, at least in the United Kingdom.

Although originally introduced as a method for testing difficult children, today ERA is restricted almost entirely to testing older school-age children and adults and the indications are essentially for the investigation of non-organic hearing loss (NOHL) as described in Chapter 27 and for medicolegal assessment in cases of occupational hearing loss (Chapter 37). In each case the object is to check the reliability or otherwise of the pure-tone audiograms which may be suspect. Young children have unfortunately proved to be unsuitable, in general, for testing by ERA for two main reasons (i) the background EEG of the immature brain of the child often contains many large, slow fluctuations which are difficult to eliminate by conventional averaging, and (ii) it is only rarely that sufficient co-operation can be ensured in the case of children most in need of such investigation. Sedation (see Chapter 34) is not particularly satisfactory and unless some anaesthetic agent can be introduced which does not suppress the V-potential it is doubtful if the V-potential can be seriously considered as a suitable method for young children. However, the discovery of a suitable anaesthetic agent, would transform the situation especially if combined with fully objective computerized analysis and evaluation of the record as will now be briefly outlined.

A method of fully objective computerized ERA has been developed as a result of the collaborative studies of this subject between the Royal National Throat, Nose and Ear Hospital and the Imperial College of Science and Technology, University of London (Sayers, Beagley, and Henshall 1974; Sayers, Beagley, and Riha 1979; Beagley, Sayers, and Ross 1979).

The impetus to this investigation was the dissatisfaction with coherent averaging as a method of extracting the V-potential, partly because the frequency content of the V-potential and the background EEG largely overlap and because in all averaging procedures undue emphasis is always placed upon single measures which deviate far from the mean, and on-line coherent averaging is no exception to this.

Attention was therefore concentrated on single 'sweeps' instead of ensembles of sweeps so that the widely deviant measures would be less emphasized than in averaging. Amplitude and power measurements proved unhelpful but analysis of the phase spectrum of the stimulated EEG record ultimately provided the key to the problem. It became quite clear that the phase spectrum is the factor which influences the *pattern* of a waveform and pattern analysis based on phase spectral analysis proved to be a valid method for detecting a pattern in single segments of stimulated EEG. The crux of this proposition is that in an ensemble of, say, 64 sweeps the phase spectrum of the relevant harmonics (H_2 to H_6) of a 0.64 s record length would be distributed randomly if there was no pattern present (e.g. subthreshold or 'control' trial with no stimulus) but that there would be significant aggregation of phases in cases where an acoustic stimulus had created a pattern in the ensemble, albeit not visible by eye in the individual sweeps. From this, despite some mathematical complexities in dealing with phase spectra, an analytical method was developed which could be used to score a series of EEG records to show whether an evoked potential was present or not and to evaluate it statistically and automatically. the technique was developed in an off-line study (using tape-recorded data) in a large computer, then on-line using a laboratory computer, the subjects in each case being a group of normals, plus some patients with impaired hearing. At present a clinical trial is under way using both a laboratory computer as well as a specially designed apparatus based on microprocessors which will both synthesize the acoustic stimulus *and* carry out the phase spectral analysis.

The results of the phase spectral method of hearing assessment can be written out and recorded in a variety of ways and one of the ways used at the Hospital mentioned is shown in Fig. 33.22. In this case the data included in

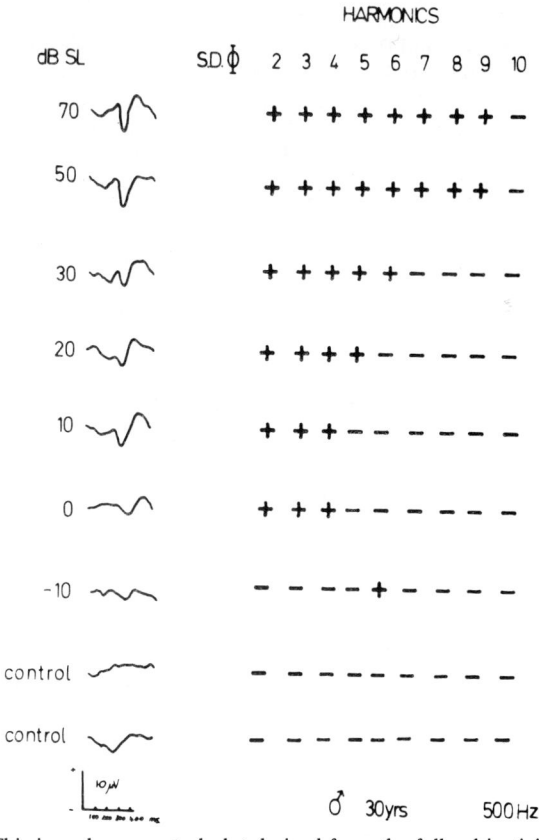

Fig. 33.22. This is a phase spectral plot derived from the fully objectivized, computerized ERA method based on analysis of the phase spectrum which is automatically evaluated by means of a fixed statistical criterion; + means significant at 0.05 or better. (Beagley, Sayers, and Ross (1979). Courtesy *Acta Otolaryngologica*.)

the writeout has been simplified considerably and *positive* means significance at the 0.05 level or better; *negative* of course means non-significance. The average V-potential is recorded alongside the significance levels for the harmonics tested. It can be seen that the sensitivity of the test is comparable with visual scoring but more important, it is entirely objective, the significance levels being evaluated automatically by the computer and observer bias is thereby completely eliminated.

REFERENCES

BEAGLEY, H. A. and GIBSON, W. P. R. (1976). Lesions mimicking acoustic neuromata on electrocochleography. In *Disorders of auditory function* (ed. S. D. G. Stephens) Vol. 2, pp. 119–26. Academic Press, London.

—— (1978). Electrocochleography in adults. In *Evoked electrical activity in the auditory nervous system* (ed. R. Naunton and C. Fernandez) pp. 259–75. Academic Press, London.

—— and SHELDRAKE, J. B. (1978). Differences in brainstem response latencies with age and sex. *Br. J. Audiol.* **12**, 69–77.

—— SAYERS, B.McA., and ROSS, A. J. (1979). Fully objective ERA by phase spectral analysis *Acta oto-lar.* **87**, 270–8.

CULLEN, J. K., ELLIS, M. S., BERLIN, C. I., and LOUSTEAU, R. J. (1972). Human acoustic nerve action potential recordings from the tympanic membrane without anaesthesia. *Acta oto-lar.* **74**, 15–22.

DAVIS H. and HIRSH S. K. (1979). A slow brainstem response for low-frequency audiometry. *Audiology* **18**, 445–61.

EGGERMONT, J. J. and SPOOR, A. (1973). Cochlear adaptation in guinea pigs (a quantitative description). *Audiology* **12**, 193–220.

ELBERLING, C. and SALOMON, G. (1971). Electrical potentials from the inner ear in man in response to transient sounds generated in a closed acoustic system. *Revue Lar. Otol. Rhinol.* Suppl. 691–707.

KHESHINACHVILI, S. N. and KEVANISHVILI, Z. S. (1974). Experience in computer audiology (ECochG and ERA). *Audiology* **13**, 391–402.

KNIGHT, J. J. (1979) Acoustic measurements. In *Auditory investigation: the scientific and technological basis* (ed. H. A. Beagely). Clarendon Press, Oxford.

PICTON T. W., OUELLETTE J., HAMEL G., and SMITH A. D. (1979). Brainstem evoked potentials to tone pips in notched noise. *J. Otolar.* **8**, 289–314.

PORTMANN, M. and ARAN, J. M. (1971). Electro-cochleography. *Laryngoscope, St. Louis* **81**, 899–910.

—— —— and LE BERT, G. (1968). Electrocochléogramme humain en dehors de toute intervention chirurgicale. *Acta oto-lar.* **71**, 253–61.

ROBINSON, K. and RUDGE, P. (1977). Abnormalities of the auditory system in patients with multiple sclerosis. *Brain* **1**, 19–40.

SAYERS, B.McA., BEAGLEY, H. A., and HENSHALL, W. R. (1974). The mechanism of auditory evoked EEG responses. *Nature, Lond.* **247**, 481–3.

—— —— and RIHA, J. (1979). Pattern analysis of auditory-evoked EEG potentials. *Audiology* **18**, 1–16.

YOSHIE, N. (1968). Auditory nerve action potential responses to clicks in man. *Laryngoscope, St. Louis* **178**, 198–215.

NOTE ADDED IN PROOF

In recording BSER, if one records the potential between the vertex and the *opposite* ear-lobe certain changes are noted: wave V is slightly prolonged in latency (0.1 ms); wave V and IV, which are often fused, separate; wave III is diminished, sometimes greatly; wave II is unaffected, and wave I is not seen.

34 Sedation and anaesthesia

J. N. T. HUTTON

In order to carry out various investigations of the auditory system it may be necessary to use sedation or general anaesthesia. General anaesthesia is required for clinical examination of the ears in very disturbed children. It is also used in transtympanic electrocochleography and recording of brainstem electrical responses and also for radiological studies. Sedation, as opposed to anaesthesia, is employed in obtaining satisfactory conditions for cortical electrical response audiometry in young children. Mentally disturbed or very nervous adults may require sedation or anaesthesia, either local or general, for electrocochleography.

CLINICAL EXAMINATION

In the vast majority of patients presenting with a suspected hearing disorder it is possible to do routine otoscopy, but in some children this may not be the case even with the greatest degree of care and patience by the audiological physician. It may be necessary to administer a general anaesthetic in order to examine mentally retarded, emotionally disturbed or hyperactive children. A simple anaesthetic with nitrous oxide, oxygen, and halothane is satisfactory, preceded by oral atropine sulphate as a premedication. A conductive deafness may be present due to impacted wax, a foreign body, or serous otitis media and facilities should be available to deal with these conditions.

ELECTROCOCHLEOGRAPHY

Recording of the cochlear potentials in response to sound may be obtained from a transtympanic electrode placed on the promontory or from an electrode placed extratympanically. In the latter case it may be possible to obtain recordings without resource to anaesthesia but the electrical pick-up of this method is only one-tenth of that obtained with the transtympanic placement. The transtympanic method giving a clear-cut biological signal is preferred and general anaesthesia is required in children for the placement of the electrode. It may also be necessary in some adults to administer either local or general anaesthesia.

Anaesthesia for children

Two methods of anaesthesia may be used for transtympanic ECochG in children—dissociative anaesthesia with Ketamine or conventional anaesthesia with nitrous oxide, oxygen, and halothane.

KETAMINE ANAESTHESIA

Ketamine is used to anaesthetize children under three years old. It has two disadvantages: recovery is prolonged and unpleasant hallucinations may occur during the recovery period. This recovery period is much shorter when the drug is administered by the intravenous route than intramuscularly but nevertheless the intramuscular route is preferred as it has been shown by Morgan, Singer, and Moore (1971) that distressing hallucinations are less frequent when the drug is given by this route. The children are fully recovered from the effects of Ketamine after four hours and the testing should take place in the morning so that it can be carried out as a day-case procedure. Vomiting may occur during recovery and so it is essential that the child is prepared as for any other general anaesthetic, and also facilities must be available in the recovery room to deal with this possible complication.

Premedication is with intramuscular atropine sulphate. Adequate dosage is essential as salivation can be copious with Ketamine. A general guide is 300 micrograms for infants under one year old and 600 micrograms for those over one year old. No sedative drugs are included in the premedication as they would prolong the recovery period, possibly necessitating overnight hospitalization. Children, however, with a history of fits are given Phenytoin on the morning of the test as epileptiform spasms can occur in susceptible cases under Ketamine anaesthesia interfering with the recordings. Five millilitres of phenytoin suspension containing 30 mg of phenytoin would be given to a three-year-old child and proportional doses for other ages.

The initial injection of Ketamine is made into the upper and outer quadrant of the buttock and the solution used contains 50 mg per ml. The Ketamine dosage requirement is related to the basal metabolic rate which in turn is related to the surface area. The surface area is calculated from the height and weight according to the formula

$$A = W^{0.425} \times H^{0.725} \times 71.84$$

where A = surface area in cm^2, W = weight in kg and H = height in cm.

One mg of Ketamine is given for each 35 cm^2 of surface area and dosages for various heights and weights are given in Table 34. Anaesthesia commences within three minutes of the injection and the average duration is 30 to 35 minutes. At the end of this period a second injection of the same dosage may be required. This is given into the vastus lateralis in order to obviate moving the child. Ketamine produces a dissociative anaesthesia without affecting the reticular activating or limbic systems and no artificial airway or support to the jaw is required. At the end of the procedure the child is taken to the adjoining recovery room where he is supervised by a nurse familiar with this type of anaesthesia. Extraneous stimuli are avoided in order to minimize hallucinations.

TABLE 34.1. *Dosage of intramuscular Ketamine in milligrams*

Weight/kg	\multicolumn{18}{c}{Height/cm}
	55	60	65	70	75	80	85	90	95	100	105	110	115	120	125	130	135	140
5	75	80	85	90	95	100	100	105	110	115	120	120	125	130	135	140	145	145
6	80	85	90	95	100	105	110	115	120	125	130	135	135	140	145	150	155	160
7	85	90	95	100	105	115	120	125	125	130	135	140	145	150	155	160	165	170
8	90	95	100	110	115	120	125	130	135	140	145	150	155	160	165	170	175	180
9	95	100	110	115	120	125	130	135	140	145	150	160	165	170	175	180	185	190
10	100	105	115	120	125	130	135	145	150	155	160	165	170	175	180	185	190	195
12	110	115	120	130	135	140	150	155	160	165	170	180	185	190	195	200	205	210
14	115	125	130	135	145	150	160	165	170	180	185	190	195	200	210	215	220	225
16	120	130	140	145	155	160	165	175	180	190	195	200	210	215	220	225	235	240
18	130	135	145	155	160	170	175	185	190	200	205	210	220	225	235	240	245	250
20	135	145	150	160	170	175	185	190	200	205	215	220	230	235	245	250	255	265
25	145	155	165	175	185	195	200	210	220	225	235	245	250	260	265	275	280	290
30	160	170	180	190	200	210	220	225	235	245	255	265	270	280	290	295	305	315
35	170	180	190	200	215	225	235	245	255	260	270	280	290	300	310	315	325	335
40	180	190	205	215	225	235	245	255	265	275	285	295	305	315	325	335	345	355
45	190	200	215	225	235	250	260	270	280	290	300	315	325	335	345	355	365	370
50	200	210	225	235	250	260	270	285	295	305	315	325	335	350	360	370	380	390
55	205	220	230	245	260	270	280	295	305	320	330	340	350	365	375	385	395	405
60	215	230	240	255	270	280	295	305	320	330	340	355	365	375	385	400	410	420

GENERAL INHALATION ANAESTHESIA

Inhalation anaesthesia is preferred for subjects over three years old. The use of an anaesthetic machine causes no interference with the recordings and the main problem is the elimination of the expired gases from the soundproofed testing room.

Atropine sulphate (600 micrograms) is given as a premedication and it is administered by the oral route mixed with a small amount of simple syrup. Sedative drugs are not usually necessary and the rapid recovery when atropine alone is used is advantageous.

Induction of anaesthesia is with nitrous oxide, oxygen, and halothane or an intravenous sleep dose of 1 per cent Methohexitone. Maintenance of anaesthesia is with nitrous oxide, oxygen, and halothane and the subject breathing spontaneously. When the third stage of anaesthesia is reached oral intubation is carried out with a plain Magill endotracheal tube. In the vast majority of cases the facility of a short acting muscle relaxant is not necessary for this procedure.

In order to protect the personnel in the soundproofed testing room from the deleterious effects of the halothane a valve described by Enderby (1972) is connected to the catheter mount and the exhaust gases conducted to the outside of the building where a silencer is attached (Fig. 34.1). There is a slight resistance to expiration with this system which is of negligible significance with older subjects but would be of importance with smaller children and therefore anaesthesia with Ketamine is preferred for those under three years old.

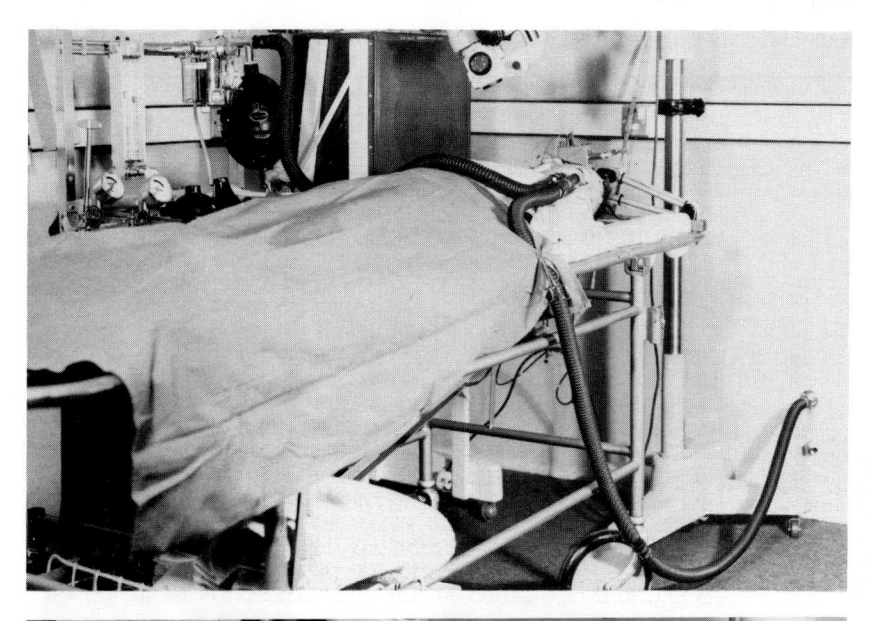

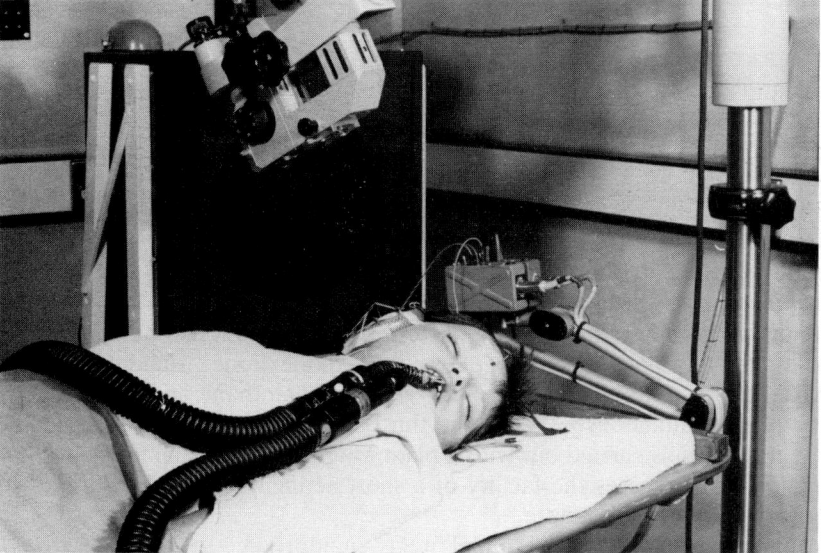

Fig. 34.1. Ducting of expired anaesthetic gas to the exterior incorporating use of the Enderby valve.

Anaesthesia for adults

LOCAL ANAESTHESIA

The majority of adults will tolerate the insertion of the transtympanic electrode without any anaesthesia but, in some, local anaesthesia may be required. Spraying the tympanic membrane with Cetacaine® is used but its effectiveness is doubtful other than that of suggestion. A more certain method of anaesthetizing the drum membrane is with Zylocaine 4 per cent using the iontophoresis method. This certainly works but is time consuming taking about 20 minutes and as it is only practicable to do one ear at a time there is considerable prolonging of the testing period.

SEDATION

Intravenous diazepam has been tried for sedation of nervous adults. The disadvantage is that, although the subject may be adequately sedated, the responses to pain are not obtunded and reaction with movement of the head may occur on piercing the tympanic membrane. A much more satisfactory technique is to inject intravenous diazepam until adequate sedation is obtained and then give an intravenous injection of 125 mg of Ketamine. There will then be no reaction to the insertion of the electrode and the subject will sleep for about an hour. There have been no hallucinatory disturbances following this régime.

BRAINSTEM ELECTRICAL RESPONSES

When a clear-cut action potential is recorded in electrocochleography it is possible at the same time to remove the transtympanic electrode, attach a vertex electrode, and record the brainstem responses. It would not appear that sedation or anaesthesia affects these responses as recognizable responses have been obtained and corresponding to threshold values with diazepam, trimeprazine, Ketamine, and halothane. By recording brainstem potentials before and after exhibiting nitrous oxide to the anaesthetic mixture the author has found a slightly worse threshold value and increased latency. This may be due to direct effect of the nitrous oxide on the brainstem nuclei or more probably to diffusion of the gas into the middle ear.

RADIOLOGICAL TOMOGRAPHY

When electrocochleography in an infant shows a complete absence of both compound action potential and cochlear microphonic it is a possibility that there is a congenital absence of the inner ear structures. This can be demonstrated by tomography but requires anaesthesia to keep the infant absolutely immobile during the exposure. In order to spare the child a second anaesthetic, it is taken to the X-ray department whilst still under the effect of the Ketamine for the tomograms to be taken.

CORTICAL ELECTRIC RESPONSE AUDIOMETRY (CERA)

CERA has the advantage over electrocochleography of being theoretically able to produce an audiogram comparable to a pure-tone audiogram. However, although the test reliability in adults is reasonable it is not possible to obtain worthwhile responses in young children when they are awake. This is especially the case when they have disabilities producing hyperactivity or poor muscular control. Occasionally it may be possible to test infants in natural sleep following a feed, but the vast majority of infants and young children will require some form of sedation. General anaesthesia is unsuitable, as the evoked response is abolished both with inhalation anaesthesia and also with intravenous anaesthesia with thiopentone.

A great variety of sedative drugs have been used in children to produce sleep for carrying out CERA testing. This fact signifies that no individual sedative drug is completely satisfactory for this purpose. Pentobarbital sodium in a dose of 5 mg per kg of body weight by mouth has been used by Rapin and Graziani (1967). It has also been used by Burian and Gestring (1971) in suppository form in a dose of 5 to 8 mg per kg of body weight. With this drug there may be changes in amplitude and latency of the responses but the threshold measurement appears to be only slightly affected. Another barbiturate, Quinalbarbitone, administered orally in a dose of 10 mg/kg body weight appears to give comparable results. Burian and Gestring also tried diazepam but this was unsatisfactory as even with intravenous injection it failed to produce sleep in 30 per cent of subjects.

The phenothiazine group of drugs appear to give more satisfactory conditions for CERA testing than the previous ones enumerated. Chlorpromazine administered in a dosage of 1 mg/kg body weight has been given by Rapin and Graziani (1967). They found that the threshold measurements were better than those with pentobarbital and also that there was no difference in threshold measurement in six babies tested both during natural sleep and in chlorpromazine-induced sleep.

Another phenothiazine—promethazine hydrochloride—has been used and given satisfactory conditions. Both Stange (1972) and Karnahl and Benning (1972) found that this drug produced less changes in the responses than diazepam or barbiturates. When drugs are administered orally there is a considerable variation with correspondingly erratic results. Beagley, Fateen, and Gordon (1972) realized this factor and administered promethazine by intramuscular injection in a dosage of 1 mg/kg body weight. The electrodes are applied about an hour after the injection and some reaction occurs from the child who then rapidly falls asleep on its mother's lap. The EEG activity shows four increasing depths of sleep and a stage of rapid eye movements. It is in the third and fourth stages of sleep, characterized by large amplitude EEG waves, that the testing is carried out. Beagley reports that in 35 cases with intramuscular phenergan it was possible in all cases to reach an estimate of threshold and in no case had the test to be abandoned.

The difficulty of obtaining satisfactory conditions with sedation for

CERA will no doubt lead to continued search for a general anaesthetic drug that does not significantly interfere with the recording of cortical responses. Enflurane shows some promise in this respect, having an effect on the EEG differing from that of other inhalation anaesthetics. Joel and Stevens (1969) obtained cortical responses to sound stimuli in dogs at all stages of anaesthesia with this drug.

REFERENCES

BEAGLEY, H. A., FATEEN, A. M., and GORDON, A. G. (1972). Clinical experience of evoked response and subjective auditory thresholds. *Sound* **6**, 8–13.

BURIAN, K. and GESTRING, G. F. (1971). Discrepancies between subjective and objective acoustic thresholds. *Arch. Klin. exp. Ohren-Nasen-u. Kehlheilk.* **198**, 73–82.

ENDERBY, G. E. H. (1972). Gas exhaust valve. *Anaesthesia* **27**, 334.

JOAS, T. A. and STEVENS, W. C. (1969). Convulsive properties of Ethrane, Fluroxene, Halothane and Chloroform anaesthesia. *Anesthesiology* **30**, 343.

KARNAHL, T. and BENNING, C. D. (1972). Effect of sedation upon evoked response audiometry: amplitude and latency vs. sound pressure level. *Arch. Klin. exp. Ohren-Nasen-u. Kehlheilk.* **201**, 181–8.

MORGAN, M., LOH, L., SINGER, L., and MOORE, P. H. (1971). Ketamine as the sole anaesthetic agent for minor surgical procedures. *Anaesthesia* **26**, 158.

RAPIN, I. and GRAZIANI, L. J. (1967). Auditory evoked responses in normal, brain-damaged and deaf infants. *Neurology, Minneap.* **17**, 881–94.

STANGE, G. (1972). The effect of sedative agents in psychotropic drugs on the acoustically evoked responses. *Arch. Klin. exp. Ohren-Nasen-u. Kehlheilk.* **201**, 294–308.

35 Radiology in audiological diagnosis

PETER D. PHELPS

Radiology may demonstrate the situation and extent of a lesion of the hearing organ and indicate the probable aetiology. The radiological examination is therefore complementary to the audiological assessment and may even suggest the type and degree of hearing loss. For instance one would expect malposition of the ossicles following head trauma to be associated with deafness which is predominantly conductive, whereas a fracture line extending through the labyrinth would indicate a dead ear. Similarly a simple unilateral congenital meatal atresia with ossicular mass and a normal middle-ear cleft and inner ear would suggest a 50–60 dB conductive hearing loss, whereas gross congenital deformity of the labyrinth with no proper cochlea denies any auditory function. When the initial audiological and radiological assessments disagree then further consideration and investigation is necessary to find out why this is the case.

The temporal bone can be examined either by conventional radiography or tomography. The former is simpler and quicker and needs only standard radiographic equipment, although the complex anatomical configuration of ear structures has led to many different projections being devised and used. In spite of this, parts of the petrous temporal bone, particularly the ossicles and oval window, cannot be adequately demonstrated. These projections, some of which are also standard skull views, are fully described in textbooks of radiology and otology. The author uses four basic projections for almost all conventional radiography of the temporal bone: the base and Towne's—which are standard skull views—the Stenvers, and the tilted lateral. The Stenvers projection is an oblique projection which gives a picture in the long axis of the petrous pyramid. It is used to demonstrate the internal auditory meatus but also shows the labyrinth and mastoid process. A lateral view with the film and the sagittal plane of the skull tilted 20° gives a good demonstration of the mastoid air-cells. Other projections are rarely used as tomography is preferred.

Tomography gives a more precise demonstration of the temporal bone and enables structures to be shown which cannot be assessed on plain radiographs. For the best results modern tomographic apparatus with multidirectional tube movement is necessary. There are many pitfalls in the interpretation of tomograms and a thorough understanding of tomographic anatomy is necessary so that the level of any particular section can be easily recognized. Sections in the coronal plane (anteroposterior, AP or posterioanterior, PA) form the basis of any tomographic examination. There are two sections in the coronal plane that are important and must be recognized; these pass through the centre of the cochlea and vestibule respectively

(Fig. 35.1). The cochlear cut shows the modiolus or central bony spiral as a 'curl' while above the cochlea is the pit for the geniculate ganglion of the facial nerve (Fig. 35.2(left)). The ossicle shown in the middle ear cavity is the malleus. The vestibular cut 2 or 3 mm posteriorly shows the oval window and also the full length of the internal auditory meatus (Fig. 35.2(right)). The ossicle is the incus and sometimes the stapes may be demonstrated. The outer attic wall, which also forms the roof of the deep part of the bony external auditory meatus is called because of its appearance 'the spur'. For simplicity all illustrations in this chapter are based on these two coronal sections.

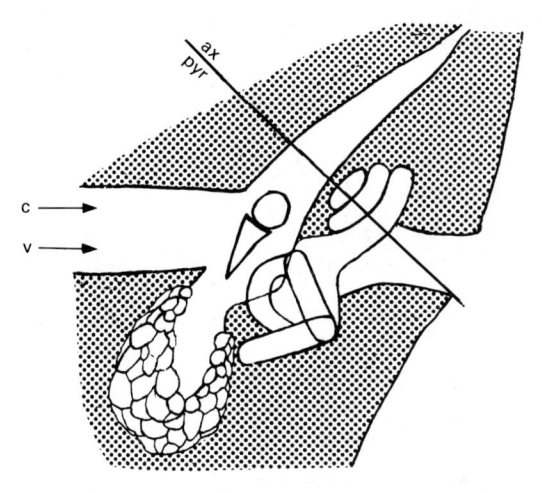

Fig. 35.1. Diagrammatic base section of the temporal bone. The levels of the two important coronal sections through the cochlea and vestibule are indicated by arrows in the external auditory meatus.

Other tomographic projections may be used to supplement the information obtained. Although these will not be discussed, it would seem appropriate in a textbook of audiology to describe the optimum tomographic demonstration of the cochlea. Generally speaking careful examination of the 'curl' of the modiolus as seen on coronal sections (Fig. 35.2(left)) is adequate for showing that the bony skeleton of the cochlea is normal. However, to demonstrate the separate coils of the cochlea, sections in the long axis of the modiolus are necessary. In practice this means using the axial-pyramidal or the base (submento-vertical) projection (Fig. 35.1). The latter gives more information about the labyrinth and internal auditory meatus and allows the two sides to be examined simultaneously; however, the patient has to maintain rather an uncomfortable position for this projection to be used. The radiology of some of the more important lesions of the temporal bone is considered in relation to the audiological investigation.

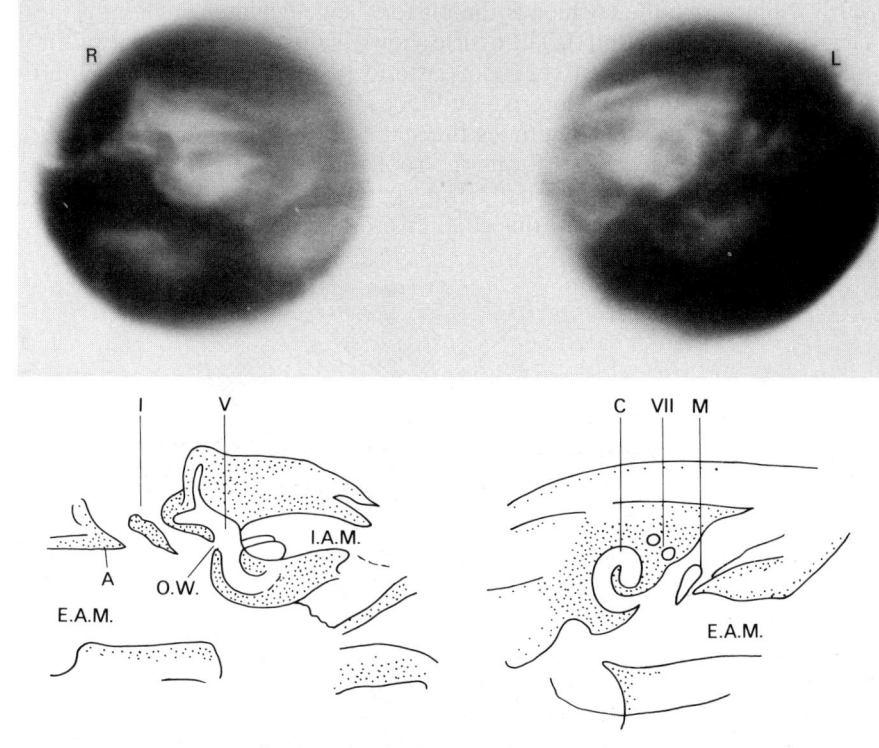

Fig. 35.2. Coronal section tomogram, at the level of the vestibule (V) on the right and the cochlea (C) on the left. O.W. = oval window, I = incus, M = malleus, A = spur or outer attic wall, VII = facial nerve, E.A.M. = external auditory meatus, I.A.M. = internal auditory meatus.

CONGENITAL DEAFNESS

Many abnormalities of the hearing organ do not involve bony structures and therefore no lesion would be demonstrated by tomography. Moreover as deafness is usually discovered in one- or two-year-old children when tomography is virtually impossible without sedation or a general anaesthetic this technique should only be used for those cases in which useful information may be obtained. Ideally electrocochleography and the tomographic examination would be performed under the same sedation but this is rarely possible in most hospitals. Suggested guidelines for selection of patients for tomography might be: (i) any syndrome known to be associated with structural deformity of the ear, in particular mandibulo-facial or craniofacial dysostosis, hemi-facial microsomia or the Goldenhar syndrome; (ii) certain spinal abnormalities including the Klippel–Feil syndrome; (iii) abnormalities of the external ears including auricular appendages and pits; (iv) after attacks of meningitis and c.s.f. rhinorrhoea (see below).

A child with an obvious ear deformity should in the author's opinion have tomograms soon after birth as these can often be obtained with minimal radiation and no sedation other than a large feed. The results, however, must be available for consideration when the hearing is assessed at a later stage.

Inner-ear leasions

In any tomographic examination for congenital deafness the state of the inner ear should be assessed first for the following reasons: (i) The level of any tomographic section is assessed from the part of the labyrinth shown on that section (see above). (ii) A severe degree of cochlear deformity (Fig. 35.3) is obviously incompatible with auditory function whatever other tests

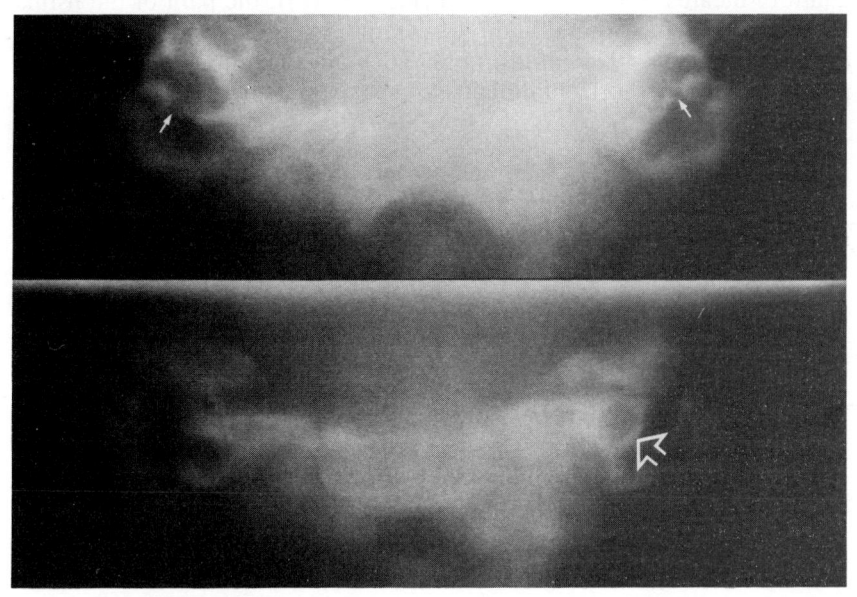

Fig. 35.3. The upper section shows dilated vestibules and lateral semicircular canals with tapering internal auditory meatuses. The arrows point to normal oval windows. The lower section shows an 'empty' cochlea sac (open arrow) on the left while on the right there is no vestige of cochlea. The middle ears are normal. The child, aged two, with failure of speech development, was sent for tomography after electro-cochleography had shown complete lack of auditory function. There is a risk of a cerebrospinal fluid fistula developing via the internal auditory meatus and oval window in this patient.

may suggest. This is important in bilateral cases, because although such a melancholy diagnosis is hard to accept, the child will have to be educated by methods not involving sound. (iii) It is possible in some cases of inner-ear deformity to assess the likely degree of deafness. For instance the commonest inner-ear anomaly shown by tomography, namely shortening and dilatation of the lateral semicircular canal, is usually associated with normal cochlea function (Fig. 35.4(b)). However, if other canals are abnormal and especially if they are absent rather than dilated then there will almost certainly be a severe degree of sensorineural deafness, even if the cochlea appears normal (Phelps 1974). Similarly there is probably a range of deformities with underdevelopment of the modiolus of the cochlea (Fig. 35.4(c)), the best known being that described by Mundini, the presence of a basal turn meaning that some degree of cochlea function is possible. (iv) There is risk of a cerebrospinal fluid fistula developing through the oval window, either spontaneously or as a result of stapes surgery, in some types of labyrinthine abnormality. The route may be via the internal auditory meatus or an abnormally wide cochlear aqueduct. A specific type of deformity with general dilatation and dysplasia of the labyrinth and a tapering internal auditory meatus has been described (Fig. 35.4(e)), the path of the fistula being through the internal auditory meatus and the empty 'cochlear sac' (Phelps and Lloyd 1978). It is probable that any dilatation of the vestibule particularly in the horizontal plane indicates a potential 'stapes gusher'.

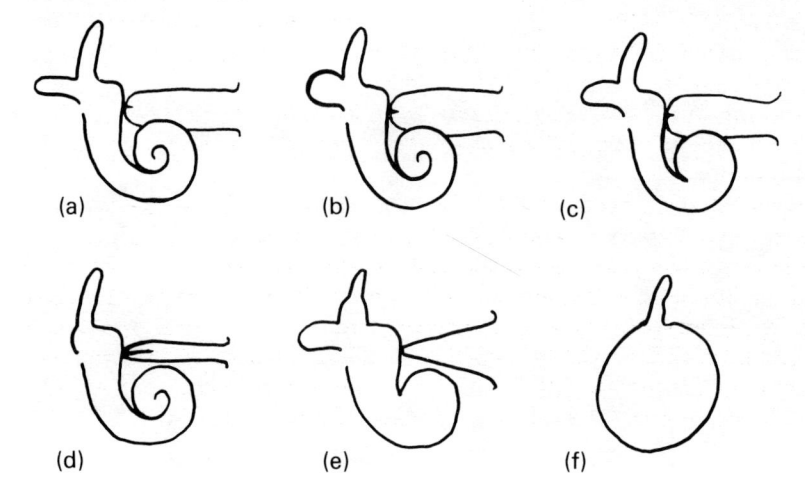

Fig. 35.4. Diagrammatic representation, based on coronal section tomograms, of some congenital inner ear deformities. (a). Normal. (b). Solitary dilatation of the lateral semicircular canal. (c). Deficient modiolus of the cochlea but with normal basal turn (Mundini defect). (d) Absent lateral semicircular canal; narrow internal auditory meatus; hypertrophid crista falciformis. (e). Dilated dysplastic labyrinth with tapered internal auditory meatus. (f). Amorphous labyrinthine sac.

Middle and external ear lesions

Tomography for congenital atresias relates to prospective surgical exploration. In bilateral cases, this is usually undertaken in children 2–3 years old if tomography shows it to be worthwhile. Unilateral lesions are now rarely explored and if the other ear is entirely normal the radiological investigation may be left until the child is old enough to co-operate.

The most important assessment is the state of the middle-ear cavity

(Phelps, Lloyd, and Sheldon 1977). In most unilateral atresias with associated deformity of the pinna, there is good pneumatization in a normally formed mastoid and the middle-ear cavity is of relatively normal shape. Even in the most severe deformities there is rarely complete absence of the middle ear and usually at least a slit-like cavity can be demonstrated lateral to the basal turn of the cochlea, although this is of little use to the surgeon. In mandibulofacial dysostosis (Treacher–Collins syndrome) the mastoid is unpneumatized and the attic and antrum are typically absent or slit-like, being replaced in varying degrees by solid bone or by the descent of the tegmen. The course of the facial nerve should be demonstrated.

TRAUMATIC LESIONS

Deafness following head injury is another situation where radiological investigation is complementary to the audiological assessment. The initial management of head injuries is concerned with intracranial lesions and any radiological investigation of the temporal bone will be done to assess such factors as damage to the facial nerve or the site of a cerebrospinal fluid fistula. However, it is now realized that traumatic hearing loss is often due to disruption of the ossicular chain and tomographic examination of the ossicles should be undertaken when there is a persistent conductive deafness following head injury.

Incudostapedial dislocation unfortunately cannot be demonstrated but the less common dislocation and displacement of the incus or very rarely the malleus is easily recognized with tomography. A simple rule to remember is that on any coronal tomographic section one sees either the malleus or the incus depending on whether the section is at the level of the cochlea or the vestibule. If two ossicles are present in a single coronal section then one of them must be dislocated (Fig. 35.5). In addition lateral and base sections may be used to show the relative positions of the ossicles.

INFLAMMATORY CONDITIONS

Opacity of the middle-ear cavity and mastoid air-cells are the first radiological signs of otitis media and are associated with some degree of conductive deafness. The development of bone destruction and 'cell-wall breakdown' is difficult to assess because of local decalcification and the loss of radiographic contrast. It is important to note the extent of pneumatization as in an acellular mastoid intracranial complications may occur without evidence of bone destruction.

Cholesteatoma of the acquired type typically causes erosion of the attico-antral region best seen on the lateral oblique radiographs. Earlier erosion and a soft tissue mass in the middle ear can be shown by tomography but this is rarely required in a straightforward case.

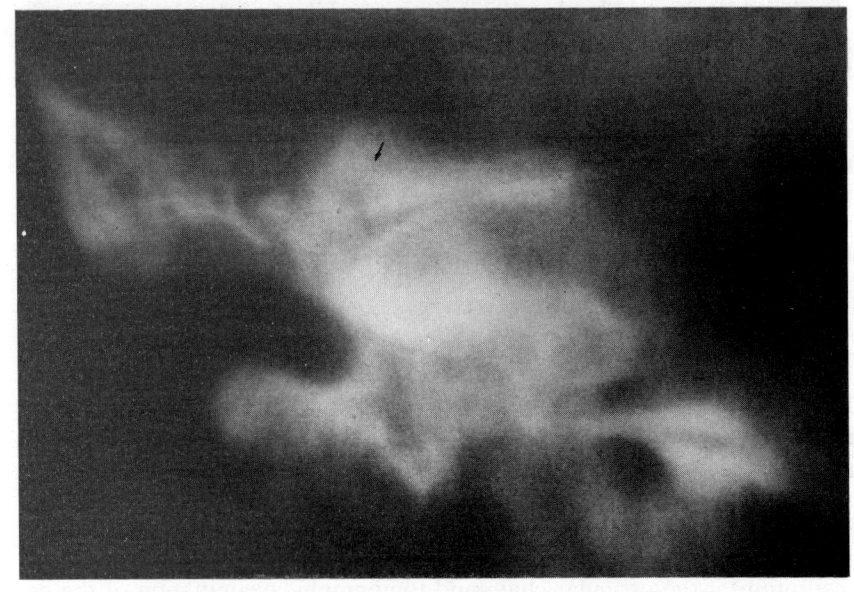

Fig. 35.5 Two ossicles are shown in this section at the level of the cochlea. The most lateral is the dislocated incus. There is also a fracture through the superior aspect of the temporal bone involving the labyrinth (arrow).

TUMOURS OF THE PETROUS BONE

Malignant tumours of the external auditory meatus or middle ear cause extensive and ragged erosion. Primary or congenital cholesteatoma usually presents with seventh or eighth cranial nerve dysfunction with a normal eardrum. A smoothly outlined defect in the petrous bone is almost pathognomonic, but other lesions such as meningioma or glomus jugular tumours can also cause extensive erosion of the petrous pyramid. Erosion of the margins of the jugular foramen may suggest a diagnosis of glomus tumours but selective angiography is necessary to confirm this.

ACOUSTIC NEUROMA

Tumours arising in the internal auditory meatus or cerebellopontine angle provide the biggest challenge in diagnosis from both a radiological and an audiological point of view. The investigation for acoustic neuromas has been altered and to some extent simplified by the introduction of computer-assisted tomography (CT). This is now the definitive investigation for angle lesions and will demonstrate all acoustic neuromas larger than 2 cm in diameter and most larger than 1 cm (Fig. 35.6). The following discussion is concerned with the selection of patients for CT and the diagnosis of acoustic neuroma when CT is negative.

Modern audiometry and vestibular examination can give strong presump-

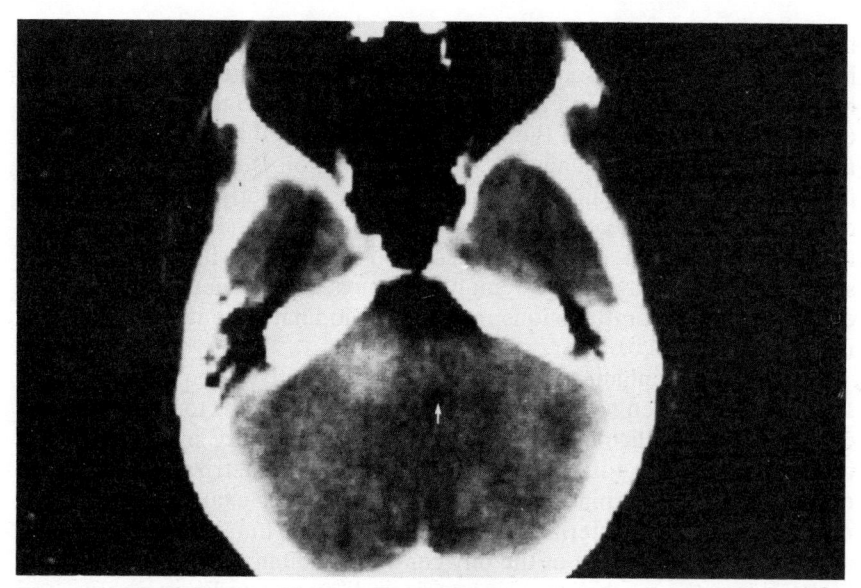

Fig. 35.6. Computerized axial tomography of the posterior cranial fossa. Contrast enhancement shows a 4 cm acoustic neuroma as a white area behind the petrous pyramid. Note the displacement of the fourth ventricle (arrow) to the opposite side.

tive evidence of a small intracanalicular neuroma but radiographic demonstration of the internal auditory meatus is necessary when there is the least suspicion of an acoustic neuroma. Expansion of the meatus may be shown as well by plain films as by tomography if there is thick bone in the petrous apex. However, extensive pneumatization may make it impossible to assess the meatus on plain films and bone erosion is better demonstrated by tomography. Flaring of the porus of the internal auditory meatus, expansion of the meatus (Fig. 35.7) or erosion of its posterior wall are very suggestive of an acoustic neuroma (Valvassori 1969). Definite erosion shown on the

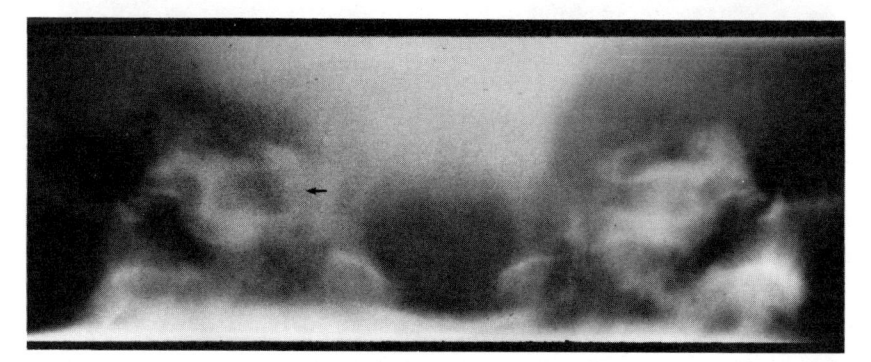

Fig. 35.7. Coronal section tomogram showing expansion of the left internal auditory meatus (arrow) by an acoustic neuroma.

lateral tomograms is almost pathognomonic of a tumour but unfortunately is not often present and some wide and asymmetrical meatuses contain no lesion. The state of the internal auditory meatus should therefore be considered in conjunction with the clinical findings, including the results of all audiometric and vestibular tests. CT examination is necessary when the index of suspicion for an acoustic neuroma is sufficiently high. A brief CT examination with one or two sections at the level of the internal auditory meatus is all that is required. These should show the position of the brainstem and fourth ventricle. To demonstrate most acoustic neuromas however enhancement with intravenous injection of iodinated contrast medium is necessary (Fig. 34.6).

If the contrast-enhanced CT examination is negative or equivocal consideration is then given to further radiological investigations to demonstrate a small or intracanalicular tumour. These procedures are invasive as they involve lumbar puncture. Air is now rarely used but metrizamide enhancement of the cerebrospinal fluid with subsequent CT examination can demonstrate the basal cisterns and outline small angle tumours. Alternatively a small quantity (1–2 ml) of the oily contrast medium myodil may be manipulated into the cerebellopontine angle and internal auditory meatus, and then demonstrated with appropriate projections or conventional tomography. A round filling defect indicates a small tumour (Fig. 35.8). Filling the meatus with myodil is the only sure way of excluding an acoustic neuroma.

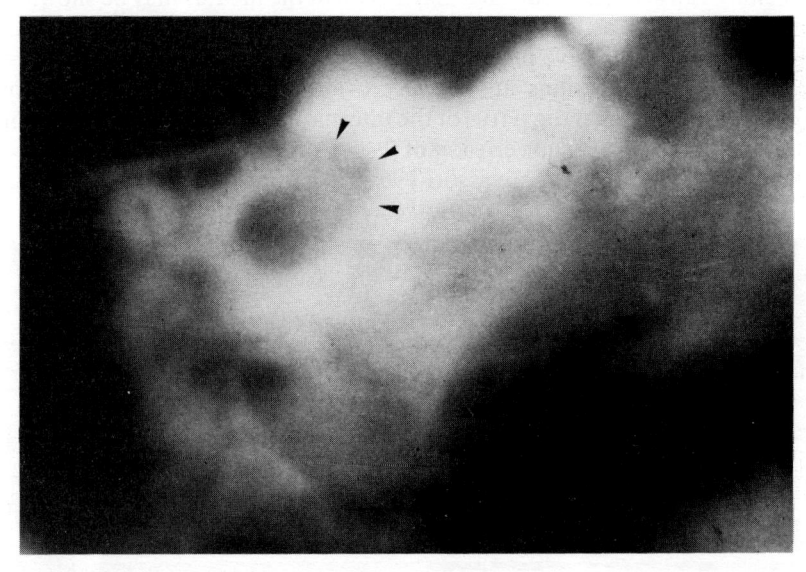

Fig. 35.8. Myodil cisternogram with Stenvers section tomogram. The internal auditory meatus has failed to fill with the contrast medium which outlines the edge of an acoustic neuroma (arrowheads)

OTOSCLEROSIS

Good quality thin section tomography using a hypocycloidal or spiral tube movement will show narrowing or obliteration of the oval window. However, radiology is of little value as a preoperative assessment in otosclerosis, as justification for 'tympanotomy stapedectomy' depends on a large air-bone gap with good sensorineural reserve. Moreover tomography will not demonstrate a small otosclerotic focus which is causing footplate fixation. Tomographic investigation may be useful in the more severe cases with some sensorineural loss. For instance it may suggest the more favourable side for exploration if this cannot be decided after the results of audiometry have been obtained. Severe obliteration of the footplate may deter the surgeon from tympanotomy in an unpromising case.

Plaques of otosclerosis if sufficiently large can be demonstrated in the wall of the labyrinth, although such a demonstration was until recently of somewhat academic interest. The success of fluoride therapy in arresting the progress of cochlea otosclerosis and the associated sensorineural deafness, means that tomography is now a valuable aid in the diagnosis and can be used to assess the effects of treatment (Shambaugh and Causse 1974). Cochlea otosclerosis usually involves the basal turn and promontory causing thickening of the bone with blurred and irregular margins (Fig. 35.9). In the early otospongiose phase considerable bone rarefaction will be demonstrated.

PAGET'S DISEASE

Extensive Paget's disease of the skull base replaces the periosteal bone of the pyramid, and eventually invades the endochondral and endosteal bone of the labyrinth causing severe sensorineural deafness. Deformity and narrowing of the internal auditory meatus often occurs.

CONCLUSION

Except for showing whether the middle-ear cleft is air-containing or opaque, radiology of the temporal bone is limited to demonstrating abnormalities of the bony architecture. Nevertheless, with the aid of multidirectional tomography it is possible to demonstrate such small structures as the stapes and the vestibular aqueduct, although interpretation of the thin tomographic sections requires much experience and anatomical knowledge. The new computerized tomography is not as good as conventional tomography for showing the fine bone detail of the temporal bone, but is now the most important investigation for tumours of the cerebellopontine angle and posterior fossa, such as acoustic neuroma, which may present with audiological problems.

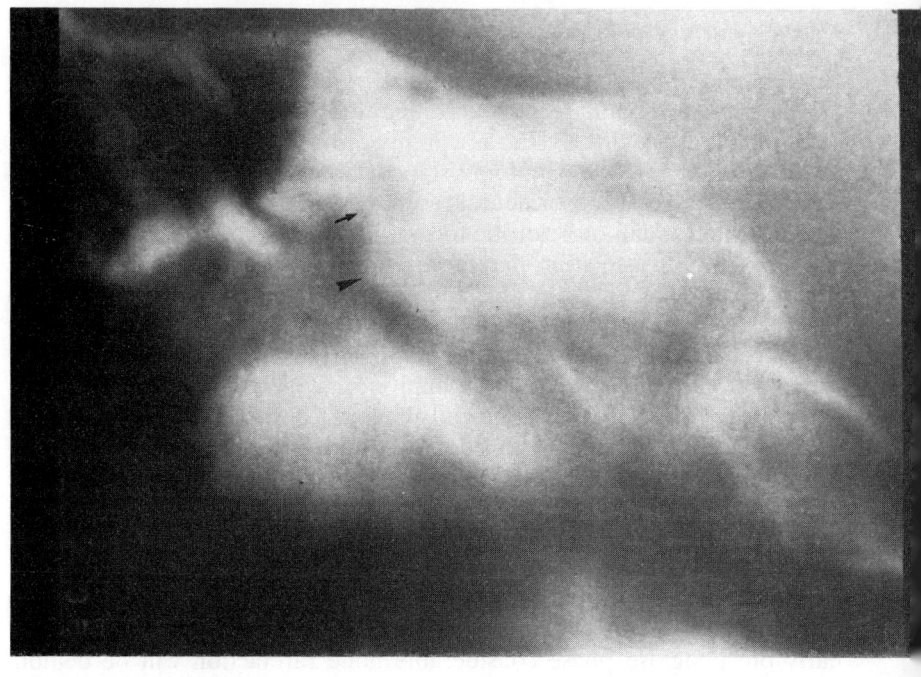

Fig. 35.9. Otosclerosis. The oval window appears normal on this tomogram (arrow) but the bone of the promontory is thickened with a 'fuzzy' margin (arrowhead) and there would seem to be encroachment on the basal turn of the cochlea.

REFERENCES

PHELPS, P. D. (1974). Congenital lesions of the inner ear demonstrated by tomography. *Archs Otolar.* **100**, 11–16.
—— and LLOYD, G. A. S. (1978). Congenital deformity of the internal auditory meatus and labyrinth associated with cerebro-spinal fluid fistula. *Adv. Oto.Rhino-Lar.* **24**, 51–7.
—— —— and SHELDON, P. W. E. (1977). Congenital deformities of the middle and external ear. *Br. J. Radiol.* **50**, 714–27.
SHAMBAUGH, G. E. and CAUSSE, J. (1974). Ten years experience with fluoride in otosclerotic (otospongiotic) patients. *Ann. Otol. Rhinol. Lar.* **83**, 635–42.
VALVASSORI, G. E. (1969). The abnormal internal auditory canal: the diagnosis of acoustic neuroma. *Radiology* **92**, 449–53.

Section 8
Forensic and Psychological Aspects of Audiology

36 Hearing conservation programmes

M. E. BRYAN and W. TEMPEST

INTRODUCTION

It has been known for some considerable time that certain occupations are associated with loss of hearing. T. R. Roger writing in the *Journal of Laryngology* in 1915 remarks that this did not only include noise deafness, but also caisson-deafness, suffered by divers, and deafness associated with lead poisoning. He goes on to mention that noise-deafness, which often affects blacksmiths, boilermakers, railway and factory employees, engineers, and others, has long been recognized both by the medical profession and by laymen.

However, it was not until about the time of the Second World War that sufficient knowledge was available for industrial medical staff to organize and run full-scale hearing conservation programmes. Hearing protection with ear plugs was developed during the First World War, and by 1925, when there was a discussion of occupational diseases of the ear, nose and throat at the British Medical Association, three proprietary ear plugs were on the market and it was also known that cotton wool soaked in Vaseline (petroleum jelly) provided protection against noise (Westmacott 1925). Audiometers were developed in the late 1920s and sound measuring equipment in the early 1930s. It was possible by 1939 for Dickson, Ewing, and Littler writing in the *Journal of Laryngology and Otology*, in discussing the effects of aeroplane noise on the auditory acuity of aviators, to give audiograms showing characteristics of noise-deafness, to give the levels of noise, in phons, from the aircraft, and to measure the amount of protection, in decibels, provided by different types of ear plug. It had already been noted, by McLachlan in 1935, that the hearing of those constantly exposed to a noise level exceeding 95–100 dB is apt to be permanently impaired. In 1940 Collier in *Outlines of industrial medical practice* was able to give practical advice for the suppression of industrial noise. In 1943 Sappington discussed the need not only for noise control but also for pre-employment and serial audiometry.

Thus by that time all the equipment and technical knowledge was available for the establishment of industrial hearing conservation programmes. We find in the Annual Report of the Chief Inspector of Factories, for 1954 (Anon 1954) a description of a hearing conservation programme being carried out in the UK at a non-ferrous tube works. In those areas where the noise exceeded 90 dB the hearing of the workers was checked regularly and any measures possible taken to reduce the noise levels at source. Where this was not possible hearing protection was issued and if serial audiometry showed subsequent deterioration the transfer of the individual was recommended.

Hazardous industries—the extent of the problem

Data on the precise extent of noise as an industrial hazard are rather sparse, but some sample surveys have been conducted in the UK by the Factory Inspectorate. The first of these, undertaken about seven years ago, suggested that around 500 000 people were regularly exposed for at least six hours per day to noise levels of 90 dB(A) or over. The total number subjected to some degree of risk is much larger than this, since the survey was limited to the occupations within the Inspectorate's purview, and there are many other workers exposed to noise in transport, mining, building, etc. who were excluded from the original survey. Further, there is reliable data (see for example Burns and Robinson 1970; Passchier-Vermeer 1968) that there is some degree of risk in exposure to noise in the 80–90 dB(A) region, involving many more workers than the half million quoted above.

Table 36.1 shows a number of examples of levels measured in various occupations. In each case the maximum permitted daily exposure is included. Table 36.2 lists the essential components of a hearing conservation programme.

THE NOISE SURVEY

The basis of any hearing conservation programme is a knowledge of the

TABLE 36.1. *Examples of measured noise levels and maximum permitted daily exposures*

Noise source	Noise level (dB(A)(Leq))	Maximum safe daily exposure†‡
'Disco music'	90	8 hr
Paper making	90	8 hr
Wood working	95	2½ hr
Four-wheel drive vehicle cab	95	2½ hr
Flour mill	96	2 hr
Earth-moving cab	97	1½ hr
Drop forging	98	1¼ hr
Weaving (dobcross looms)	100	48 min
Pop group (performers)	100	48 min
Steel fabrication	103	24 min
Glass bottle making	106	12 min
Steel rolling mill	110	5 min
Stainless steel polishing	115	1½ min
Riveting	117	1 min
Fettling (iron casting)	118	46 s
Diesel engine testing	120	30 s
Propellor chipping	132	2 s

† Without hearing protection.
‡ Department of Employment (1972).

TABLE 36.2. *Essentials of hearing conservation programmes (HCP)*

Operation	Function
Noise survey	Identification of hazardous areas/occupations
Noise control	Reduction of noise at source.
	Enclosure of noise source/operator to reduce noise to safe levels. Use of sound absorbers
Hearing protection	Where noise control is not possible, the provision, fitting and maintenance of ear plugs/muffs for personnel at risk, together with their education in the hazards of noise
Industrial audiometry	To monitor the effectiveness of hearing protection. Pre-employment and serial audiometry to determine the noise-sensitive workers
Organization of HCP	Co-ordination of work of medical, safety, and occupational hygiene staff involved.
	Education of management and workforce.
	Referral and re-deployment of workers with hearing loss/damage
Legal aspects	Statute and Common Law, legal liability. Likely legislation

hazard, i.e. the noise exposure of the individual workers. To obtain this knowledge a noise survey is necessary and it is appropriate here to outline the procedures involved.

NOISE MEASUREMENT

When the noise sources are static and operate continuously, as is often the case in factories with fixed machinery, it is necessary to use a sound level meter to 'map' the noise levels and record them on a plan of the area involved. The ordinary sound-level meter is designed to measure sound level in decibels (in almost all cases on the 'A' scale, known as dB(A)). The meter consists basically of a microphone, an amplifier, an attenuator to set the range of measurement, and a meter, pointer or digital, to display the resulting level. Meters can be divided into three categories: simple instrument 'indicators' (not meeting the British or International standards), 'industrial' (to BS 3489 and IEC 123), and 'precision' (to BS 4197 and IEC 179). The simple instruments are intended to provide a guide to levels, while industrial grade meters are appropriate to most noise measurement and evaluation carried out in industry. Precision grade meters offer a better standard of accuracy particularly if the noise source involves very high or low frequencies, and are especially valuable if noise levels are being measured for any legal purpose. Fig. 36.1 shows three meters, covering a range of prices from £50 for the cheapest indicator to over £1000 for a precision instrument.

As mentioned above, the sound-level meter is appropriate to the measurement of steady continuous noises, where it is simply set up in the sound field, and the indicated level is recorded. It may be noted that meters are normally calibrated with the microphone facing the sound source.

Where noise levels are variable, it is necessary to use a more sophisticated

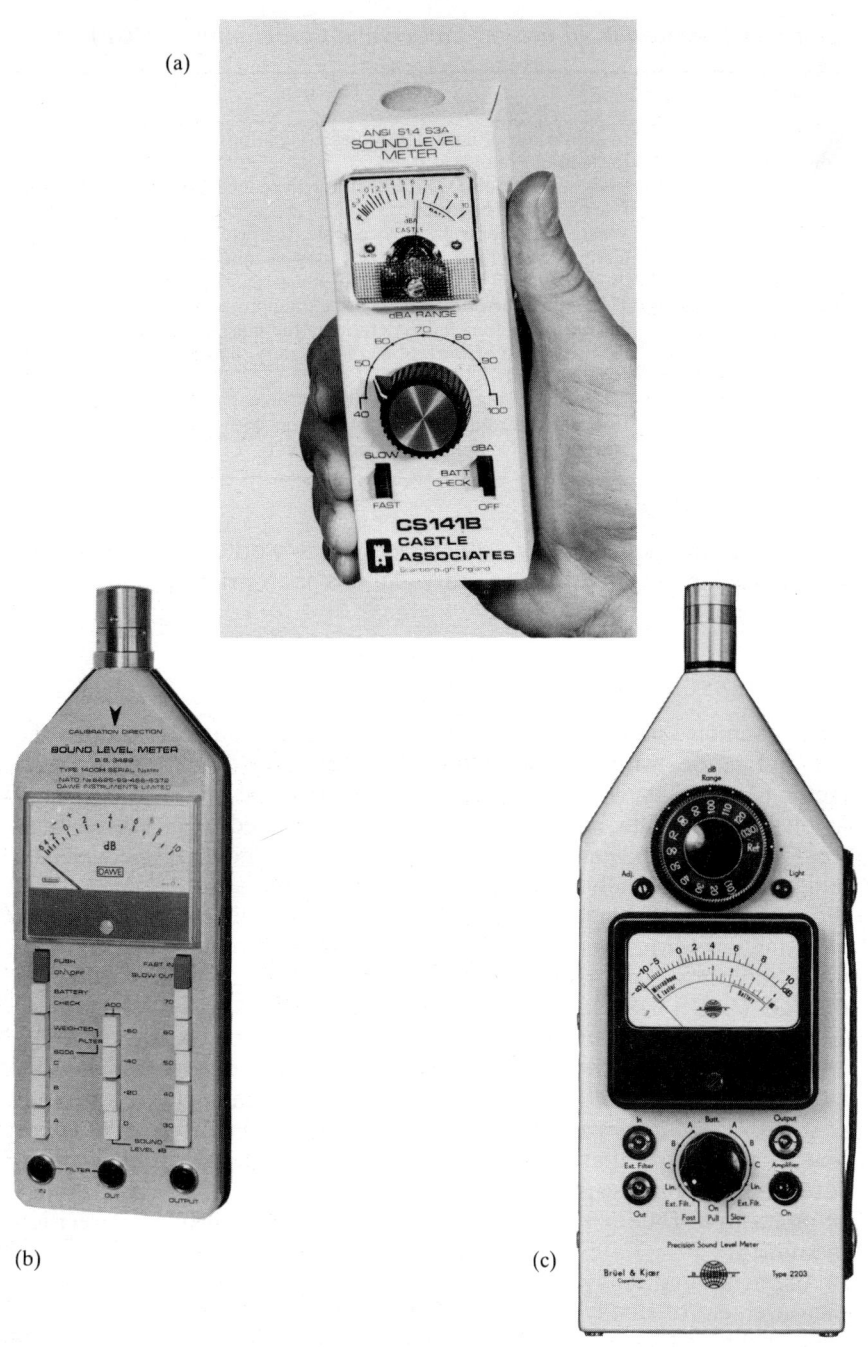

Fig. 36.1. (a). A small sound level meter to ANSI S1.4 S3A (Castle Associates). (b). An industrial grade sound level meter to BS 3489 (Dawe Instruments). (c). A precision grade sound level meter to BS4197 (Brüel and Kjaer).

instrument to obtain a measure of the average. In Britain (and other western European countries) this usually takes the form of an integrating or averaging meter, which measures the equivalent continuous dB(A) weighted level (Leq). Leq is the continuous steady-sound level which would feed as much (A-weighted) energy into the listener's ear as does the varying sound. An integrating meter can be used both for impact noises (such as hammering) and for noises with a cyclic or random variation which are often found in mechanized industrial processes.

Owing to their inherent complexity, integrating meters are necessarily more expensive than direct reading instruments, but since they will measure continuous, variable, or impact noise, they have a much wider utility. Some of the more sophisticated meters, an example of which is shown in Fig. 36.2, will operate as a direct-reading meter, and simultaneously compute the Leq level which is displayed digitally. Examples of situations in which an

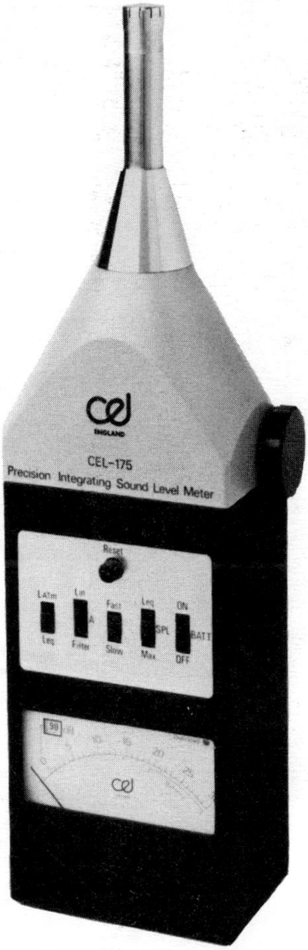

Fig. 36.2. A precision integrating sound level meter (Computer Engineering).

834   *Hearing conservation programmes*

integrating meter is essential are the measurement of the noise level from percussive tools, and from irregular hand-finishing procedures such as fettling, where the worker uses a series of different tools in succession.

With an integrating meter it is normally possible to obtain a measurement of the level of noise exposure by measuring one cycle of the process involved, however, there are cases where the cycle is very long, or the work rather variable, and it is necessary to measure over a long period. To meet this situation, noise dosimeters (Fig. 36.3) have been developed, which can

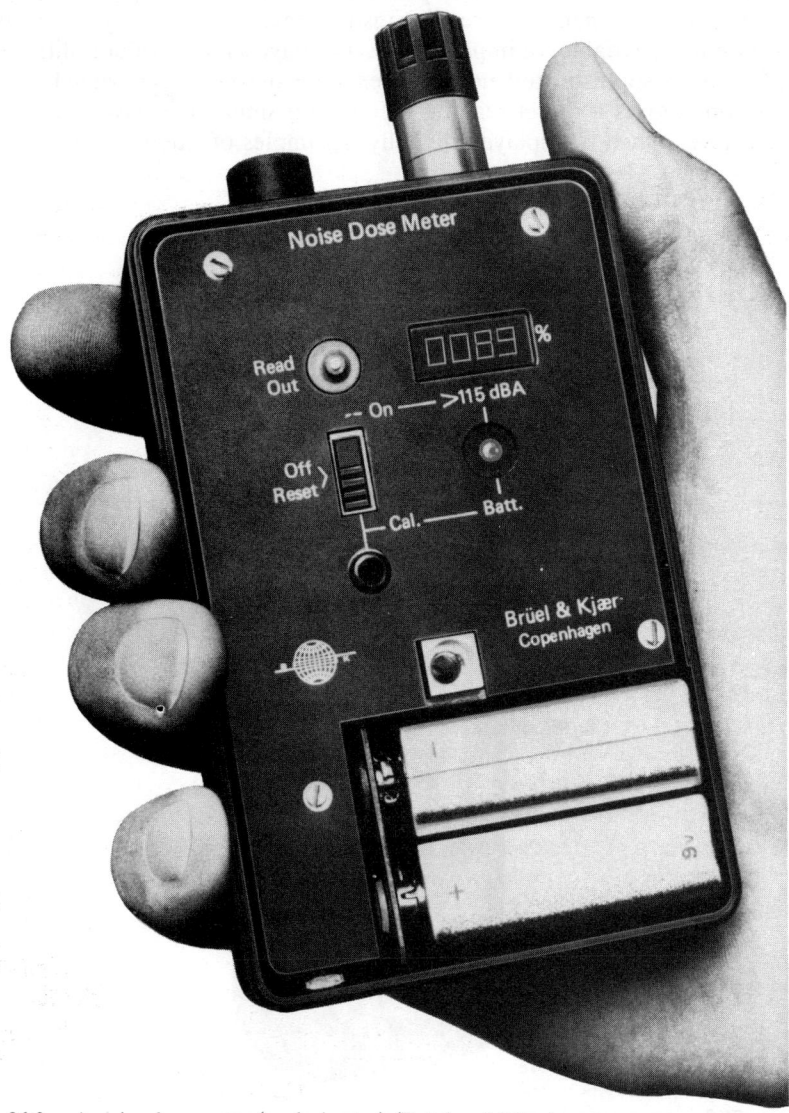

Fig. 36.3.   A noise dose meter (or dosimeter) (Brüel and Kjaer).

fit in the pocket, with a microphone mounted on the lapel or helmet. The dosimeter is designed to be worn for the full working day or shift and will indicate the total noise dose received at the end of this period.

Noise control

Noise control is the first, and most fundamental step in any hearing conservation programme. The basic approach to noise control is to reduce the noise at its source. This may pose a problem in mechanical, hydraulic, or aeronautical engineering, and is in general outside the scope of the present chapter.

Where the noise cannot be reduced at source some form of external noise reduction is required, and this can often be most effectively achieved by enclosure. To be effective, enclosure must be complete, and if the noise reduction is to be considerable, must be massive. For example to obtain a reduction of 45 dB a single brick wall (11 cm) or its equivalent in mass per unit area is needed. The principle of operation of the 'massive' enclosures is that rigid walls will reflect most of the sound back towards the source.

Where a noise source is totally enclosed, the increased reverberation of sound will increase the noise level within the enclosure. This will increase the hazard to those who must work within the enclosure, and also decrease the effectiveness of the enclosure itself. This can usually be remedied by the use of sound absorbent material inside to line the walls.

In many cases where a substantial noise reduction is required, the only practicable approach is enclosure, but it is sometimes better to apply this to the man rather than the machine, by providing 'sound-proof refuges' within the working environment.

The value of noise absorbing materials is, by comparison with enclosures, limited to those cases where a fairly modest improvement is required. It is rarely possible to reduce noise levels by more than 10 dB by the use of sound absorption. A further limitation to the value of absorbers mounted on walls and ceilings, is that they serve mainly to reduce the general level of reverberant sound in the room; they have very little effect on the noise level at the ears of the worker, who is close to the noise source. The question is often raised as to whether it is possible to reduce machinery noise by mounting 'absorbers' above the noise sources. In practice such 'absorbers' act like absorbent on walls and can achieve a modest reduction only.

A further technique to reduce noise is the use of 'screens', these can provide some reduction in noise (usually less than 15 dB) and to become more effective must be joined together to form a complete 'enclosure'.

The problem of reducing noise at source is primarily one for the manufacturers of machinery. It is discussed briefly in the *Code of Practice for Reducing the Exposure of Employed Persons to Noise* (Department of Employment 1972). It is understood that the draft of a much more detailed *Code of Practice on Machinery Noise* is to be released shortly and that this will contain proposals on the measurement of noise from machinery and the labelling of machines which can produce hazardous noise levels.

HEARING PROTECTION

Any firm with hazardous noise levels should attempt to reduce these using one or more of the methods outlined in the section on noise control. The use of personal hearing protection by means of plugs or muffs, together with monitoring audiometry is a 'second best' approach to the problem. Clearly some noisy processes do not lend themselves to noise control techniques. The use of hand tools such as in metal fabrication or forming, fall into this category. Effective reduction of noise levels can only be achieved by redesigning the process. An interesting example is the use of riveting for joining steel plates. This has been traditionally one of the worst sources of occupational hearing loss with levels often in excess of 115 dB(A). Fortunately the use of hot riveting in heavy steel fabrication has largely been replaced by welding which has lower levels of noise (around 85–105 dB(A)). Unfortunately in many situations noise reduction is not possible without redesigning the process and it is necessary to supply hearing protection to the workforce and to educate them in its use. It is a sad fact that although as long ago as 1886, Barr recommended that apprentices entering boilermaking in the Glasgow Shipyards should be advised by their foreman to wear hearing protection, this sensible advice is not always followed more than 90 years later. Barr considered both cotton wool smeared with Vaseline and the 'Ward Cousins' hollow india-rubber plug to be of value in protecting the hearing from noise.

It was not until the Second World War that the circumaural ear covering (muff) was developed in the UK by Mallock-Armstrong in conjunction with Rolls Royce Ltd. and the RAE Farnborough, for protection while testing jet-turbine aero engines (Anon 1946). Since then many more firms have begun manufacturing both muffs and plugs which have become lighter and more comfortable and able to give greater attenuation of unwanted sound.

Typically, modern plugs are suitable for protection in noise levels up to about 100–5 dB(A) while ear muffs are adequate in levels as high as 115–20 dB(A).* The use of plugs and muffs combined will give slightly greater protection still, but the theoretical maximum protection is around 40 dB and is determined by the transmission of sound to the inner ear through the temporal bone. The correct procedure for determining whether a particular type of protector is suitable for a given noise environment is set out in Appendix 4 of the Department of Employment's *Code of Practice for Reducing the Exposure of Employed Persons to Noise* (1972). This method requires the attenuation of the plug or muff to be known, as a function of frequency, and there is now a British Standard procedure by which this should be measured (British Standards Institution 1974). There is not, however, any standard for hearing protectors. Martin (1977) gives attenuation characteristics of 26 hearing protectors tested in accordance with the

---

* Some modern semi-disposable ear plugs, however, such as the EAR plug or the Decidamp are made of dense foam plastic which fit snugly into the ear canal and one size of plug fits almost all users. Their attenuation properties are as good as that of some ear muffs.

British Standard method. Perhaps the best known example of a non-disposable ear plug is the V51-R solid rubber plug manufactured by the Mines Safety Appliance Co. Ltd. since the late 1940s. This comes in five sizes, from extra small to extra large, and requires fitting by an experienced person. As well as the semi-disposable (EAR or Decidamp) type of plug mentioned above there is the personalized ear plug made of silicone rubber. These are made by curing a plug to fit each particular individual's ears. The oldest and possibly best known example of disposable ear plug is that made from fine glass-down and marketed as Bilsom Down. Originally the user had to make up his own plug, but this was wasteful of material and required a certain skill. Bilsom have, since 1971, marketed a pre-formed plug known as Bilsom Propp. A more recent innovation is the introduction of Bilsom Propp Plast with a thin plastic sheath covering the plug to prevent any tendency for it to break up in the ear canal.

Ear muffs consist of rigid plastic ear shells, filled with a foam lining to improve attenuation, a tensioning headband, and a soft seal, which helps the shell conform to the side of the head. This seal may either be of foam plastic or liquid filled (glycerine and water). The latter type of seal provides better attenuation but tends to be less robust and more expensive. Ear muffs can be obtained for fitting to safety helmets or for wearing with such protective head gear. They can also be fitted with a communication receiver, which can be a small radio receiver tuned to music or messages. One such system employs an inductive loop around the factory floor. There may be some slight loss of attenuation compared with conventional muffs but they are popular with the workforce, particularly the younger workers.

There is little doubt that there is considerable resistance to the wearing of hearing protection and strenuous efforts are required by safety staff to get a high rate of usage. Below are some of the reasons why it is difficult to persuade the work force to wear protection.

TABLE 36.3. *Workers objections to hearing protection*

Causes	Complaints
Physical discomfort (ear muffs)	Tension of headband Perspiration in hot environments Coldness with fluid seals
Poor communication (muffs and plugs)	Inability to hear machinery noise Inability to hear warning signals Difficulties in man-to-man communication Feeling of disorientation

There is little doubt that modern ear muffs are not as uncomfortable as some of the earlier types available, for instance, they tend to be lighter in weight. Muffs have been developed where the mechanical pressure decreases with time of wear. Perspiration is a real problem in some traditionally hot environments. Attempts have been made to overcome this by supplying a cloth cover for the seal.

On the communication side the problems of hearing protection are largely illusory. It has been found that it is possible to hear just as well, if not better, while wearing hearing protection in noise than when it is not worn. There is, however, a slight tendency for a speaker to lower the level of his voice (Martin, Howell, and Lower 1976), but perseverance in wearing protection should result in adaptation to the new condition. It is true that workers with existing hearing losses will have some small difficulty in communicating in noise (Linderman 1976) while wearing protection.

The above problems mean that it is absolutely essential that any members of a workforce who are required to wear hearing protection should have adequate instruction. This must include not only how to use the device but also how it should be maintained. There should also be checks to ensure that the protection is being worn correctly and is not damaged. Before the protection is issued the reasons for its use should be fully explained, and managers and supervisors should encourage its use by personal example. Visual aids, tape and slide programmes, and films are available for those safety staff organizing talks and seminars on the dangers of noise (Health and Safety Executive 1971). Section 7 of the *Code of Practice for Reducing the Exposure of Employed Persons to Noise* (Department of Employment 1972) lays down advice on the selection, inspection, and maintenance of ear protectors as well as stressing the need for education and joint consultation.

Any provision of hearing protection should be backed up by a programme of monitoring audiometry (Bryan and Tempest 1980). Not only does this provide an opportunity to check the effectiveness of the protection, but also enables the nurse, occupational hygienist, nursing sister, or doctor to explain to the worker, on a one-to-one basis, the risks he runs in not wearing protection. It will also be possible to put over the idea that the protection should be worn continuously in noise, and, unlike wearing safety spectacles, removal, even for a few minutes per day (Else 1973), does not slightly reduce the protection but can be enough to invalidate it for that day.

INDUSTRIAL AUDIOMETRY

There can be little doubt in the mind of anyone involved in the settlement of Common Law claims for hearing damage due to occupational noise exposure that if firms were engaged in the regular screening of their employees' hearing, very few of the claims would succeed or even be brought to court. All too often a firm carries out a noise survey, institutes what noise control is practical, and provides hearing protection, but no attempt is made to monitor the effectiveness of the hearing protection and consequently hearing losses are allowed to develop undetected until the firm and its insurers are involved in costs of £10 000s in defending and trying to refute such claims. On the other hand, any firm with an on-going audiometry programme of testing the hearing of their workers at risk can easily refute any charge that there has been any deterioration during their employment. A recent Common Law case concerning the hearing damage received by a docker was lost by the plaintiff because the firm was able to supply a pre-employment audiogram thus establishing there had been no deterioration of hearing in their employment.

It has long been accepted that industrial audiometry both in the UK and abroad is an integral part of any hearing conservation programme. This usually involves the determination of a base-line audiogram before employment and annually thereafter in order to detect any deterioration of hearing which may be occurring in those workers exposed to noise above 85–90 dB(A). Those persons showing a measurable deterioration should be referred to the Medical Officer, who then makes a decision whether it is necessary to move them to areas with lower noise levels, or whether they can be adequately protected without re-deployment.

Guidance on the categorization of audiograms of industrial workers is laid down in the HM Government's discussion document *Audiometry in Industry* (Health and Safety Executive 1978).

Industrial audiometry is essentially the screening of the hearing of the workforce at risk, carried out by pure-tone air conduction testing.† It might seem more logical to use speech audiometry as we are essentially concerned with the measurement of handicap in the understanding of speech. However, speech audiometry is not, at present, sufficiently standardized as to procedure, use of material, or assessment of results to make it the preferred method of assessment. Noise damage does not produce a characteristic speech audiogram as is the case in pure-tone audiometry. Fig. 36.4 shows a typical pure-tone audiogram obtained in a noisy industry for a 60-year-old press operator who has worked in noise levels of 95–100 dB(A)(Leq) for 27 years. There is extensive hearing damage above 2 kHz maximal around 6–8 kHz. This man has a slight handicap for understanding speech under noisy conditions (Tempest 1977). The growth of hearing damage with noise exposure is illustrated in Fig. 36.5 which shows the mean audiogram for groups of female workers who have spent different periods from 1–2 years to 35–9 years in noise levels of 101 dB(A). The loss occurs after 1–2 years, initially around 4 kHz, and spreads to lower and higher frequencies with increasing exposure (Taylor, Pearson, Mair, and Burns 1965). This figure excludes the loss of hearing due to presbycusis, which is usually additive to the hearing damage and results in increased handicap in the fifth decade of life onwards. Because we are essentially concerned with the earliest detection of loss and deterioration due to noise the highest accuracy is required in industrial audiometry. Frequent calibration of the audiometer and careful

---

† This may be carried out using either a manual or self-recording audiometer. Both methods if employed correctly should give identical results and neither method has been shown to be superior in accuracy (Bryan and Tempest 1976). The choice of type of audiometer used is determined by the number of workers which is to be tested per year. Generally a throughput of more than 200–300 audiograms each year would be carried out by use of self-recording audiometers.

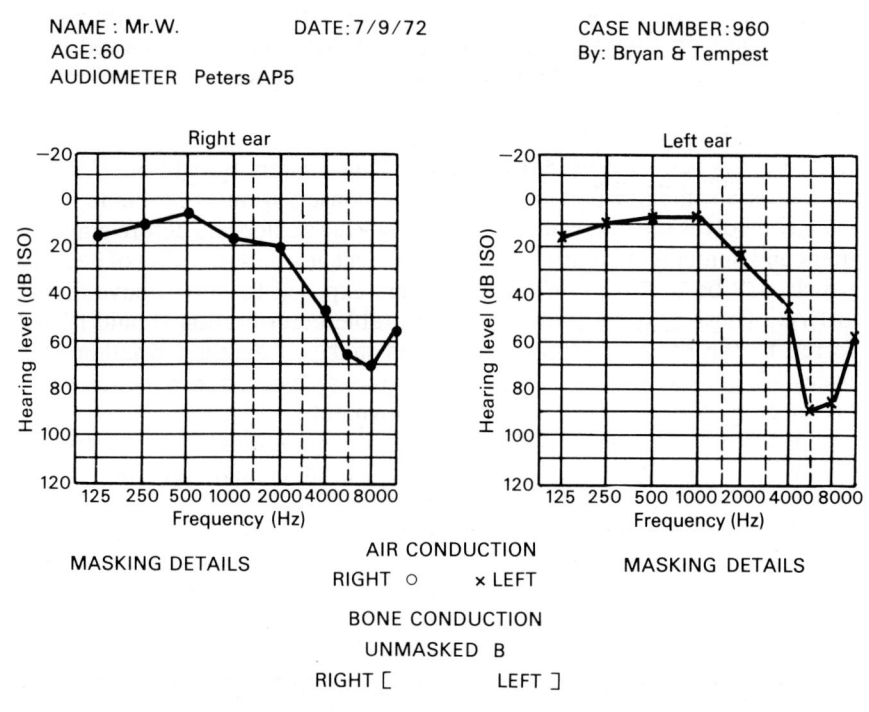

Fig. 36.4. The pure-tone audiogram of a 60-year-old man who has spent 27 years working in noise levels of 95–100 dB(A).

control of ambient noise in which the testing is carried out are essential. Guidance on these matters is given both in *Industrial audiometry* (Bryan and Tempest 1976) and *Audiometry in industry* (Health and Safety Executive 1978). Usually it will be necessary to carry out testing in an acoustic booth (Fig. 36.6) because the noise levels in industrial medical centres are rarely low enough to enable audiometric thresholds to be determined down to 0 dB re ISO zero.

Good testing technique is of equal importance to adequate calibration procedures and environmental control. Therefore if a firm's medical staff are to carry out the screening, as is usually the case, they should have received adequate training in all aspects of industrial audiometry. This should include not only practical experience in obtaining audiograms, but lectures on care and maintenance of equipment, assessment of audiograms, and also on other aspects of hearing conservation. Several universities and other institutions now run such training courses and the British Society of Audiology have prepared a syllabus to which such courses generally conform. The setting up of audiometric test facilities probably costs (at 1979 prices) of the order of £2400–3600. It is difficult to estimate the actual overall cost when industrial medical staff are used in the programme, and clearly

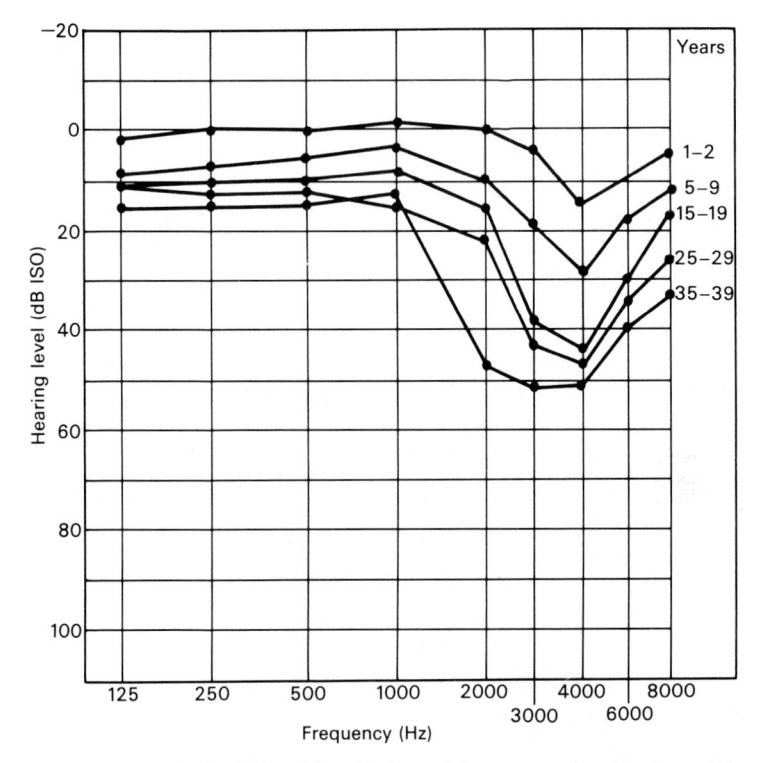

Fig. 36.5. Growth of noise-induced hearing loss with exposure time in a group of weavers exposed to 101 dB(A). (From Taylor et al. 1965.)

one of the factors which has to be taken into account is loss of production while workers are being tested.

Smaller firms may prefer to contract out to outside organizations the screening of their workforce. A number of commercial organizations specialize in carrying out industrial audiometry on a contract basis on their clients' premises using mobile testing facilities. At 1979 prices the cost of such services are around £10/man/audiogram.

Current progress

It is unfortunate that, despite all the above knowledge, the establishment of hearing conservation programmes in this country has been very slow indeed, and it is perhaps only in the last decade that most large firms have taken effective action. That knowledge and liability for protecting the workers hearing exists in industry (Bryan and Tempest 1971) is evidenced by the fact that since 1972, many thousands of them have successfully made Common Law claims against their employers (and insurers) for occupational hearing loss. Indeed, many more claims are to be expected as it has been estimated that some one million workers in the UK labour in levels in excess of the

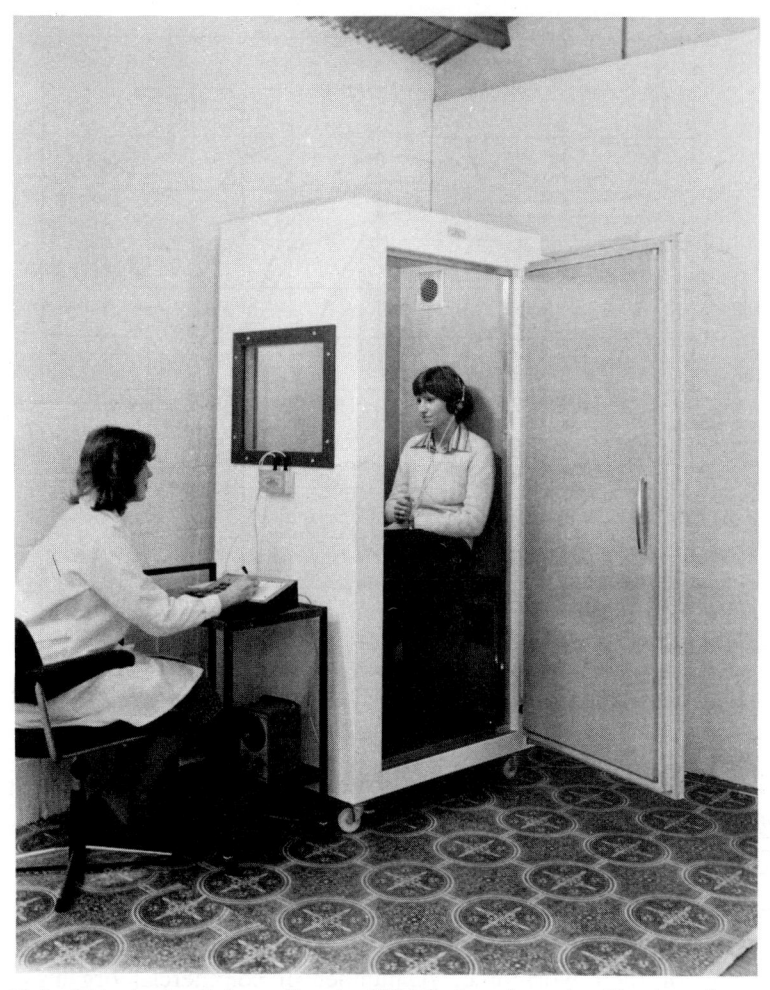

Fig. 36.6. Listening booth for audiometry (Whittingham Acoustics, Manchester).

commonly accepted safe level of 90 dB, and we find typically half of these, whose hearing we assess, have marked hearing damage and some handicap.

Legal aspects

The law becomes involved in industrial noise in two ways: through laws and regulations designed to control and reduce noise, and through the payment of compensation to those whose hearing has been destroyed by noise. This latter topic is dealt with in another section of this book, and the present discussion is concerned only with the former aspect.

The Health and Safety at Work Act

The Health and Safety at Work Act (1974) imposes general duties on employers etc. to take action to ensure the health and safety of persons at work. In this respect it follows the lines of the previous Factories Acts and does not make explicit legal requirements on noise control. The Factories Acts, and now the Health and Safety at Work Act, are frequently referred to in common law actions for compensation for occupational deafness, since a breach of the Acts may be regarded as evidence of negligence. However, the specific question of whether the Acts can be correctly construed as including a prohibition on hazardous noise levels has never been fully tested in Court.

For one occupation only, the Woodworking Machinery Regulations were made in 1974, giving legal force to a series of provisions in general similar to those proposed in the *Code of Practice for Reducing the Exposure of Employed Persons to Noise.*

In 1974, when the woodworking regulations came into force, some consideration had already been given to the question of general noise legislation applying to all occupations. This led to the publication of a report by the Industrial Health Advisory Sub-committee on Noise entitled, *Framing Noise Legislation.* This report recommended legislation under the Health and Safety at Work Act, which would, in general, follow the lines of the Code of Practice. It would include obligations on employees to wear ear protection in situations where this was necessary. It would also oblige machinery designers, manufacturers, importers etc to provide a warning to purchasers if their machines were likely to produce hazardous noise.

At the time of writing (1979) no date for noise legislation has been announced, although it is reported that discussions are in progress between various interested parties. It has also been suggested in some circles, that the 90 dB(A) criterion, recommended in the *Code of Practice* and in *Framing Noise Legislation*, might be lowered, in order to provide a greater degree of protection.

'The Code of Practice'

In 1972 the Department of Employment issued the *Code of Practice for Reducing the Exposure of Employed Persons to Noise* (Department of Employment 1972). Although not possessing the force of law, this is a most valuable guide to some aspects of hearing conservation. It sets out a number of recommendations. Basically they are:
  (i) That the aim should be to reduce noise exposure by noise control.
  (ii) When this is not practical, that ear protectors should be provided and their use ensured.
  (iii) That areas with hazardous noise levels should be identified and marked.
  (iv) That employed persons should use and maintain the measures adopted for noise control and (if appropriate) use ear protectors when provided.

In addition the *Code of Practice* sets a maximum acceptance level for continuous exposure of 90 dB(A) for an eight-hour day, together with appropriate equivalent levels for shorter and longer exposures. The Code is also careful to point out that 90 dB(A) is not a 'desirable' sound level, and that, where it is reasonably practicable it is desirable for sound to be reduced to lower levels.

REFERENCES

ANON. (1946). Aural protection, defence of the ear against jet-turbine noise. *Aircraft Production.* August 6.
—— (1954). *Annual Report Chief Inspector of Factories.* Cmnd. 9605. HMSO, London.
—— (1974). *The Woodworking Machinery Regulations.* Statutory Instrument No. 903/1974. HMSO, London.
BARR, T. (1886). Enquiry into the effects of loud sounds upon the hearing of boilermakers and others who work amid noisy surroundings. *Proc. Glasgow Phil. Soc.* **17**, 223.
BRITISH STANDARDS INSTITUTION (1962). *Sound level meters (industrial grade).* BS 3486 and Amnd. 4825 (1963).
—— (1967). *A precision sound level meter.* BS 4197 and Amnd. 1871 (1976).
—— (1974). *Method of measurement of attenuation of hearing protectors at threshold.* BS 5108.
BRYAN, M. E. and TEMPEST, W. (1971). In Noise damage liability—evidence as to the state of knowledge. *Occupational hearing loss* (ed. D. W. Robinson) p. 143. Academic Press, London.
—— and —— (1980). *Industrial audiometry.* Bryan and Tempest, Noise Consultants, 469 Walshaw Road, Bury, Lancs.
BURNS, W. and ROBINSON, D. W. (1970). *Hearing and noise in industry.* HMSO, London.
COLLIER, H. E. (1940). *Outlines of industrial medical practice.* Edward Arnold, London.
DEPARTMENT OF EMPLOYMENT (1972). *Code of practice for reducing the exposure of employed persons to noise.* HMSO, London.
DICKSON, E. D. D., EWING, A. W. G., and LITTLER, T. S. (1939). The effects of aeroplane noise on the auditory acuity of aviators. *J. Lar. Otol.* **54**, 531.
ELSE, D. (1973). A note on the protection afforded by hearing protectors. *Ann. occup. Hyg.* **10**, 415.
HEALTH AND SAFETY EXECUTIVE (1971). *Noise and the worker.* Health and Safety at Work, Booklet 25. HMSO, London.
—— (1974). *Framing noise legislation.* HMSO, London.
—— (1978). *Audiometry in industry.* Discussion Document. HMSO, London.
INTERNATIONAL ELECTROTECHNICAL COMMISSION (1961). *Recommendations for sound level meters*, Publication 123. Geneva.
—— (1973). *Precision sound level meters*, Publication 179. Geneva.
LINDEMAN, H. E. (1976) Speech intelligibility and the use of hearing protectors. *Audiology* **15**, 348.
MCLACHLAN, N. W. (1935). *Noise, a comprehensive survey from every point of view.* Oxford University Press.
MARTIN, A. M. (1977). The acoustic attenuation characteristics of 26 hearing protectors evaluated following the British Standard Procedure. *Ann. occup. Hyg.* **20**, 229.
—— HOWELL, K., and LOWER, M. C. (1976). In Hearing protection and com-

munication in noise. *Disorders of auditory function* (ed. S. D. G. Stephens) Vol. II, p. 48, Academic Press, London.

PASSCHIER-VERMEER, W. (1968). *Hearing loss due to exposure to steady-state broad-band noise*. Report 35, Institute for Public Health Engineering TNO, Netherlands.

ROGER, T. R. (1915). Noise-deafness: a review of recent experimental work and a clinical investigation as to the effects of loud noise upon the labyrinth of boilermakers. *J. Lar. Rhinol. Otol.* **30**, 91.

SAPPINGTON, C. O. (1943). *Essentials of industrial health*, J. B. Lippincott, Philadelphia.

TAYLOR, W., PEARSON, J., MAIR, A., and BURNS, W. (1965). Studies of noise and hearing in jute weaving. *J. acoust. Soc. Am.* **38**, 113.

TEMPEST, W. (1977). The assessment of hearing handicap. *J. Soc. occup. Med.* **27**, 134.

WESTMACOTT, F. H. (1925). Discussion on occupational diseases of the ear, nose and throat and their prevention. *Br. med. J.* **ii**, 886.

37 Industrial hearing loss: compensation in the United Kingdom

W. TEMPEST and M. E. BRYAN

INTRODUCTION

In the United Kingdom, there are three possible routes to compensation for noise-induced hearing loss. One of these, the compensation of servicemen for hearing loss sustained in the Armed Forces, is outside the scope of the present discussion. The other routes are an action at Common Law for damages, which is open to all workers, and Industrial Injuries Compensation, which is payable only to certain employees who have been employed in the prescribed occupations.

The basis of the Common Law actions is the principle that damages are awarded for injuries which arise owing to negligence, and the various stages in the procedure can be summarized as follows: The plaintiff must first establish that he has suffered some loss, this means a significant loss of the ability to hear, resulting in a handicap, and may further include a direct financial loss (i.e. a loss of earnings). The establishment of loss of hearing normally relies primarily on a medical opinion, plus the plaintiff's own description of the degree of handicap. A loss of earnings claim will usually result from the fact that the claimant has been dismissed or moved to a quieter occupation in order to protect him from further hearing damage, and has therefore suffered a loss of wages. In some instances a plaintiff may argue that he has voluntarily changed his employment to protect his hearing, or that he has refused promotion because his hearing loss would have prevented him from properly coping with the duties that promotion would entail.

The medical evidence, that the hearing loss is due to noise, must in many cases be supported by evidence as to the level of noise experienced during employment, and this noise exposure needs to be related as accurately as possible to the degree of hearing loss.

If it can be successfully established that the hearing loss is due to noise, and that the noise exposure occurred at work, then the first two stages of the claim have been completed. The next stage is to establish that a degree of negligence existed on the part of the employer in permitting the noise exposure to occur, and in failing to protect the employee from its effects. To prove negligence, it is necessary to show that the defendant had knowledge of the hazard, or at least if he did not himself have knowledge, that a reasonable and prudent employer would have had knowledge. If the case refers only to the last few years, then it is easily established that knowledge of industrial noise and its effects was widespread throughout industry, as was knowledge of protective measures such as ear plugs and ear muffs. In such a case it is not likely that the evidence of negligence would be seriously contested. If, however, the claim refers to a much longer period of time, say 20 to 30 years, then it becomes increasingly difficult to establish that employers were cognisant of noise and its effects. In such a case it may be successfully argued that no liability exists for the earlier part of the period of exposure, and any damages awarded will be reduced accordingly.

If the action reaches the stage that loss has been established, that it is due to noise at work, and that the employer has been negligent, then it will normally result in the award of damages, assessed according to the degree of handicap incurred. One important issue which often arises is that of contributory negligence. If hearing protection has been made available, but not worn regularly, then it can be argued that the plaintiff has, to some extent, failed to protect himself, and that his award should be reduced. The contributory negligence concept is well established, and often applied in accident cases generally.

The brief outline given above is intended to give an overall view of the main features of Common Law actions for occupational deafness. It is perhaps appropriate here to look in a little more detail at some of the features of the system.

The role of the medical consultant

The medical evidence is normally provided by an ear, nose, and throat consultant, who examines the plaintiff and provides an opinion as to the extent of any hearing loss and its cause. The diagnosis is initially based on the pure-tone audiogram, which, if a diagnosis of NIHL is to be supported, must show at least a fair resemblance to the classic shape, with a 'notch' in the 4–6 kHz region of frequency. The degree of resemblance required to sustain the diagnosis is clearly a matter of professional judgement, based largely on experience. If the audiogram is typical of noise-induced loss, then the rest of the diagnosis is mainly a process of elimination. Audiological tests, such as bone conduction, speech, and impedance audiometry can be used to investigate any conductive element in the loss. Other standard tests can be used if a retrocochlear lesion is suspected. An examination of the patient will give some evidence as to any former or active disease. A detailed medical history should bring out any history of disease in childhood, or any hereditary factors, and of any injury to the head or ears. The medical history (with medical records, if available) may show whether any ototoxic drugs have ever been administered.

If all the evidence points towards noise as the most probable cause of hearing loss, the doctor is often faced with the problem of trying to relate the loss to the noise exposure in present or past employment, or possibly during other exposure, for example during military service. The evaluation of the audiogram must also consider the extent to which presbycusis will have contributed to the hearing loss.

In practice, the quantitative evaluation of the audiogram is, for the otologist, very difficult, since there is rarely sufficient data available as to the levels of noise exposure. At this point it is often necessary to call upon the services of a noise consultant to measure and/or estimate the plaintiff's exposure to noise.

THE ROLE OF THE NOISE CONSULTANT

The task of the noise consultant is to obtain the best possible estimate of the noise exposure experienced by the claimant in the course of his work. In most cases this begins with a visit to the place of work, and a direct measurement of the noise levels. If these are steady and continuous, this will require only a sound level meter, while for variable level and impact noises some form of integrating meter will be needed. In some instances the direct measurement of noise levels is not possible since the process has been discontinued and a best estimate must be obtained by reference to data obtained elsewhere, or by reference to published data.

The noise data, together with a detailed employment history, makes it possible to calculate the total noise exposure received during employment, and, if necessary, to apportion this exposure between different employers or periods of employment.

The task of relating the total noise exposure to the measured hearing loss has been greatly facilitated by the publication, in 1970, of the report *Hearing and Noise in Industry* by Burns and Robinson. This work, which was based on an extensive study of hearing loss and noise exposure, put forward the concept of a 'noise immission level' (NIL) to provide a single-figure measure of total noise exposure over a period of time. The NIL is defined by:

$$\text{NIL} = L_A + 10 \log_{10} T$$

where L_A = noise level in dB(A) and T = exposure duration in years. Defined in this way NIL is a logarithmic unit which evaluates the total A-weighted noise energy to which the ear has been subjected in the period of time T. The definition of NIL can be easily extended to take into account different noise levels for different periods of time. The concept of NIL was based on the experimental findings, in their survey, that the main determinant of hearing loss was the noise immission level, since a short exposure to high noise levels gave the same hearing loss as a larger exposure to a lower level if the two exposures were equal in terms of NIL.

Starting from a value for NIL, Burns and Robinson's data permit a calculation of the expected NIHL audiogram for a person of average liability to noise damage, or for a person with any specified degree of susceptibility above or below the average. Susceptibility is expressed in the form of a percentile distribution, 1 per cent implying an extremely high liability to damage, and 99 per cent an extremely low liability. In addition to the NIHL term, the calculation includes a term to take into account presbycusis.

With the aid of Burns and Robinson's data it is quite practicable to make a judgement as to whether the measured audiogram is reasonably compatible with the noise exposure history. Other valuable data on the relationship between noise exposure and hearing loss are available in the report by Passchier-Vermeer (1968).

LIABILITY

The establishment of negligence on the part of the employer relies largely on the plaintiff showing that, at the time of his injury, it was recognized that loss of hearing and resulting handicap could result from the noise associated with his occupation, and that his employer either knew of the hazard, or, as a reasonable employer should have been aware of it. It is also highly relevant to his case if the plaintiff can show that action (e.g. noise reduction, personal protection, or audiometric tests) could have been taken to prevent his hearing being damaged.

These questions of the state of knowledge of the hazard, and of practical steps to counteract it, must be decided largely by reference to the relevant literature and it is appropriate briefly to survey this topic.

Knowledge

It has long been known among medical men at least, that in certain trades and professions, the workers became permanently hard of hearing and that this is due to the intense noise levels involved. It was noted by Bernardino Ramazzini, the father of occupational medicine, in 1713 that deafness was an occupational hazard of millers who 'were hard of hearing due to the noise of wheels and millstones and coppersmiths grew completely deaf when they were old'. Charles Turner Thackrah, a Leeds clinician, who decided to devote his life to studying preventive medicine, wrote in 1831 that he found deafness among ships' carpenters, frizzers (who worked up the nap on cloth), and shear grinders. The *Lancet* of 1830–1 contained the observations of Dr John Fosbroke that deafness is caused by sudden explosion of cannon and by continued noise, such as blacksmith's deafness. In 1886 Barr reported that only 9 per cent of the boilermakers (riveters, caulkers, platers, and 'holders on') he studied in the Glasgow shipyards, had normal hearing compared with 79 per cent of letter carriers (postmen) and 46 per cent of iron moulders (foundrymen). Roger examined some 48 cases of occupational deafness in 1915. Two were blacksmiths, one an engineer (locomotive driver?), one a brass finisher, and the remaining 44 were boilermakers and riveters. The hearing was below normal in 85–95 per cent of these cases while 56 per cent gave a history of tinnitus and 10 per cent of giddiness. The fact that deafness was caused by certain occupations was first mentioned by the factory inspectorate in 1908 (Anon 1908). Besides citing boilermaking this report also stated that deafness was brought on by the conditions of employment prevalent in the occupations of hammering metal sheets and cylinders, use of pneumatic tools, the beetling of cloth, engine driving, and firing guns. McKelvie found nerve deafness or noise deafness in 6.7 per cent of 1101 Lancashire weavers. No cases were found in those working for less than ten years while 30.1 per cent of those with 41 to 50 years of service were deaf (Anon 1927).

Animal experiments by Wittmaack (1907) and Yoshii (1909) had established at the beginning of the twentieth century, that noise deafness is due to the degeneration of the organ of Corti in the inner ear. Thus by the time occupational diseases of the ear, nose, and throat were discussed, at the meeting of the section of Laryngology, Otology, and Rhinology of the British Medical Association, in 1925 (Westmacott 1925) a good deal of evidence was available among the medical profession as to the occupations involved, the characteristics, and the site of lesion of industrial hearing loss. Consequently, most general medical textbooks, those specializing in diseases of the ear, nose, and throat, and those on diseases of occupation made at least passing reference to occupational hearing loss from about that time. See for instance, Bezold and Siebenmann (1908), Legge (1934), Ballenger and Ballenger (1938), Collier (1940), and Scott Stevenson (1943). However, it is another matter as to the date at which the lay person became aware of the hazards of working in intense noise. It could be argued that in those occupations traditionally regarded as deafening the hazard was well known to the workers. Certainly there is evidence that they have always attempted to protect their hearing by plugging up their ears with wool, india rubber, or plasticine (Barr 1886; Chippendale 1866; Anon 1908; Roger 1915; Westmacott 1925), though it would seem that the employees were more concerned with reducing the painful sensation of the noise rather than in preventing destruction of the hearing.

It is common usage to describe a loud noise as being 'deafening'! This may or may not be implying an awareness by the public of the hazard to hearing of excessive levels of noise. By the 1930s there must have been some knowledge by the general public that excessive noise caused deafness. Walter Greenwood, wrote in 1933, in his classic novel of working-class life in Salford, *Love on the Dole*, of a local forge that the thump of a forging hammer made one giddy and that the din in the riveting shop was insufferable. He goes on to add that every man was stone deaf after a spell of six months there! The *Cassell's Modern Encyclopaedia* (Hammerton 1935) mentions, under the entry for 'deafness', that 'Occupational deafness accounts for many cases of nerve deafness.'

In the United Kingdom the public's interest in noise was aroused by, among other things, the growth in the number of motor vehicles on the roads in the 1930s. The then Minister of Transport appointed a Technical Committee under the chairmanship of Sir Henry Fowler and the Anti-Noise League was formed under the chairmanship of Lord Horder (McLachlan 1935). Several non-medical text books on noise were published in this period (Bartlett 1934; McLachlan 1935; Davis 1937). All three dealt with occupational deafness due to noise.

However it was not until after the Second World War that concern about ever increasing levels of noise both in the environment but particularly at work led first to articles in the press (Evans 1947; Anon 1953; Challen and Hickish 1958; Anon 1955a; Anon 1955b) and to questions and a debate (1953, 513, 1101) in Parliament (Parliamentary Debates, 1955, 546, 2665). This was followed by government action in setting up the Wilson committee on noise which reported in 1963 (Committee on the Problem of Noise 1963). This led, as far as occupational deafness is concerned, to the publication, by the Ministry of Labour, of a guide to employers, *Noise and the worker* (1963), where advice was given on how to recognize and deal with a noise problem along the lines laid down in the Chapter 36 of this book. It would not be unreasonable to put the date of knowledge of the responsible layman, with regard to the hazard to hearing from excessive noise, in the period of the late 1950s to the early 1960s (Bryan and Tempest 1971).

PRACTICAL STEPS

In Chapter 36 we outlined the development of the means to detect hazardous noise levels, to introduce noise control procedures, to provide hearing protection, and to carry out screening audiometry. Personal protection by way of ear plugs has been in use since the end of the nineteenth century (Chippendale 1866; Barr 1886) and available commercially from Mallock-Armstrong from the First World War onwards in the form of their ear defender. This was available in seven sizes and while primarily intended for protection against gun fire, it was also advertised as supplied to aircraft, motor-engine, and boiler works. Although we understand these ear plugs were used by ship's propeller chippers in the 1930s, where the noise levels were in the 120–130 dB(A) region, the use of hearing protection was not generally taken up by industry until after the Second World War. Despite this it was possible for Dickson, Ewing, and Littler in 1939 to measure the attenuation given by several different types of ear protection. They were concerned with the hazards to aviators from aeroplane noise and not only gave details of measurement of noise levels from aero engines but also audiograms showing the typical 4 kHz 'notch'. This illustrated the point that as well as hearing protection both sound level meters and audiometers were available in the 1930s. Hazardous noise from such sources as riveting, boilermaking, and aero engines had been measured and it was known what levels were hazardous (McLachlan 1935; Sappington 1943; Davis 1937). However, it was not until after the Second World War that we find evidence in the UK of industry instigating hearing conservation programmes (Anon 1954; Davies 1962).

Since the early 1950s there has been a steady and welcome increase in interest amongst larger companies in carrying out noise control and hearing conservation programmes. This would appear to bear out an opinion expressed in 1971 (Bryan and Tempest 1971) that a large firm employing specialists to look after the health of its employees should have become aware of the hazard to hearing from noise no later than the early 1950s. This would be particularly true of those firms in the traditionally noisy industries involving such operations as riveting, stamping, forging, chipping, and weaving.

Those firms with no medical officer or safety officer would seem to have to be judged against a background of general knowledge. It would be increasingly difficult for an employer to put up a convincing defence of ignorance towards the end of the 1950s. It seems very likely that by 1963 all but the smallest firms would have had the dangers of noise brought to their notice and consequently would be liable under Common Law.

The small firm, employing less than several hundred men, and using some new noisy process, might be able to put up a convincing demonstration of ignorance into the late 1960s. But their credibility would be small since the activities of the Factory Inspectorate and the publication in 1972 of the government's *Code of Practice for Reducing the Exposure of Employed Persons to Noise* (Department of Employment 1972).

COMMON LAW ACTIONS HEARD IN COURT

Owing to the high cost of litigation, only a very limited number of cases have been heard in the English courts. Not all cases are reported, but it seems likely that the total does not exceed ten to date. The first, and one of the most important cases was that of Berry v. Stone Manganese Marine. Mr Berry was by occupation a propeller chipper and had worked in noise levels of 115–20 dB(A) for 15 years. He had suffered a substantial hearing loss and in the hearing it was not disputed that his loss was due to his exposure to occupational noise. The defendants accepted that, in this very noisy occupation knowledge of the hazard to hearing was current as far back as 1957. The case was a fairly long and complex one, the major line of defence being that hearing protection, firstly plugs and later muffs, had been offered to the defendant, who had failed to wear them regularly. Judgment was given for Mr Berry and damages were assessed at £2500 (in 1971). No reduction was made for contributory negligence on the part of Mr Berry but, due to the Limitations Acts, only half the assessed damages were awarded and the plaintiff received £1250 for the hearing loss incurred since April 1967.

The other case of particular interest was heard in 1975. In this action Mr McCafferty claimed damages from the Metropolitan Police. Mr McCafferty had been employed as a ballistics expert and was frequently required to test-fire various guns, revolvers, sawn-off shotguns, etc. He was employed by the Police in London from 1965, and in 1973, after a routine audiometric test showed signs of severe acoustic trauma, his employment was prematurely terminated when he was only 58. He brought an action against his employers, claiming damages for loss of hearing and for loss of earnings owing to his premature retirement. The main issues in the case were those of negligence by the employer and contributory negligence on the part of Mr McCafferty. The Judge concluded that, before 1965, the dangers of damage to hearing from gunfire were known to the armed services, and information could have been obtained from them. It was contested by the defence that the plaintiff was himself negligent, as a ballistics expert, in failing to make enquiries about hearing hazard when the test-firing range was being designed. This contention was rejected and Mr McCafferty was awarded a total of £10 000, comprising £850 for hearing loss and tinnitus, and £9150 for loss of salary due to premature retirement. The Metropolitan Police subsequently appealed against this award, but the appeal was rejected.

A recent case heard in Manchester (John Bailey v. ICI Ltd., Manchester Crown Court 1979) resulted in a man being awarded an additional element of damages for the possibility that his future employment prospects might be worsened by his hearing handicap. In this instance Mr Bailey, aged 35 years, was awarded £7000 for his loss of hearing plus a further £1500 for what the Judge described as 'a sort of single payment' insurance premium in case there is any possibility of error on my part in assessing the Plaintiff's future.'

While English cases are almost invariably heard by a single Judge, civil actions in Northern Ireland are usually heard before a jury, which is responsible both for deciding liability and assessing the amount of damages. The Northern Irish procedure often leads to much higher awards than the English, and several cases have gone to trial in Northern Ireland. In one of these, Darby v. Short Bros. and Harland and the Ministry of Aviation Supply (1972) the plaintiff received £27 000 (which included a substantial award for loss of potential earnings). Other more recent cases have followed the same pattern of high awards.

OUT-OF-COURT SETTLEMENTS

Large numbers of claims for occupational deafness are now being put forward, mainly in the heavy industries, and at least 99 per cent are settled out of Court. The current level of awards is in the range £600 to about £6000. Many of these cases are negotiated in batches and a number of 'grouping schemes' have been put forward, or are in process of negotiation. In a large proportion of these claims there is no dispute about the liability or the level of noise, and a medical report is all that is needed to support the case.

HISTORY OF COMPENSATION UNDER STATUTE LAW

Compensation for occupational hearing loss resulting from boilermaking noise was considered as long ago as 1907 in the United Kingdom by the departmental committee on Compensation for Industrial Diseases. The committee commented that Boilermaker's Deafness was unquestionably an injury due to employment and was widely prevalent among men working in the incessant noise of the shipbuilding yards or the boilermakers' shop (from the use of pneumatic hammers for riveting and boring holes). It did not, however, prevent a man from continuing at his trade and it could not therefore give rise to claims for compensation on the grounds of incapacitation.

Under the 1946 National Insurance (Industrial Injuries) Act it was no longer necessary for a worker to be incapacitated by a disease from his employment to be awarded compensation. In future social disability was adequate grounds for compensation. So diseases such as occupational deafness became eligible under the Act though in fact it was not until 1975 that it became a prescribed disease. (Department of Health and Social Security 1974.)

At the end of 1962, the Minister of Pensions and National Insurance announced in the House of Commons that he had agreed to give financial sponsorship to the extent of £65 000 to a programme of research into the effects of industrial noise on workers' hearing (Anon 1962). This followed a recommendation of the Industrial Injuries Advisory Council. The Medical Research Council and the National Physical Laboratory were allocated the responsibility and the research was conducted under the leadership of Dr D W Robinson of the National Physical Laboratory and Professor W Burns of Charing Cross Hospital Medical School. The exact terms of reference are set out in their report *Hearing a Noise in Industry* (Burns and Robinson 1970) already mentioned.

In October 1969 the Secretary of State for Social Services asked the Industrial Injuries Advisory Council to consider whether there were degrees of hearing loss due to noise which satisfied the conditions for prescription under the National Insurance (Industrial Injuries) Act of 1965. The Council's report (Department of Health and Social Security 1973) was presented to Parliament in October 1973. The findings of the Joint MRC/NPL Survey (Burns and Robinson 1970) led directly to the enquiry by the Council and it duly recommended in the report that occupational deafness should be prescribed under the Industrial Injuries Act and that the scheme should be started as soon as possible. The scheme was to apply only to a limited number of processes in the metal manufacturing and shipbuilding and repairing industries.

From 3 February 1975 disablement benefit became payable for deafness resulting from noise at work. (Department of Health and Social Security 1974). On this date a 'limited scheme' was brought into effect and applied only to three occupations. These were defined as occupations involving: (i) the use of pneumatic percussive tools or high-speed grinding tools in the cleaning, dressing, or finishing of cast metal or of ingots, billets, or blooms; or (ii) the use of pneumatic percussive tools on metal in the shipbuilding or ship repairing industries; or (iii) work wholly or mainly in the immediate vicinity of drop-forging plant or forging press plant engaged in the shaping of hot metal.

The other conditions to be satisfied in putting forward a valid claim are that the claimant must also (i) have been employed in one or more of the prescribed occupations for a combined total of not less than 20 years, and (ii) disablement benefit shall not be paid in respect of a claim for occupational deafness which is made later than 12 months after the claimant has ceased to be employed in an occupation prescribed in relation to occupational deafness. The degree of disability is assessed by the 'DHSS' procedure (see next section), with the further condition that the hearing loss must be 50 dB or greater in the better ear.

At the inception of the scheme it was made clear that the reason for its limited scope arose from the limited capacity within the National Health Service to undertake the necessary audiological examinations. It was decided that these should not exceed 10 000 per annum. In practice, the first three years of operation (up to 31 October 1977) produced only 5500 cases in total and the possibility of an expansion of the scheme became apparent.

The scheme was amended in 1980 (SI 377/1980). The principal change proposed is the extension of the range of prescribed diseases to include (i) the use of pneumatic percussive tools in general where they are used on metal, or in drilling coal or rock, (ii) workers in the textile industry in weaving sheds or on texturing machines, (iii) nail making and nail cleaning processes, and (iv) the use of plasma spray guns for the deposition of metal.

ASSESSMENT OF HEARING HANDICAP DUE TO NOISE INDUCED HEARING LOSS

As a result of the large number of industrial workers in the United Kingdom making claims for compensation for loss of hearing due to noise damage there is considerable interest in schemes for giving them adequate and fair compensation. This depends upon the ability to make reliable assessments of the degree of hearing handicap which their occupational noise exposure has produced. This handicap is usually considered in terms of the disability in understanding the spoken word in a variety of situations.

There are several different approaches to the problem of assessing handicap which results from noise induced hearing loss. They fall into three categories; the use of: (i) pure-tone audiograms, (ii) speech audiograms, and (iii) questionnaires. In (i) various combinations of hearing level, at different frequencies from the pure-tone air-conduction audiogram are averaged over the speech frequency range. Among the better known procedures are those proposed by the American Academy of Ophthalmology and Otolaryngology (1959) (0.5, 1, 2 kHz), United Kingdom Department of Health and Social Security (1973) (1, 2, 3 kHz) (as used in the assessment of claims under the Industrial Injuries scheme), the British Occupational Hygiene Society (0.5, 1, 2, 3, 4, 6 kHz) (Committee on Hygiene Standards 1971), the Dundee index (2, 4, 6 kHz) (Pearson, Kell, and Taylor 1973), and the British Standards Scheme (1, 2, 3 kHz) (British Standard Institution 1976). The handicap is proportional to the amount by which the average hearing level exceeds that for normal hearing subjects and is usually expressed on a scale from 0–100 per cent. Generally each scheme has a 'fence' which the average hearing loss has to exceed before the subject is deemed to have a handicap.

In (ii) the response of the subject to some sort of standard speech material, i.e. word lists or sentences, is determined as a function of sound level and compared with that of normal hearing subjects. The test can be carried out in the quiet or against a background of noise (Lindeman 1971) and in freefield or monaurally using headphones.

In (iii) the subject completes a questionnaire designed to assess his or her hearing handicap under a variety of 'everyday conditions' in such differing circumstances as communicating with family and friends, at public meetings, on the telephone and watching television (Noble and Atherley 1970; Pearson et al. 1973).

Clearly the most widely used procedures for the assessment of handicaps are those based upon the pure-tone audiogram. It might be thought that the use of speech audiometry would give superior results because handicap in understanding speech is basically what is being assessed. However, for a variety of reasons, this has not proved to be the case. An excellent review on the limitations of speech audiometry is given by Coles, Markides, and Priede (1973).

There seems to be relatively little support for the self-assessment approach of determining handicap for noise-induced hearing loss by means of questionnaire. Its protagonists claim it is superior to the use of the pure-tone audiogram (Noble and Atherley 1970), but there may be possibly an inherent bias against such a method because it is a more subjective test than either pure-tone audiometry or speech audiometry and has fewer inbuilt safeguards against cases of non-organic hearing loss.

Following Giolas (1970), hearing handicap might be defined as 'any disadvantage in the activities of everyday living which derives from hearing impairment'. While few would dissent from this definition there is clearly considerable difference of opinion as to how this handicap should be measured (American Academy of Ophthalmology and Otolaryngology 1959; Noble and Atherley 1970; Lindeman 1971; Committee of Hygiene Standards 1971; Department of Health and Social Security 1973; Pearson et al. 1973; British Standards Institution 1976).

It is also disquieting that many workers who have noise-induced hearing loss are coming forward and making claims for compensation under Common Law, when, according to most of the schemes based on pure-tone audiometry, they should not have any handicap because their average hearing loss does not exceed the appropriate 'fence' (Tempest 1978). Such persons frequently state that they can understand normal conversation on a one-to-one basis, in the quiet, but are unable to join in group discussions, e.g. at Union meetings, etc. or are at a loss in the pub, or at the social club where there is a background of noise. This led Tempest (1977) to propose a seven-point category grouping scheme mainly for use in litigation arising from claims for noise-induced hearing loss.

Ideal measures of hearing handicap resulting from noise-damaged hearing should we feel take into account the fact that such people may be disadvantaged in the following situations:

Speech in the quiet
Speech in noise—clubs, public houses, parties, discotheques
Round table discussions—committee meetings

TABLE 37.1. *Seven-point category grouping scheme for use in litigation arising from claims for noise-induced hearing loss*

High-frequency hearing level at 4 and/or 6 kHz(dB)†	Average hearing level at 0.5 1, and 2 kHz(dB)‡	Group	Brief description of handicap
less than 25	0–25	O	No handicap
25 or more	0–25	I	Slight handicap in noise
NA	25–40	II	Slight handicap for faint speech
NA	40–55	III	Mild handicap, affects normal speech
NA	55–70	IV	Marked handicap, affects loud speech
NA	70–90	V	Severe handicap, affects amplified speech
NA	more than 90	VI	Total deafness

† For the better ear.
‡ For the better ear; if the average for the poorer ear exceeds the better ear by 25–40 dB, add 5 dB to the better ear. If the average for the poorer ear exceeds the better ear by more than 40 dB, work out grouping the better ear and then raise to the next higher group.

Public entertainment—theatre, cinema, church, bingo, etc.
Watching television/listening to radio
Use of the telephone

These situations not only require an understanding of what is being said (intelligibility) but also where the sound has originated from (directionality) as well as an ability to 'keep up with the conversation'. It is well known that the directional relation between a speech sound and an interfering noise or other speech sounds has a great influence on the intelligibility of speech. The phenomenon called the 'cocktail party effect' is associated with this effect. Hochberg (1962) indicated that auditory localization ability might be important for job performance and safety in many industries. Davis and Silverman (1960) have made the point that the reduction in localization ability might contribute to a feeling of unsafeness that could lead to psychological maladjustment. The auditory system's spatial role should therefore be considered when assessing hearing handicap.

Until a great deal more research has been carried out to determine the various factors involved in establishing handicap we are forced to use such imperfect tools already referred to in this section. However, a series of experiments carried out at Salford University have already established the importance of directionality and response time as well as intelligibility in determining handicap due to noise-induced hearing loss (Hogstaat 1977; Bryan 1978). This work has also shown it is possible to predict handicap, with a high degree of accuracy, from the pure-tone audiogram using the hearing loss at frequencies of 1, 2, and 6 kHz.

Combined handicap in the quiet, in noise, and by self-assessment questionnaire CQDOL is given by the equation:

CQDOL = 0.23 HL 1 kHz + 0.69 HL 2 kHz + 0.54 HL 6 kHz − 24. This result raises the interesting and important point that the hearing loss at 6 kHz is as important as the loss at 2 kHz and more important than the loss at 1 kHz in determining the handicap experienced by subjects with noise induced hearing loss. Of the existing handicap schemes only the Dundee Index (Pearson *et al.* 1973) and the BOH scheme (Committee on Hygiene Standards 1971) involve the use of 6 kHz.

APPENDIX 37.1

APPENDIX 37.1. *DHSS Handicap Assessment Scheme*
The percentage disablement due to a binaural hearing loss may be read directly from the table below. This table is applicable only to cases of occupational deafness (Prescribed Disease No. 48) and not to deafness caused by any other condition. The pure-tone hearing levels refer to the 1, 2, 3 kHz average (HL) dB.

1, 2, 3 kHz Pure-tone average HL   WORSE EAR

Pure-tone HL	dB	50–53	54–60	61–66	67–72	73–79	80–86	87–95	96–105	106+
B	50–53	20	22	24	26	28	30	32	34	36
E	54–60	22	30	32	34	36	38	40	42	44
T	61–66	24	32	40	42	44	46	48	50	52
T	67–72	26	34	42	50	52	54	56	58	60
E	73–79	28	36	44	52	60	62	64	66	68
R	80–86	30	38	46	54	62	70	72	74	76
E	87–95	32	40	48	56	64	72	80	82	84
A	96–105	34	42	50	58	66	74	82	90	92
R	106+	36	44	52	60	68	76	84	92	100

A presbycusis correction is made by means of a 0.5 per cent deduction from the assessment at age 65 with a further deduction of 0.5 per cent for each year over 65.

REFERENCES

ACADEMY OF OPHTHALMOLOGY AND OTOLARYNGOLOGY (1959). *Trans. Am. Acad. Ophthal. Otolar.* **63**, 236–8.
ANON. (1908). *Annual Report: Factories and Workshops*, p. 206. HMSO, London.
—— (1927). *Annual Report: Factories and Workshops*, Cmnd. 3144, p. 107. HMSO, London.
—— (1953). Noise in industry. *Scope* 42, October. Creative Journals, London.
—— (1954). *Annual report of the Chief Inspector of Factories*, p. 134. HMSO, London.
—— (1955a). Noise dangers in industry. *The Times*, 29 April.
—— (1955b). Living in bedlam. *The Manchester Guardian*, 3 December.
—— (1962). *Annual Report of the Chief Inspector of Factories on Industrial Health*, Cmnd. 2129, p. 11. HMSO, London.
BALLENGER, W. L. and BALLENGER, H. C. (1938). *Diseases of nose, throat and ear*. Lea and Febiger, Philadelphia.
BARR, T. (1886). Enquiry into the effects of loud sounds upon the hearing of

boilermakers and others who work amid noisy surroundings. *Proc. Glasgow phil. Soc.* **17**, 223.

BARTLET, F. C. (1934). *The problem of noise*. Cambridge University Press, London.

BERRY V. STONE MANGANESE MARINE LTD. (1972). Knights Industrial Reports **12**, 13–35.

BEZOLD, F. and SIEBENMANN, F. R. (1908). *Textbook of otology* (trans. J. Holinger). Chicago Medical Books, Illinois.

BRITISH STANDARDS INSTITUTION (1976). *Estimating the risk of hearing handicap*. BS5330, London.

BRYAN, M. E. (1978). Assessment of handicap. Paper read at North of England Branch, British Society of Audiology, Manchester, April.

—— and TEMPEST, W. (1971). In *Occupational hearing loss* (ed. D. W. Robinson) p. 143. Academic Press, London.

BURNS, W. and ROBINSON, D. W. (1970). *Hearing and noise in industry*. HMSO, London.

CHALLEN, J. R. and HICKISH, D. E. (1958). Noise and the worker. *The Times Review of Industry*, 3 August, **12**, 9.

CHIPPENDALE, J. (1866). Letter. *Lancet* **ii**, 170.

COLES, R. R. A., MARKIDES, A., and PRIEDE, V. (1973). In *Disorders of auditory function* (ed. W. Taylor). Academic Press, London.

COLLIER, H. E. (1940). *Outlines of industrial medical practice*. Edward Arnold, London.

COMMITTEE ON HYGIENE STANDARDS (1971). *Hygiene standard for wideband noise*. Pergamon Press, Oxford.

COMMITTEE ON THE PROBLEM OF NOISE (1963). *Noise: Final Report* Cmnd. 2056. HMSO, London.

DARBY V. SHORT BROS. AND HARLAND LTD. AND MINISTRY OF AVIATION SUPPLY (unsupported). High Court in Northern Ireland. Quoted in *Daily Telegraph*, 6 June 1972.

DAVIES, D. LL. (1962). In *The control of noise*. NPL Symposium, No. 12, p. 311. HMSO, London.

DAVIS, A. H. (1937). *Noise*. Watts, London.

DAVIS, H. and SILVERMAN, S. R. (1960). *Hearing and deafness*. Holt and Rinehart, New York.

DEPARTMENT OF EMPLOYMENT (1972). *Code of practice for reducing the exposure of employed persons to noise*. HMSO, London.

DEPARTMENT OF HEALTH AND SOCIAL SECURITY (1973). *Occupational deafness*, Cmnd. 5461. HMSO, London.

—— (1974). *Benefits paid for occupational deafness*. Leaflet NI 207.

DEPARTMENTAL COMMITTEE ON COMPENSATION FOR INDUSTRIAL DISEASES (1907). *Report*. Cmnd. 3495. HMSO, London.

DICKSON, E. D. D., EWING, A. W. G., and LITTLER, T. S. (1939). The effects of aeroplane noise on the auditory acuity of aviators: some preliminary remarks. *J. Lar. Otol.* **54**, 531.

EVANS, E. J. (1947). Noise in the factory. *The Times Review of Industry*, 6 February.

FOSBROKE, J. (1830–1). Practical observations on the pathology and treatment of Deafness, No. II. *Lancet* **i**, 645.

GIOLAS, T. G. (1970). The measurement of hearing handicap: a point of view. *Maico Audiological Library Series* **8**, 6.

GREENWOOD, W. (1933). *Love on the Dole*. Jonathan Cape, London.

HAMMERTON, J. A. (c. 1935). *Cassell's Modern Encyclopaedia*, p. 321. Cassell, London.
HOCHBERG, I. (1962). Auditory localisation of speech and its presumed underlying factors. Doctoral thesis, Pennsylvania State University, USA.
HOGSTAAT, K. E. (1977). Evaluation of hearing handicap due to noise induced hearing loss. M.Sc. thesis, University of Salford, UK.
LEGGE, T. (1934). *Industrial maladies*. Oxford University Press.
LINDEMAN, H. E. (1971). Relation between audiological findings and complaints by persons suffering from noise-induced hearing loss. *Am. Indust. Hyg. Ass. J.* **32**, 447–52.
MCCAFFERTY V. METROPOLITAN POLICE DISTRICT RECEIVER (1977). All England Law Reports **2**, 756–76.
MCLACHLAN, N. W. (1935). *Noise, a comprehensive survey from every point of view*. Oxford University Press, London.
MINISTRY OF LABOUR (1963). *Noise and the worker*. Safety, Health and Welfare Series, No. 25. HMSO, London.
NOBLE, W. G. and ATHERLEY, G. R. C. (1970). The hearing measurement scale: a questionnaire for the assessment of auditory disability. *J. audit. Res.* **10**, 229–50.
PASSCHIER-VERMEER, W. (1968). Hearing loss due to exposure to steady-state broad-band noise. Report 35, Institute for Public Health Engineering, TNO, Netherlands.
PEARSON, J. C. G., KELL, R. L., and TAYLOR, W. (1973). An index of hearing impairment derived from the pure tone audiogram. In *Disorders of auditory function* (ed. W. Taylor). Academic Press. London.
RAMAZZINI, B. (1713). *De Morbis Artificium*. Padua. [1964 Edition entitled *Disease of workers*. Hafner, New York.]
ROGER, T. R. (1915). Noise deafness: a review of recent experimental work, and a clinical investigation into the effect of loud noise upon the labyrinth, in boilermakers. *J. Lar. Rhinol. Otol.* **30**, 91.
SAPPINGTON, C. O. (1943). *The essentials of industrial health*. Lippincott, Philadelphia.
SCOTT STEVENSON, R. (1943). *The ear, nose and throat in the services*. Oxford University Press.
STATUTORY INSTRUMENT No. 377 (1980). The Social Security (Industrial Injuries) (Prescribed Diseases) Regulations 1980. HMSO, London.
TEMPEST, W. (1977). The assessment of hearing handicap. *J. soc. occup. Med.* **27**, 134–7.
—— (1978). Noise exposure and hearing loss. *Ann. occup. Hyg.* **21**, 51–6.
THACKRAH, C. T. (1831). *The effects of arts, trades and professions on health and longevity*. [1957 Edition. Livingstone, London.]
WESTMACOTT, F. H. (1925). Discussion on occupational diseases of the ear, nose and throat and their prevention. *Br. med. J.* **ii**, 886.
WITTMAACK, K. (1907). Uber Schadigung des Gehossdurch Schalleinwirkung. *Z. Ohrenheilk*. 54. 37.
YOSHII, U. (1909). Experimentelle Untersuchungen uber die Schadigung des Gehororgans durch Schalleinwirkung. *Z. Ohrenheilk* **58**, 201.

38 Compensation for industrial hearing loss: the practice in the United States

ARAM GLORIG

LEGAL AND LEGISLATIVE DEVELOPMENTS

Historical background

Hearing loss is an affliction which has existed throughout the history of mankind. It occurs in all walks of life and is due to many causes. Hearing problems received little attention in the past because, until the development of the audiometer within the past 30 years, there was no means of measuring hearing acuity with any degree of accuracy. The partial losses which constitute no appreciable handicap or disability and which are predominant in the overall picture were seldom recognized.

That workers in noisy occupation develop a greater than average decrease in hearing sensitivity has been known for more than 100 years. Attention was focused upon occupational exposures as a result of the industrial evolution which occurred during and after the Second World War and the resultant increase in the number of persons exposed to intense noise, both in industry and in the military forces.

Prior to 1948, hearing loss, either partial or total, was not regarded as a significant factor in workmen's compensation. Some claims occurred but these were due primarily to traumatic injuries from such causes as blasts, concussions, blows to the head, and foreign objects or infections in the ears. Such injuries have generally been covered under the existing Workmen's Compensation laws, either as schedule disabilities or on the basis of wage loss.

In years past noise-induced hearing loss was not ordinarily considered compensable for several reasons. Usually, many years of exposure are necessary to cause a significant hearing loss. The development of the impairment is slow and insidious making it impossible to identify a specific date of injury. Seldom is a wage loss involved, and, in general, the disability schedules in the Workmen's Compensation laws were not construed as applicable to occupational diseases. Where hearing loss was compensable as an occupational disease, claims were limited by such factors as requirements that there be a wage loss or that the hearing loss be total, or restrictive provisions for establishment of a date of injury.

Noise-induced hearing loss of the type which develops after years of exposure has been treated as an occupational disease in several states which have thus far enacted specific legislation to deal with the subject, viz. in Missouri it is specifically defined as a disease; in Wisconsin and New York it is treated under the occupational disease sections of the laws, and in Georgia it is considered to be trauma.

Significant legal precedents

The situation described above was placed in a different light by precedents established during the years 1948 to 1959. Although no attempt will be made in this article to describe in detail the history of these cases, attention will be called to some of the important points which have a significant bearing upon the probable course of events in other states. These cases involved claimants who were still engaged in their usual occupations and who had suffered no loss of wages as a result of the hearing loss.

NEW YORK

The precedent in this state was established in the case of Slawinski v. J. H. Williams & Co. in 1948. Although the New York Workmen's Compensation law contained a schedule for loss of hearing this had been construed as applicable only to accidental injuries. The law defined 'disablement' in connection with occupational diseases as 'the state of being disabled from earning full wages at the work at which the employee was last employed'. The New York Workmen's Compensation Board ruled, however, that the schedules in the law applied to both accidental injuries and occupational diseases and that Slawinski was entitled to a schedule award for partial loss of hearing even though he had not been disabled from earning full wages at his usual employment. The ruling of the Workmen's Compensation Board was upheld by the Appellate Division of the Supreme Court of New York and later by the Court of Appeals.

WISCONSIN

The precedent in Wisconsin was established in the case of Wojcik v. Green Bay Drop Forge Company filed in 1951. The Wisconsin law covered occupational diseases and required disability for the disease to be compensable. Establishment of disability was accomplished by defining 'date of injury' as the last day of work for the last employer whose employment caused disability. The Industrial Commission of Wisconsin ruled, however, that the 'date of injury' was the last day of work before the filing of the claim. Under this interpretation it held that Wojcik was entitled to a schedule award for partial loss of hearing even though he was still employed and had lost no wages. The ruling of the Industrial Commission was eventually upheld by the Wisconsin Supreme Court.

THE LONGSHOREMEN'S PRECEDENT

The legal precedent under the United States Longshoremen's and Harbor Worker's Compensation Act was established in 1955 in the case of Travelers Insurance Company, Todd Shipyards et al. v. Cardillo. The Longshoremen's Act makes no distinction between accidental injury and occupational disease and defined 'injury' as 'accidental injury or death arising out of and in the course of employment and such occupational disease or infection as arises naturally out of such employment'. In contesting the claim, Travelers argued that the disability schedules did not apply to occupational diseases and that to be compensable an occupational disease had to result in a wage loss or loss of earning capacity. The court held that occupational loss of hearing was compensable under the schedules even though there was no wage loss involved.

MISSOURI PRECEDENT

In 1959 the Missouri Supreme Court ruled on the case of Marie v. Standard Steel Works. In reversing an award by the Missouri Industrial Commission, the lower courts had held that loss of hearing due to prolonged exposure to noise was not an occupational disease within the meaning of the law. The Supreme Court in reversing the lower courts cited the precedents established in Wisconsin and New York and held that loss of hearing due to noise exposure is an occupational disease, compensable under the disability schedules.

THE MARYLAND DECISIONS

Exceptions to the pattern indicated above are found in two 1959 cases in the State of Maryland. The Maryland Workmen's Compensation law provides in Section 22A that to be compensable an occupational disease must result in the worker being incapacitated from performing his usual work at full wages. The two cases in which rulings were made on this point were Vinson v. Bethlehem Steel Company, decided in the Superior Court of the City of Baltimore, and Belschner v. Anchor Post Products, decided in the Court of Appeals. In both cases the courts held that under the Maryland Workmen's Compensation law no compensation can be paid under the schedules for an occupational disease as long as the claimant is not actually incapacitated from performing his work and suffers no wage loss.

THE GEORGIA PRECEDENT

Significant in its implications is the 1962 decision of the Georgia Court of Appeals in the case of Shipman v. Lockheed Aircraft Corporation. The Georgia law in Section 114–102 states that *injury* and *personal injury* . . . 'shall mean only injury by accident and shall not, except as hereinafter provided, include a disease in any form'. Section 114–405 includes a schedule of benefits for total loss of hearing in one or both ears.

In Section 114–803 the law defines occupational diseases. The definition states that . . . 'the term "occupational disease" shall include only those diseases hereinafter listed in this section . . .'. The list of diseases which follows does not include loss of hearing. The defendants argued that loss of hearing due to prolonged exposure to noise was an occupational disease. The court ruled, however, that the loss of hearing was the cumulative effect of a succession of traumatic injuries suffered by impingement of each sound impulse upon the ear. It therefore held that the injury was compensable under the accidental injury provisions of the law. Also, the Court accepted medical evidence presented in this case that a 51 per cent hearing impairment in one ear constituted for all practical purposes a total loss of industrial use of that ear. The Georgia Supreme Court declined to review the case.

LEGISLATIVE PRECEDENTS

Although estimates vary, it is certain that the working population includes several million individuals with less than normal hearing. These hearing losses have accumulated throughout the years and no financial provision has been made for settlement of the claims that could develop if all were free to file claims and collect benefits at any desired time. The situation is further complicated by the fact that the existing hearing losses may be due only in part to occupational exposure. In many cases there are no records by which causal relationships can be established as between present employment, past employment, and non-occupational causes. Employers are reluctant to accept responsibility for hearing losses which may be due to non-occupational causes or which existed prior to their employment of the worker. Difficulties are encountered when attempting to devise a system of compensation for occupationally induced hearing losses fair to the employer and which will not work against the employment of workers with pre-existing losses.

In the legislative treatment which has emerged in several of the states the above mentioned factors have been taken into consideration. Before describing the legislative precedents which have appeared, the basis for several of the significant provision will be commented upon briefly below. Where medical and scientific factors are involved, more complete explanations will be included for reference in the technical sections to follow.

If all workers with some degree of hearing 'loss' or impairment were free to file claims for compensation at any desired time the result could be a mass influx of claims with chaotic results. The so-called six months waiting period is recognized generally as the most satisfactory method of dealing with this situation. Under such a provision no claim may be filed for noise-induced hearing loss until six consecutive months after the worker's last exposure to injurious noise. It therefore spreads out the filing of claims but protects the worker's right to establish a claim when his hearing loss results in disablement or impairment or earning capacity or when he is no longer employed in a noisy occupation.

The prevailing medical opinion is that the criterion for handicap due to hearing loss should be the loss of ability to hear speech and that minor deviations from the so-called normal hearing level create no such handicap. Because of the present limitations of speech audiometry, the practice is to estimate the hearing level for speech from pure-tone audiometric tests. Based upon these considerations, both the American Academy of Ophthalmology and Otolaryngology and the American Medical Association recommend a formula in which the pure-tone hearing thresholds or losses are measured at the frequencies of 500, 1000, and 2000 Hz on an audiometer calibrated according to American Standard 224.5–1951 (American Standards Association, New York). Average losses of 15 dB or less constitute no compensable hearing impairment, and losses of 81.7 dB (nominally 82 dB) or more represent total loss of hearing for speech. When the 1969 American National Standards Institute audiometric reference levels are used, these numbers become 25 dB and 92 dB.

It is recognized that some hearing loss, due to non-occupational causes develops with increasing age. Commonly referred to as 'presbycusis', these losses are due in part to the physiological changes due to age itself and in part to harmful noises which are common in a modern social environment. Although the organized medical groups have not recommended an allowance for this factor in compensation systems, the American Academy of Ophthalmology and Otolaryngology suggests that this is a legal determination to be considered by the legislatures or the compensation administrative agencies. In its Guide for Evaluation of Hearing Impairment appears the following statement: 'At this time the Subcommittee on Noise makes no specific recommendation regarding a correction for a shift in the hearing threshold due to age, because the relation of presbycusis to noise-induced hearing loss is not yet fully understood.' It is generally agreed, however, that no correction for presbycusis is necessary since no compensation is paid until the average hearing level is greater than 25 dB.

WISCONSIN

Legislative activity in Wisconsin was precipitated by the Wojcik case in 1953, and the filing of some 500 claims, most of which were against one employer. Pending further study of this matter, an interim law was enacted in 1953 under which occupational loss of hearing was compensable only on the basis of wage loss. Subsequently, an agreed bill was introduced and enacted in 1955. Full details of the Wisconsin provisions will be found in Section 102.555 (Wisconsin Statutes 1957). The major points are summarized briefly below:

1. Occupational hearing loss, partial or total, is compensable as a schedule from that applied to hearing loss resulting from accidental injury.
2. The last employer who exposes the worker to injurious noise is liable for previous hearing loss shown to have existed prior to his employment of the worker.
3. No claim for benefits under the schedule may be filed until six consecutive months of removal from noisy employment after the date of injury, which is defined as any one of the events described below:
    (i) Transfer because of occupational deafness to non-noisy employment;
    (ii) Retirement;
    (iii) Termination of the employer–employee relationship;
    (vi) Layoff, provided the layoff is complete and continuous for one year, in which case the six consecutive months' period may commence within the last six months of layoff.
4. Separate provision is made for compensating an employee who, because

of occupational deafness, is transferred to other noisy employment and thereby sustains actual wage loss, subject to a maximum of $3500.
5. The formula for measurement and evaluation of hearing loss is not included in the law. This subject is treated under an administrative ruling of the Wisconsin Industrial Commission which prescribes the formula recommended by the American Academy of Ophthalmology and Otolaryngology and the American Medical Association. It will be discussed on page 870.

NEW YORK

Developments in New York followed the same pattern as in Wisconsin. Claims activity was precipitated by the Slawinski decision in 1948. Some 400 claims were filed within a short time, mainly against two employers. Disposition of these cases was delayed by an administrative ruling of the New York Workmen's Compensation Board that the degree of disability could not be determined until after at least six months' separation from exposure to injurious noise. This ruling was based upon a medical opinion in one case; medical opinion would be the determining factor on this point in other states where there is no legislation dealing with occupational hearing loss. In 1958 the legislature enacted specific legislation to deal with occupational loss of hearing. Although there are technical differences, the basic intent of the law follows the precedent established by the 1955 Wisconsin amendment. Partial or total loss of hearing due to noise exposure is treated as a schedule disability under the Occupational Diseases section of the law. Compensation for occupational loss of hearing becomes due and payable six months after separation from work for the last employer who at any time exposed the worker to harmful noise, and the last day of such six months' separation from work is defined as the date of disablement. The formula for the measurement and evaluation of hearing loss is the subject of an administrative ruling by the New York State Workmen's Compensation Board, and, as in Wisconsin, follows in general the recommendations of the American Academy of Ophthalmology and Otolaryngology and the American Medical Association. Full details of the New York provisions will be found in Sections 49–aa to 49–gg inclusive, Article 3–A of the New York law as amended effective 1 July 1958.

A major point of difference between the Wisconsin and the New York laws lies in the area of apportionment of liability. The Wisconsin law relieves the employer of liability for hearing losses shown to have existed prior to employment. The New York law makes the last employer liable to the employee for the total compensable hearing loss. However, if a pre-existing hearing loss is disclosed and the employer complies with certain specified requirements it enables him, when a claim is eventually filed, to secure proportionate reimbursement from prior employers who may have, within the previous three years, also exposed the worker to noise.

MISSOURI

Following the precedents established in Wisconsin and New York, the Missouri legislature in 1959 amended the Workmen's Compensation law to provide specifically for occupational loss of hearing. Full details will be found in Section 287.197 in the Missouri law as amended effective 29 August 1959. The amended law follows closely the pattern established in Wisconsin. It specifically defines noise-induced hearing loss as an occupational disease compensable as a schedule disability, requires six consecutive months of separation from noise exposure before filing a claim, and relieves the last employer of liability for pre-existing hearing loss. A separate schedule providing benefits lower than those provided for accidental injuries is included.

There are two points on which the Missouri law differs significantly from the Wisconsin and New York laws. First, it includes as a statutory requirement the formula for measurement and evaluation of hearing losses. Second, as part of this formula, it requires an allowance for the average hearing losses that accompany age in the population (presbycusis). The formula requires that for compensation purposes the hearing thresholds be measured at the three frequencies of 500, 1000, and 2000 Hz. From the average losses in these three frequencies 0.5 dB per year of age over age 40 is deducted for 'presbycusis'. Average losses of 15 dB (ASA) or 25 dB (ANSI) or less after the deduction constitute no compensable hearing impairment. Above this point, 1.5 per cent hearing disability is allowed for each additional dB of hearing loss, reaching 100 per cent at 82 dB (ASA) or 92 dB (ANSI).

OTHER LEGAL AND LEGISLATIVE ACTIVITIES

With a few major exceptions significant claims activity has been concentrated in the states or jurisdictions mentioned previously. In California, a moderate but increasing number of claims have been filed within the past 15 years. Limited numbers of claim have appeared in other states such as Minnesota, Hawaii, Connecticut, Oregon, and Washington.

Legislation similar to the Wisconsin, New York, and Missouri laws has been introduced in several other states, for example Rhode Island, New Jersey, Michigan, and Pennsylvania. On the other hand, amendments to the laws which would have added occupational loss of hearing to the schedules without the special requirements embodied in the Wisconsin, New York, and Missouri laws have been proposed but not enacted in Arizona, Colorado, Illinois, and Massachusetts, as well as other states.

Legislation similar to the Wisconsin, New York, and Missouri Acts has been recommended in the Workmen's Compensation and Rehabilitation section of the Program of Suggested State Legislation, published in 1963 by the Council of State Governments. The committee which drafted the recommendations was made up of experts in workmen's compensation and included representatives of Industry, Labor, Insurance, and State Workmen's

Compensation Administrative Agencies. The report includes essentially the provisions concerning occupational loss of hearing contained in the Missouri legislation. Included are a six months' waiting period, measurement of the hearing threshold levels at 500, 1000, and 2000 Hz, low and high 'fences' at 15 and 82 dB ASA, (25 and 92 dB ANSI) and allowance of 0.5 dB per year of age over 40 for the hearing losses that accompany age (presbycusis) as in the Missouri law.

Concerning formulae for evaluation of hearing losses it is interesting to note that in 1961 all of the Canadian provinces adopted rating schedules based upon disability rather than impairment. Included in the schedules are a six months' waiting period, measurement of the hearing losses at the three frequencies of 500, 1000, and 2000 Hz and a presbycusis allowance of 0.5 dB per year for each year of age over 50. Average hearing losses of less than 25 dB are not compensable and losses of more than 70 dB are construed as total hearing disability. Under the system which prevails in the Canadian provinces, the hearing loss ratings are applied to a schedule of percentage disabilities to the whole body.

Impairment or disability formulae

Where workmen's compensation benefits for hearing loss are paid under the disability schedules, some formula must be used to convert the hearing losses in decibels as shown by the audiometric test to a percentage of the disability benefits payable for total loss of hearing. Prior to the audiometer, percentage hearing loss ratings were based upon whispered or spoken voice tests, tuning-fork tests, or watch-tick tests. Although none of these tests is today recognized as having any value in establishing a quantitative measurement of hearing, the spoken voice test is commented upon briefly below as a matter of historical interest.

SPOKEN VOICE TESTS

The spoken voice test was used widely for many years, particularly in the military service. In the test, the distance at which the subject could hear spoken or whispered voice was recorded as a fraction, the numerator of which was the distance in feet at which the subject could hear the voice, the denominator being the distance at which a normal ear would hear the same voice. 20/20ths was commonly used to represent normal hearing. A table or formula was used to convert the fractional measurement to a percentage hearing loss. Because of the variables involved, these tests permitted no objective measurement results and comparison of tests made at different times, in different rooms, and by different testers were of little value.

Relatively few states have adopted a mandatory formula for rating hearing impairment or disability. In states where there is no such requirement the examining otologist may presumably apply any formula which he may desire. The result is that any one of several different formulae may be used in various localities. Those most likely to be encountered are described below.

FLETCHER POINT 8 FORMULA

Introduced in 1929 the Fletcher point 8 formula was used commonly for many years and will still be encountered in some jurisdictions. This formula marked the introduction of one basic concept which has endured throughout the years, namely, that ability to hear everyday speech is indicated by the average hearing levels at the three 'speech' frequencies of 500, 1000, and 2000 Hz. To determine the percentage loss of hearing for speech under the point 8 formula, the average of the hearing levels in the three speech frequencies is multiplied by 0.8. The resultant percentage is applied to the schedule for total loss of hearing to determine the number of weeks of compensation benefits payable. Each ear is rated separately since the formula contains no binaural rating provision.

The reason for multiplying the average hearing level by 0.8 may explained briefly. The maximum effective range of hearing was estimated to be from zero to about 125 dB. The maximum range of commerically available audiometers was about 100 dB. Thus, the individual with a 50 dB hearing loss had lost not 50 per cent of his potential hearing but 50/125ths. The ratio between decibels and percentage was, therefore, in the nature of 0.8 to 1. A 50 dB loss would be equivalent to 40 per cent of total hearing capacity.

The point 8 method was subject to two major criticisms. First, any deviation from the so-called normal hearing level was recorded as a loss even though well within the range of normal hearing. Second, the maximum hearing loss measurable on the audiometer (about 100 dB) resulted in only an 80 per cent loss rating.

1947 AMA METHOD

The so-called 1947 AMA method was published by the American Medical Association in 1942, modified in 1947, and used extensively until replaced by the AAOO–AMA formula in 1961. The formula makes use of measurements at four frequencies (500, 1000, 2000, and 4000 Hz). The measured losses at each of the four frequencies are not averaged, each frequency being weighted separately according to its assumed importance in hearing speech, and the four percentages added to arrive at the total percentage hearing loss for the ear. The relative importance assigned to total loss at each frequency is: 15 per cent at 500 Hz; 30 per cent at 1000 Hz; 40 per cent at 2000 Hz; and 15 per cent at 4000 Hz. In determining the binaural percentage loss, the hearing in the better and poorer ears is weighted in the ratio of 7 to 1. Percentage loss ratings started at 10 dB in each of the four frequencies, reaching the maximum rating at 90 dB at 500 Hz, and at 95 dB at each of the remaining three frequencies involved. The progression between the minimum and maximum ratings mentioned above was not linear; the percentages were weighted to give greater importance to a loss of a given number of decibels in the middle intensity range. Application of the AMA formula is illustrated in Table 38.1.

TABLE 38.1. *Hearing loss formula—illustration of AMA method. (Based on (Fowler and Sabine (1947))*

Loss (dB)	Percentage Losses			
	500 cps	1000 cps	2000 cps	4000 cps
0				
5				
10	0.2	0.3	0.4	0.1
15	0.5	0.9	1.3	0.3
20	1.1	2.1	2.9	0.9
25	1.8	3.6	4.9	1.7
30	2.6	5.4	7.3	2.7
35	3.7	7.7	9.8	3.8
40	4.9	10.2	12.9	5.0
45	6.3	13.0	17.3	6.4
50	7.9	15.7	22.4	8.0
55	9.6	19.0	25.7	9.7
60	11.3	21.5	28.0	11.2
65	12.8	23.5	30.2	12.5
70	13.8	25.5	32.2	13.5
75	14.6	27.2	34.0	14.2
80	14.8	28.8	35.8	14.6
85	14.9	29.8	37.5	14.8
90	15.0	29.9	39.2	14.9
95		30.0	40.0	15.0
100				

Explanation
1. *Unilateral (one ear) hearing loss determination*: for each of the four frequencies included, determine from the table above the percentage loss corresponding to the loss in decibels shown in the column at the left.
2. Add the percentage losses as indicated above to determine the total percentage loss for the ear.
3. *Binaural (both ears) hearing loss determination*: multiply the total percentage loss in the better ear (with the least loss) by 7, add the total percentage in loss in the worse ear, and divide by 8. The result is the binaural percentage loss. This is shown below as a formula:

$$\frac{(\text{Total \% hearing loss, better ear} \times 7) + (\text{Total \% hearing loss, worse ear} \times 1)}{8} = \text{Combined or binaural hearing loss}$$

AAOO–AMA FORMULA

In 1955 a joint committee of the American Academy of Ophthalmology and Otolaryngology and the American Medical Association recommended development of a new formula for evaluating hearing loss. The primary reason advanced by the joint committee in support of its recommendation was as stated below in its report. (The references to the 'AMA method' refers to the 1947 AMA formula.)

Actually, the AMA method is fairly satisfactory for calculating percentage capacity to hear speech for persons who have conductive hearing losses in which the losses are not very different for different frequencies. For persons with nerve deafness, however, and particularly for those in whom hearing for low and middle tones is good but the hearing for high tones is poor, the results often are in conflict with the clinical evidence.

The development of a new formula was undertaken by the Subcommittee on Noise of the American Academy of Ophthalmology and Otolaryngology. The formula eventually recommended by this group was approved by the Committee on Conservation of Hearing and published by the Academy in 1959 (Committee on Conservation of Hearing 1959). Subsequently, with editorial modifications, the formula was approved and published by the American Medical Association in August 1961. Since the AAOO–AMA formula is the most widely recognized and likely to be universally adopted, it will be described in some detail and referred to hereafter simply as the AAOO formula.

The AAOO formula is based upon impairment rather than disability. In publishing the formula, the Academy distinguished between these two terms in a footnote which is quoted below:

'Impairment' is here used as defined in 'Guides to the Evaluation of Permanent Impairment', approved by the Committee on Medical Rating of Physical Impairment, *Journal of the American Medical Association*, September 27, 1958, Volume 168, Number 4, Page 475. 'Impairment', as defined by the American Medical Association, denotes a medical condition that affects one's personal efficiency in the activities of daily living. It is recognized that 'disability', as used in various workmen's compensation laws, involves nonmedical factors, since it may be related to actual or presumed reduction in ability to remain employed at full wages. Permanent impairment is, therefore, a contributing factor to, but not necessarily an indication of, the extent of a patient's permanent disability within the meaning of the workmen's compensation laws.

The principles upon which the AAOO formula is based and its application are explained in the four paragraphs excerpted below from the 1959 report from the Committee on Conservation of Hearing mentioned above. Similar explanations appear in the 1961 statement by the American Medical Association, also mentioned above.

Ideally, hearing impairment should be evaluated in terms of ability to hear everyday speech under everyday conditions; the term 'impairment' will be used hereinafter in this sense only. The ability to hear sentences and repeat them correctly in a quiet environment is taken as satisfactory evidence of correct hearing for everday speech. Because of the present limitations of speech audiometry, the hearing level for speech should be estimated from measurements made with a pure-tone audiometer. For this estimate, the Subcommittee recommends the simple *average* of the hearing levels at the three frequencies, 500, 1000 and 2000 Hz.

In order to evaluate the hearing impairment, it must be recognized that the range of impairment is not nearly as wide as the audiometric range of human hearing. Audiometric zero, which is presumably the average normal hearing threshold level is not the point at which impairment begins. If the average hearing level at 500, 1000 and 2000 Hz is 15 dB or less ASA, (or 25 dB or less ANSI), usually no impairment exists in the ability to hear everday speech under everyday conditions. At the other extreme, however, if the average hearing level at 500, 1000 and 2000 Hz is over 82 dB ASA (or 92 dB ANSI), the impairment for hearing everyday speech should be considered total. The Subcommittee on Noise recommends the following formula: for every decibel that the estimated hearing level for speech exceeds 15 dB (or 25 dB ANSI), allow 1.5 per cent up to the maximum of 100 per cent. This maximum is reached at 82 dB ASA (or 92 dB ANSI).

At this time, the Subcommittee on Noise makes no specific recommendation regarding a correction for a shift in the hearing threshold due to age, because the relation of presbycusis to noise-induced hearing loss is not yet fully understood.

The Subcommittee on Noise recommends that any method for the evaluation of impairment include an appropriate formula for binaural hearing which will be based on the hearing levels in each ear tested separately. Specifically, the Subcommittee on Noise recommends the following formula: the percentage of impairment in the better ear is multiplied by five (5). The resulting figure is added to the percentage of impairment in the poorer ear, and the sum divided by six (6). The final percentage represents the binaural evaluation of hearing impairment.

CALIFORNIA VARIATION OF AAOO FORMULA

Effective from 1 March 1962, the California Industrial Accident Commission adopted a formula based upon the AAOO formula but containing one variation. The only difference is that the percentage impairment ratings are based upon the hearing level measurements in the four frequencies, 500, 1000, 2000, and 3000 Hz. The sum of the hearing levels in the four frequencies is divided by four to determine the average hearing level.

Since in noise-induced hearing losses the loss at 3000 Hz is invariably greater than 500, 1000, or 2000 Hz, this formula develops a substantially higher impairment rating than the basic formula described above. This departure from the principles recommended by the medical organizations mentioned above is reported to have been made as an administrative decision by the Industrial Accident Commission. Fortuitously, California adopted a formula in 1962 which has recently (1978) been approved by the AAOO and the American Council on Otolaryngology to replace the previous formula. The only difference as mentioned above is the addition of 3000 Hz used in calculating the average hearing level. The proposed formula is the same as the old one in all other respects.

Allowance for hearing losses that accompany age

Whether an allowance should be made in compensation cases for the hearing losses that accompany age (presbycusis) has been a controversial question. Contrary to often stated impressions, the American Academy did not take a position against such an allowance when the AAOO formula was published. In the introductory statement accompanying the presentation the formula was presented as a guide for the evaluation of hearing impairment *regardless of the cause or causes of such impairment*. Inclusion of the footnote shown under the previously quoted statement of the AAOO formula makes it clear that the viewpoint of the Subcommittee was that the question of liability for this portion of the loss is a legal problem to be resolved by the legislatures or the administrative agencies. A similar viewpoint by the American Medical Association is obvious in the statements contained in a preface to the *Guides to the evaluation of permanent impairment—ear, nose, throat, and related structures* to which reference has been made above.

Most investigators in the field of hearing loss concede that age-induced hearing losses are common throughout the population and that some allowance should be made. However, it is usually stated that questions remain to be resolved before a satisfactory method of making such an allowance can be determined. As evidence of this viewpoint, a comment contained in Glorig (1960) is quoted below:

Threshold shift that accompanies aging is of interest medicolegally because it is found in the general population. Certain amounts of shift accompany age, in groups of persons not exposed to occupational noises. It is reasonable, then, to assume that some sort of correction of loss of hearing due to aging should be allowed in compensation cases. Because of the complexity of the problem, however, it is impossible at this time to designate a correction that can be said to be scientifically valid.

The presbycusis values referred to in the footnote to the description of the AAOO formula quoted above are shown in Table 38.2.

TABLE 38.2. *Hearing losses that accompany age—men. (Presbycusis losses as shown in four selected publications)*

Losses in the three speech frequencies (500, 1000, and 2000 Hz. Age in years.)

1. From Figure 2, American Standards Association (1954)

Age	35	40	45	50	55	60	65
Average dB loss	0.6	2.6	4.3	6.0	8.3	10.7	13.0

2. From Glorig, Grings, and Summerfield (1958)

Age	35	40	45	50	55	60	65
Average dB loss	2.0	3.3	4.5	6.3	8.0	10.0	12.0

3. From Table XXII, Glorig, Wheeler, Quiggle, Grings, and Summerfield (1954)

Age	35	45	55	65
Average dB loss	4.0	6.3	7.2	15.6

4. From Figure 4, Corso (1963)

Age groups	34–40	43–9	51–7	59–65
Average dB loss	1.7	7.0	7.4	11.8

BINAURAL RATING

The formulae currently approved by leading medical organizations are designed to rate impairment of ability to hear speech. It is recognized that total loss of hearing in one ear does not reduce the ability to hear speech by 50 per cent if the hearing in the other ear is within normal limits. Medical opinion is that such a loss would result in a hearing handicap in the range of 15–20 per cent.

Recognizing the above concept, the formula currently approved by both the American Medical Association and the American Academy of Ophthalmology and Otolaryngology recommends that the final rating be based upon the combined hearing ability in the two ears; the better ear is assumed to be worth five times as much as the poorer ear. To determine the final rating, therefore, to the percentage loss in the poorer ear is added five times the percentage loss in the better ear and the total divided by six; the result represents the percentage of the schedule benefit for total loss of hearing in both ears which should be allowed in compensation cases. The binaural formula has a significant effect upon the final rating only where there is a substantial difference in the hearing threshold levels in the two ears.

Factors in claim evaluation

When a claim for occupational loss of hearing is filed, evaluation as respects compensability rests upon a number of variable factors. The legal, medical, and technical factors which may be involved have been summarized in preceding sections. Other than in the few states that have enacted legislation to deal specifically with noise-induced hearing loss, or where judicial precedents have been established, it is impossible to predict the outcome of a claim based upon any given set of circumstances. Conclusions rest upon thorough knowledge of the applicable laws, regulations, and legal precedents in the jurisdiction involved.

Variations in laws and regulations

Claims in substantial numbers have appeared in relatively few states. Opinions have been expressed that occupational loss of hearing may be held compensable under the laws of more than half the states. In any given case, however, the probabilities would be affected by variable requirements, some of which are indicated below.

In some states occupational hearing loss may be compensable only on the basis of actual wage loss (Maryland is an example). Noise-induced hearing loss, however, seldom incapacitates the worker from earning full wages at his usual occupation. Where the occupational hearing loss is compensable as a schedule disability, wage loss is, of course, not a factor. In some states, however, the impairment is compensable only in cases involving total loss of hearing, as in Illinois and Pennsylvania. In other states the impairment may be compensable when due to accidental injury but not when due to prolonged exposure to noise, generally recognized as an occupational disease (examples are Texas and Kansas). Prolonged exposure to noise seldom, if ever, results in a profound or total loss of hearing. Also, occupational hearing loss due to prolonged exposure to noise is not recognized in otological circles as a condition that causes temporary total disability.

Under the laws of all states, loss of hearing resulting from a traumatic injury would be compensable. There have been cases, however, where a hearing loss due to prolonged exposure to noise has been held to be compensable as an accidental injury. An example is the Shipman case in Georgia. In this case the court held that the hearing loss was the cumulative result of a series of traumatic injuries caused by the impingement of each sound impulse upon the ear.

Subject to variable legal requirements, some of which have been mentioned above, two basic questions are important in the evaluation of the claim. These are: (i) is noise-induced (occupational) loss of hearing partial or total, compensable as a schedule disability under the applicable laws, and (ii) is the injury attributable to the occupation? With these general qualifications in mind, some specific suggestions may be made concerning subjects to be considered in claim evaluation.

Date of injury

The establishment of a 'date of injury' within the meaning of the applicable law may have an important bearing upon the worker's eligibility to file a claim against the employer. The requirements in this respect have been established definitely in jurisdictions which have special occupational disease loss of hearing provisions. In other states, the occupational disease provisions in the laws may relate the payment of benefits to the 'last day of work', to 'incapacitation', or 'the beginning of disablement', the injury being treated under the provisions applicable to the last date on which the employee was exposed to allegedly injurious noise and whether the exposure has ceased because of transfer to other work, termination of employment, strike disablement, or any other cause. If the exposure has not ceased, it should be determined when the employee first visited the doctor and was told that he had a hearing loss presumably due to noise exposure.

Evaluation of the hearing loss

HISTORY

Most important in the diagnostic procedure is careful attention to the worker's medical, occupational, and family history. In some cases, it may be found that the hearing loss existed prior to the worker's employment but was not realized until disclosed by audiometric tests. In other cases, it may be disclosed that the worker's hearing had been impaired by non-occupational causes such as otological and infectious diseases, noise exposure or toxic drugs. A history of military exposure to gunfire or jet engine noise, for example, will indicate that some loss of hearing is to be expected regardless of industrial noise exposure.

HEARING TESTS

The otological examination and hearing test will determine the extent of the hearing loss and whether it is of a type which may be attributable to noise exposure. The tests will involve a complete ear, nose, and throat examination followed by air-conduction and bone-conduction audiometry, in addition to speech reception and discrimination tests. In some cases the otologist may, as an aid to diagnosis, employ additional test procedures such as recruitment tests, tone decay tests, etc.

WHEN TO TEST

Hearing tests in compensation cases should be made as long as possible after the last exposure to noise. The time required for full recovery from temporary threshold shift (auditory fatigue) varies among individuals; opinions differ among experts concerning the maximum period for stabilization of hearing in any given individual. In a number of medical reports statements have appeared that *average* recovery time for auditory fatigue is about 16 hours. It should be emphasized that this is only an average figure which would not necessarily apply to any given individual. Also, this statement applies to relatively minor hearing losses; the higher the loss the longer the recovery time. Some authorities feel that about 48 hours' separation from noise is adequate for maximum recovery; others estimate the necessary recovery time at varying periods ranging from three to six months.

Wisconsin, New York, and Missouri have enacted statutory requirements that a claim may not be filed until at least six months after the last exposure to injurious noise. These provisions are, however, based upon other factors in addition to possible recovery to hearing.

Glorig (1960) stated with reference to noise-induced hearing losses that 'Temporary changes may be defined as those which result from an acute insult and recover to the resting threshold within a few days, from 10 to 14 at the most'. With reference to hearing loss resulting from blows to the head, often difficult to distinguish from noise-induced loss, Glorig stated 'it is wise to allow a period of at least six months to elapse before making a diagnosis of permanent threshold shift due to a blow on the head'.

The 1953 report of the New York Committee of Consultants on Occupational Loss of Hearing stated:

Until such time as the above discussed research evidence is available on which to base a precise answer, your Committee is of the opinion that the present policy of the Board in this matter should be continued, namely, that appraisal of permanency of an occupational hearing loss be made after an interval of not less than 6 months after the cessation of exposure to the injurious noise.

Based upon the above mentioned factors it is obvious that final evaluation of hearing should be based upon hearing tests made at least 14 days after the last exposure to noise. Wherever possible, greater assurance of maximum stabilization of hearing will be obtained by basing the hearing evaluation upon tests made after a longer period of separation from noise, preferably from two to four weeks after the last exposure.

SUMMARY

The foregoing has presented a few historical facts and the status of compensation for hearing loss as it has been for a number of years. But owing to the changing nature of compensation in all respects, reciting what legislation and regulation exists now is not necessarily the same as it will be one year from now. Much is happening regarding hearing loss and its relation to compensation. There is a committee set up by the federal government to study the question and provide recommendations that will unify the system throughout the country. A glance at Table 38.3 should convince anyone that this is essential. There is absolutely no consistency among the states with respect to monetary considerations, methods of calculation of percent impairment, allowance for presbycusis, etc.

TABLE 38.3. *Summary of several aspects of the compensation laws in all states. (From Fox 1976)*

Jurisdiction	Is occupational hearing loss compensable in jurisdiction?	What is the maximum compensation (one ear)? ($)	What is the maximum compensation (two ears)? ($)	What method/formula is used for determining hearing loss?	Is there a waiting period?	Is deduction made for Presbycusis?
Alabama	Yes	5406	16 526		No	
Alaska	Yes	7280	28 000	ME	No	
Arizona	P	11 000	33 000	AMA	No	P
Arkansas	Yes	2660	9975	ME	No	No
California	Yes	3157	21 770	AMA (3000 Hz)	No	
Colorado	Yes	2940	11 676	ME	No	Yes
Connecticut	Yes	6552	19 656	ME	No	No
Delaware	Yes	5625	13 125	ME	No	No
District of Columbia	Yes	16 552	63 660	AMA	No	P
Florida	Yes	4480	16 800	ME	No	Yes
Georgia	Yes	5700	14 250	AMA	6 Mo.	No
Hawaii	Yes	8684	33 400	AMA	No	Yes
Idaho	Yes		14 437	AMA ME	P	
Illinois	Yes				No	No
Indiana	Not decided	4500	12 000	ME	No	No
Iowa	Yes	7350	25 725	ME	No	P
Kansas	Yes	3093	11 341	ME	No	No
Kentucky	Yes	7200	14 976	AMA	No	No
Louisiana				ME		
Maine	Yes	7070	28 282	AMA	6 Mo.	Yes
Maryland	Yes		14 655	AMA	6 Mo.	Yes
Massachusetts	No	4500	12 000	ME	No	P
Michigan	Yes			ME	No	P
Minnesota	Yes	11 475	22 950	ME	No	No
Mississippi	Yes	2520	9450	ME	No	No
Missouri	Yes	3200	11 840	AMA	6 Mo.	Yes
Montana	Yes	2940	14 700	AMA	6 Mo.	Yes

TABLE 38.3. *Summary of several aspects of the compensation laws in all states. (From Fox 1976) (cont.)*

Jurisdiction	Is occupational hearing loss compensable in jurisdiction?	What is the maximum compensation (one ear)? ($)	What is the maximum compensation (two ears)? ($)	What method/formula is used for determining hearing loss?	Is there a waiting period?	Is deduction made for Presbycusis?
Nebraska	No	5000	10 000	AMA	No	No
Nevada	Yes				No	No
New Hampshire	Yes	7644	31 458	AMA	No	No
New Jersey	Yes	3000	8000	old AMA	No	No
New Mexico	No	3918	14 694	ME		No
New York	Yes	5700	14 250	AMA	6 Mo.	No
North Carolina	Yes	10 220	21 900	AMA	6 Mo.	No
North Dakota	Yes	2000	8000	ME AMA	Yes	No
Ohio	Yes	2325	11 625		No	Yes
Oklahoma	Yes	5000	10 000	ME	No	
Oregon	Yes	4200	13 440	Modified AMA	No	
Pennsylvania	Yes	11 220	48 620	ME	No	
Puerto Rico	Yes	2250	9000	ME	No	
Rhode Island	Yes	765	4500	AMA	Yes	
South Carolina	Yes	7628	15 733	ME	P	
South Dakota	Yes	4400	13 200	ME	No	
Tennessee	Yes	6375	12 750	ME		
Texas	Yes		10 500		P ME	
Utah	Yes	Only trauma	10 323	ME	Yes	
Vermont	No	4732	19 565	ME	No	
Virginia	Yes	8100	16 200	Modified AMA	No	
Washington	Yes	2400	14 400	AMA	No	
West Virginia	Yes	10 380	31 340	AMA	P ME	
Wisconsin	Yes	2 052	12 312		No	
Wyoming	Yes	4720	9440	ME	Yes	
US Department of Labor	Yes	28 360	109 030			

ME: medical evaluation; AMA: American Medical Association; P: possible.

Compensation for hearing loss in this country can produce a serious economic impact over the next ten years unless a reasonable system for handling the multitude of claims that will inevitably be filed during that time. The cost of compensation for noise-induced hearing loss can run into billions of dollars if the existing situation is allowed to continue.

REFERENCES

AMERICAN STANDARDS ASSOCIATION (1954). The relations of hearing loss to noise exposure. Report of Exploratory Subcommittee Z24-X-2.
COMMITTEE ON CONSERVATION OF HEARING (1959). Guide for the evaluation of hearing impairment. *Trans. Am. Acad. Ophthal. Otolar.* **63**, 236–8.
CORSO, J. F. (1963). Age and sex differences in pure-tone thresholds. *Archs Otolar.* **77**, 396.
FOWLER, E. P. and SABINE, P. E. (1947). Tentative standard procedure for evaluating the percentage loss of hearing in medico-legal cases. *J. Am. med. Ass.* 133, 396–7.
FOX, M. S. (1976). Workman's compensation hearing loss statutes in the U.S. and Canada. *Natn. Saf. News.*
GLORIG, A. (1960). Impaired hearing. In *Traumatic medicine and surgery* (ed. P. D. Cantor) Vol. 3, p. 158. Butterworth, Washington.
—— GRINGS, W., and SUMMERFIELD, A. (1958). Hearing loss in industry. *Laryngoscope, St. Louis* **68**, 447–65.
—— WHEELER, D. E., QUIGGLE, R., GRINGS, W., and SUMMERFIELD, A. (1954). Wisconsin State Fair Hearing Survey. Statistical treatment of clinical and audiometric data. *Trans. Am. Acad. Ophthal. Otolar.* Suppl.
NEW YORK WORKMAN'S COMPENSATION BOARD (1953). Report of the Committee of Consultants on Occupational Loss of Hearing, p. 11.

39 Compensation for industrial hearing loss: the practice in Canada

PETER W. ALBERTI

INTRODUCTION

The compensation of industrial injuries, including hearing loss, is a Provincial responsibility in Canada, administered by appointed Workers Compensation Boards in each of the ten Provinces and two Territories. Law courts are involved only exceptionally, to arbitrate points of law, but not to give awards.

The Boards assess whether there is an acceptable claim and decide the size of the award to be made. An award once made may be appealed by employer or employee and, if need be, re-appealed to a quasi-judicial board-appointed appeal tribunal. Claims are settled fairly quickly, but from the standpoint of noise claims, less emphasis is placed on exposure risk factors than if an adversary legal system was involved.

Workers Compensation Boards

The Boards are appointed by the Provincial government, usually under the aegis of the Ministry of Labour, but are semi-autonomous Crown Corporations, not Government departments. They act as industrial insurance companies. Employers are obliged to pay a premium for each worker if the work force exceeds a very small number, which may vary from Province to Province, but is always below ten. For smaller work forces subscription is voluntary. The workman does not contribute. The Boards are designed to be fiscally self-supporting, receiving no funds from taxation and therefore the charges bear a close relationship to other insurance premiums less the profit margin. The assessments are based on industries, and within industries upon previous claims experience. Thus, an employer with all his work force seated in an office will be charged a lower premium than a mine operator. The basic premium for any group is determined by the total number of claims from that group in the preceding three-year period, but if a particular plant has a bad accident record, then its premiums will be loaded, i.e. there is a no-fault incentive to a safe record. The parallelism with insurance companies is only superficial, for the Boards are quasi-judicial bodies with powers equal to the Supreme Court of the Province in relation to the procuring of evidence. Compensation payments may be temporary—as for an acute injury—or permanent. If the latter they may be paid as a lump sum in the case of smaller awards, or as lifelong pensions with larger awards. Most hearing loss awards are permanent.

The boards are headed by a Chairman, assisted by a number of deputy commissioners or members, usually lay people, who act as a corporate board of directors. The senior professionals are the Medical Directors, who are assisted in the larger Provinces by full-time physicians undertaking pension assessments and rehabilitative therapy.

The author polled the Medical Directors of the Boards concerning hearing claims practice to obtain information for this chapter. The results are incorporated here and are gratefully acknowledged.

Geography

The situation in Canada is difficult to follow without appreciating its geography. The country is huge and the population sparse. The four Maritime Provinces, Newfoundland, Prince Edward Island, Nova Scotia, and New Brunswick, have a combined surface area twice that of the United Kingdom, and a total population of just under that of either of Canada's two biggest cities—Toronto and Montreal. Details of size and population are given in Table 39.1 and Fig. 39.1. The physical size determines to some extent what is feasible in terms of providing comprehensive compensation services, and one cannot put the numbers of claims into perspective without a knowledge of population density.

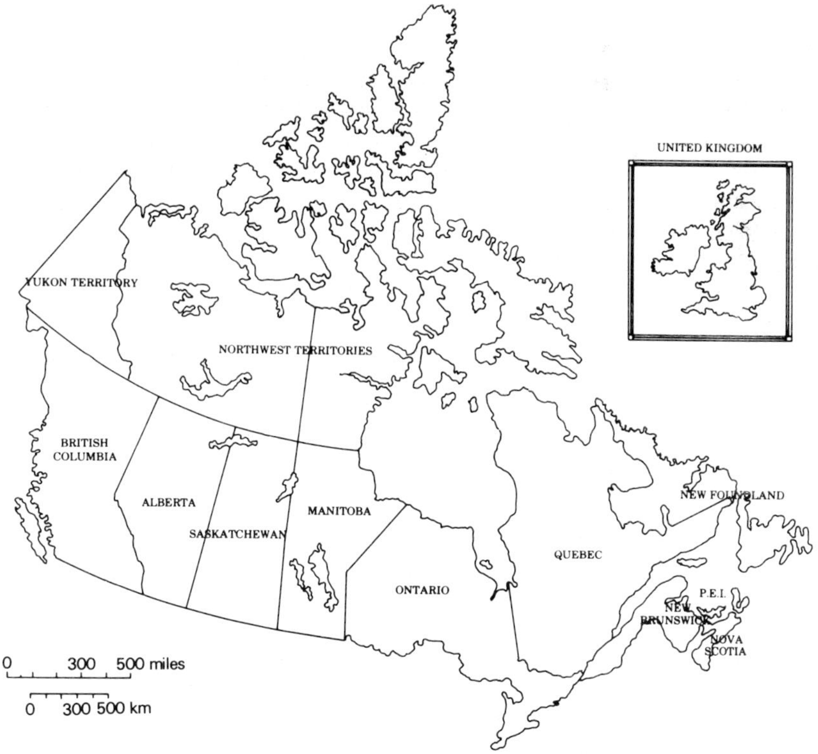

Fig. 39.1. Map showing the size of Canadian provinces compared with the United Kingdom.

TABLE 39.1. *Population and size of Canadian Provinces compared with the UK*

Province	Population (1976)	Surface area (sq. miles)
Alberta	1 838 000	255 285
Br. Columbia	2 466 600	366 255
Manitoba	1 021 500	251 000
Newfoundland	557 700	156 185
New Brunswick	677 300	28 354
N. W. Territories	42 600	1 304 903
Nova Scotia	828 000	21 425
Ontario	8 264 000	412 582
PEI	118 200	2184
Quebec	6 234 500	594 860
Saskatchewan	921 300	251 700
Yukon	21 800	207 076
Dominion of Canada	22 992 600	3 851 809
United Kingdom	>50 000 000	94 214

History

Acute hearing loss caused by trauma has been compensable as long as workmen's compensation boards have existed. Compensation for hearing loss caused by chronic exposure to intense sound came later; the provinces vary widely in the date that compensation first became available, ranging from Saskatchewan in 1930, to the Northwest Territories in 1974 (Table 39.2). In practise chronic hearing loss was not a major compensation problem until the mid-1970s.

TABLE 39.2. *Date that compensation first became available*

Province	Date hearing loss from noise first compensible	Date of first claim
Alberta	pre-1942	not available
Br. Columbia	1975	1976
Manitoba	not available	1965
Newfoundland	1967	1976
New Brunswick	1968?	1968?
N. W. Territories	1974	1975
Nova Scotia	1965	not available
Ontario	1947	1950
Quebec	not available	not available
PEI	not available	not available
Saskatchewan	1930	not available
Yukon	not available	1973

PHILOSOPHY

The philosophy underlying compensation generally determines what happens to claims. Whether impairment (a deviation from the normal), handicap (an impairment sufficient to cause social difficulty) or disability (an inability to earn a full living), is to be compensated, clearly affects how hearing loss, measured in decibels, is converted into percentage pension, expressed in dollars. The compensation boards are charged to provide a partial award to compensate for loss of earning capacity. There is supposed to be no compensation for pain and suffering, damage or loss of enjoyment of life. Thus the underlying philosophy originally was to compensate a disability and to ignore social handicap and minor impairments. However, in Canada, as elsewhere this philosophy has not been applied to hearing loss, with confusing consequences.

Until approximately 1973 in most Canadian provinces compensation was paid to an eligible claimant only if he had stopped working in noise. If he was still employed in quiet surroundings this usually, but not always implied a loss of earning power, but more often compensation was only paid upon retirement. This completely negated the general philosophy of compensation for clearly compensation was being paid for loss of quality of life in retirement rather than loss of earning power. In the poll of the Chief Medical Officers of the Boards, the answers received covered a wide spectrum. The Chief Medical Officer of Nova Scotia summarizes the actual situation in most provinces:

> Workmen's compensation was basically put into effect to compensate individuals for loss of earnings in relation to disabilities arising in the course of their employment. Since then, however, it has become much more broad in scope and permanent disability awards regarding all types of occupational diseases and injuries do try to take into account the social implications as well as the claimant's ability to earn a living, etc. However, I believe that the basic concept of compensating a man regarding his ability to earn a living probably should be kept as the main point, although this certainly must not be allowed to completely control the basic outcome in compensation awards.

The Director of Medical Services of the Worker's Compensation Board of Saskatchewan has summarized the dilemma concerning hearing:

> In as much disability awards are paid to workers whose earning capacity is not impaired by the hearing loss, we are presumably attempting to compensate for handicap. For those of us who are engaged, daily, in the assessment of 'permanent disability', it seems essential that disability awards must, eventually, be broken down into two components. One component we call total body impairment or handicap, and the other component is loss of earning power. We do this to a certain extent at the present time, but we are aware that there are serious inconsistencies in our present practice.

It is clear that the Canadian provinces are no different from many other countries, where this particular question is under considerable debate. The matter is well discussed by Noble (1978) and by Suter (1978).

In 1973 Ontario changed its legislation covering the compensation of hearing loss and allowed claimants to be compensated for hearing loss even though they continued to work at risk. This opened a floodgate of claims. All provinces now allow workmen to continue in noise, and to receive compensation. Thus compensation for hearing loss moved from compensation for loss of earning power (at least during the working lifetime), to compensation for a physical impairment, although as will be seen later, the impairment has to be quite marked to the point of being handicapping before it is considered severe enough to be worthy of pension.

Rating scale

The basis for the rating scales in all areas of the country is pure-tone audiometry, although the details vary. Glorig was commissioned by the Compensation Board of Ontario in the 1950s to devise a hearing compensation scale, which in a much modified version is still used today. At that time audiometric calibration was to ASA standards. He recommended that pensions be awarded when hearing loss averaged at frequencies 500, 1000, and 2000 Hz exceeded 25 dB (ASA). The same figures were used by the American Academy of Ophthalmology and Otolaryngology in their rating scale (1959) but by then ASA had given way to ISO and the Ontario table was rewritten to take note of the calibration changes, and so that pensions started at 35 dB (Table 39.3). The better ear carried a weighting of 5:1, with one ear total deafness rated at 3 per cent, and the hearing loss was graded in 5 dB averaged steps. In 1972 a revision of the schedule raised the award for total deafness in one ear to 5 per cent. In case a measurement falls between 5 dB steps rounding is upwards. The scale is not linear, for after an initial loading it rises by quite small increments in the low range of hearing loss,

TABLE 39.3. *Table used by Ontario Compensation Board for converting hearing loss into PD*

ISO average hearing loss (dB)*	better hearing ear	plus	Worse hearing ear
35–6	2.0		0.4
37–41	3.5		0.7
42–6	5.0		1.0
47–51	7.0		1.4
52–6	9.0		1.8
57–61	11.5		2.3
61–6	14.0		2.8
67–71	17.0		3.4
72–6	20.0		4.0
> 76	25.0		5.0

*Average threshold loss at 0.5 1, 2, and 3 kHz.
PD = sum of PD for better and worse hearing ears.
Remove 0.5 dB from average for each year of age older than 60 years.
Total hearing loss in one ear with no loss in the other equals 5 per cent PD.

and quite sharply in the upper range. Total bilateral hearing loss however is only rated 30 per cent of total body disability (Pensionable Disability—PD), reached at a hearing loss of 80 dB.

A presbycusis correction of 0.5 dB/a was originally applied for each year above the age of 50, but in the early 1970s it was moved upwards by a decade, i.e. was only applied from the age of 60 at the same level, 0.5 dB/a. 3 kHz was also added to the frequencies averaged. At present therefore, pensions are based on a four-frequency average 500, 1000, 2000, and 3000 Hz weighted equally with a 5:1 weighting for the better ear and interpreted by the same table as previously, shown as Table 38.3. It has been shown that with the sloping high-frequency loss characteristic of chronic noise exposure the numbers pensioned under the Ontario four-frequency average starting at 35 dB is virtually identical to the AAOO three-frequency average (Alberti, Morgan, Fria and LeBlanc 1976) starting at 25 dB, (which has now been replaced by a four-frequency average, starting at 25 dB!).

The provinces of Alberta, Manitoba, Newfoundland, New Brunswick, Nova Scotia, and Saskatchewan use the same tables as Ontario as do the Northwest Territories and Yukon. British Columbia and Quebec compensate on a three-frequency average, 500, 1000, and 2000 Hz: the former with a 4:1 weighting for the better ear starting at 28 dB, and reaching the maximum at 68 dB (Table 39.4), the latter with a 5:1 weighting and a range from 25 to 65 dB (Table 39.5).

TABLE 39.4. *PD hearing loss table—British Columbia*

Loss of hearing (dB) measured in each ear	Percentage of total disability		
	Ear most affected	plus	Ear least affected
0–27	0		0
28–32	0.3		1.2
33–7	0.5		2.0
38–42	0.7		2.8
43–7	1.0		4.0
48–52	1.3		5.2
53–7	1.7		6.8
58–62	2.1		8.4
63–7	2.6		10.4
> 68	3.0		12.0

Complete loss of hearing in both ears equals 15 per cent total disability.
Complete loss of hearing in one ear with no loss in the other equals 3 per cent of total disability.
The loss of hearing is the average threshold at 500, 1000, and 2000 Hz.

The scale for British Columbia, like that of Ontario, is non-linear, with small PD increments for relatively minor hearing losses but greater increments for higher losses. In contrast the Quebec scale is essentially linear, and therefore relatively more generous at low hearing losses than either British Columbia or Ontario. This is a matter of some significance as most

TABLE 39.5. *PD hearing loss table—Quebec*

Loss of hearing (dB)*	Better hearing ear	plus	Worse hearing ear
25	2.5		0.5
30	5.0		1.0
35	7.5		1.5
40	10.0		2.0
45	12.5		2.5
50	15.0		3.0
55	17.5		3.5
60	20.0		4.0
65	25.0		5.0

*Average pure-tone threshold 500, 1000, and 2000 Hz; remove 0.5 dB from average for each year of age older than 59 years.

hearing loss claims fall in the lower portions of the PD scales. The maximum PD for hearing loss in British Columbia is 15 per cent, in Quebec it is 30 per cent. Quebec uses the same presbycusis corrections as Ontario. The other Provinces vary in their application of this correction. In British Columbia and Nova Scotia it is not applied, New Brunswick applies it sparingly.

The following illustrative case shows how these various factors affect the final PD figure in the Provinces.

Illustrative case

A 66-year-old retired gold miner establishes a claim for industrial hearing loss. No other cause for deafness is found. The length of exposure (36 years) is sufficient and noise levels are accepted as potentially harmful. His loss is sensorineural, bone conduction thresholds equalling air conduction thresholds, which are:

Thresholds (Hz)	250	500	1000	2000	3000	4000	6000	8000
Right ear	20	25	40	55	70	80	85	85
Left ear	15	20	30	50	70	75	80	80

How would he fare in the various Provinces?
British Columbia. Average three-frequency hearing loss: left ear 33 dB, right ear 40 dB. No presbycusis correction is applied. From Table 39.4, PD = 2.7 per cent.

Ontario. Average four-frequency hearing loss: left ear 42 dB, right ear 47 dB. Presbycusis correction of 0.5 dB/a above age 59 applied to each ear. Compensable loss left ear 39 dB, right ear 44 dB. From Table 39.3, PD = 4.5 per cent.

Alberta, Nova Scotia, Newfoundland. Similar calculations as Ontario except no presbycusis correction applied. Compensable hearing loss therefore 42 dB in left ear and 47 dB in right ear. From Table 39.3, PD = 6.4 per cent.

Quebec. Three-frequency average hearing loss, left ear 33 dB, right ear 40 dB. A presbycusis correction of 0.5 dB/a above the age of 59 is applied. The compensable hearing loss is therefore 30 dB in the left ear and 37 dB in the right ear. From Table 39.5, PD = 7.0 per cent. (Had the presbycusis correction been omitted the PD would be 9.5 per cent)

Cash value

The cash value of pensions is affected both by the annual value and the numbers of years for which it is paid. Canadian provinces, with the exception of British Columbia, equate a total hearing loss with 30 per cent whole-body disability if the hearing loss is chronically produced. This figure on first sight seems harsh, but in reality is probably fairly generous. Unlike many States in the US where pensions for hearing loss are paid for a finite time, the Canadian pensions are paid for life and are paid even though the workman continues to work in a noisy environment. The average age of claimants in Ontario is 55 years, and their life expectancy at that age 20 years. Thus, an average pension is paid for 20 years. The monetary basis is as follows: 100 per cent PD is equated with 75 per cent of a workman's earnings in the last full year in which he was employed. There is however a maximum to the scale which varies from province to province, but in round figures is not less than $16 000 ($12 000 in Newfoundland). Thus 100 per cent PD represents up to $12 000 annually tax free (often reached in well unionized industries) and 30 per cent PD—the maximum paid in most provinces for total hearing loss—is worth $3600 ($2700 in Newfoundland) annually. In practice the overwhelming majority of hearing losses produced by noise are much less than this, and the mean PD of a large series of claimants in Ontario is approximately 7 per cent. This is equivalent in cash terms to a maximum of approximately $850 per year or $17 000 in the man's lifetime. In British Columbia payments are much lower. Alberta, Quebec, New Brunswick, and Saskatchewan tend to make one-time lump sum payments for PD awards of less than 10 per cent—the majority of hearing claims, the amount being based on the estimated cost of an annuity paying a similar amount as the lifetime pension. In an inflationery economy this system is less costly to the boards. If a worker's hearing worsens (and he continues to work in noise) he may claim a further evaluation, which may lead to a further payment.

Traumatic hearing loss

Acute traumatic hearing losses are usually treated more generously than chronic losses. Ontario and Quebec give up to 60 per cent PD for acute bilateral complete hearing loss, as do Alberta, Manitoba, Nova Scotia, New Brunswick, and the two Territories. During rehabilitation the temporary award is 100 per cent. In Newfoundland total deafness is awarded a period of total temporary benefits which is then followed, after appropriate rehabilitation, by a 30 per cent disability pension. Clearly, this type of accident is rare, and if it occurs is usually overshadowed by other physical injuries, which would be compensated at their own and possibly greater rate. In Saskatchewan, although there has never been a claim for acute sudden hearing loss, theoretically the claimant would be paid 100 per cent until rehabilitated and then 60 per cent for life, possibly supplemented to 100 per cent on wage loss. As these claims are so few, the author believes they would be treated generously on an ad hoc basis in most Provinces.

Tinnitus compensation

Boards are cautious about compensating for tinnitus because the symptom does not produce a lack of earning power and becasue of the difficulty in measuring it. Most will reluctantly give some funds towards tinnitus if there is a coexistent compensable hearing loss. The newly introduced tinnitus masking devices are being considered as benefits under compensation, although the evidence for their effectiveness in industrial hearing loss is rather vague.

NUMBER OF CLAIMS

The total number of claims has risen greatly in many parts of the country. The figures are particularly startling when population size is taken into account. The number of claims naturally exceeds the number pensioned. The former give an indication of the additional workload on hearing testing centres, and the latter the monetary cost of the pensions.

On a province-by-province basis there are no figures available for Alberta, although it is stated that the number of claims there is small—certainly less than 50 per year (perhaps due to the requirement for one month away from industrial noise before evaluation can take place—see below). By contrast, in British Columbia where the population is larger but comparable, there were 1484 claims in 1976 and a similar number in 1977, leading to 210 pensions in 1976 and 572 pensions in 1977. In Manitoba since 1965 there have been 477 claims; 201 have been accepted. The number of claims averaged about 20 per year from 1966 to 1973, but have since risen to nearer 100 claims per annum. However, the numbers pensioned only reached double figures in 1973, with 19, 27, 51, and 34 in the years 1974–7 respectively. In Newfoundland there have been 13 claims for chronic noise exposure, four have been pensioned and 13 claims for accidental hearing loss due to head injury of which 12 are pensioned. In New Brunswick there have been 225 claims of which 82 qualified for regular monthly pensions. It is possible others were settled with lump sum payments, but annual figures are not available and thus it is impossible to tell whether or not the number of claims is increasing. In the Northwest Territories the first claim was received in 1975; there have been 20 in all, four of which were referred to other provinces as being due to noise exposure elsewhere, 11 have been processed, three pensioned and two rejected. The others are under review. In Nova Scotia there were between 20 and 30 claims per year, of which approximately 75 per cent are pensioned.

The total claims in Ontario are proportionately greater than in any other province, including British Columbia, as shown in Table 39.6. Both the numbers of claims and numbers pensioned have increased dramatically. The claims have increased approximately ten-fold (ten in 1954, 100 in 1964, 996 in 1974) in each of the first two decades since the first claim was received, and in 1977 alone exceeded 2400. The numbers pensioned exceeded 1300 in

TABLE 39.6. *Claims and awards 1961–77*

Year	British Columbia		Ontario		Quebec	
	Claims	Awards	Claims	Awards	Claims	Awards
1961–5			312	62		
1966–70			862	238		
1971–4			2320	969		
1975	NA	NA	1519	639	960	385
1976	1484	210	2463	1066	1597	165
1977	1500	572	2405	1364	1843	1140

1977. In Quebec there has been an equally dramatic recent rise in claims and pensions: 960 claims with 385 pensioned in 1975; 1597 claims with 167 pensioned in 1976; 1843 claims with 1140 pensioned in 1977. The discrepancy between claims and pensions in 1976 is due to the time taken to complete the total assessment, in many Provinces often several months.

In Saskatchewan the numbers pensioned for hearing loss have risen from three in 1973 to 22 in 1975 and 43 in 1977. In the Yukon Territory there have been only two claims, one a miner who was pensioned and assessed on the basis of work in another province, and the second a hunting guide who was exposed to rifle blast in the course of his occupation.

Thus, in Canada in 1977 there were approximately 6000 claims and 3500 pensions awarded (or cash settlements) for hearing loss caused by chronic exposure to noise. The significant rise in claims in the past five years is clearly a cause for concern, and is stretching the existing hearing test facilities to the limit. Part of the rise is due to more general Union and public awareness of the existence of pensions for hearing loss caused by noise, part by highly unionized industries becoming concerned with health in the workplace. The claims so far have come largely from the mining, steelmaking, lumber and timber, and paper industries, all well unionized. There was an enormous rise in claims when it became possible to obtain a pension for hearing loss and yet continue working in noise.

There are still untapped reservoirs of hard-of-hearing workmen, who if their unions became alert, will keep the numbers of claims high for some years to come. The whole of the Canadian automobile industry, much of which is centred in Southern Ontario, has yet to start claiming in any great numbers; with a work force of approximately 50 000 it is likely to swell the numbers of pensioners. A major problem exists with the transient element of the work force, e.g. the construction industry, largely consisting of immigrant workers, hired on a seasonal basis and not necessarily aware of their rights.

It is thus anticipated that the numbers of claims will continue to rise for some time before dropping, as a result of the hearing conservation programmes established in the last decade.

CLAIM EVALUATION

Hearing testing for pension evaluation requires a greater degree of accuracy than diagnostic audiometry, because in certain ranges of hearing each decibel is worth a significant sum. Facilities undertaking this type of work should be equipped not only with conventional audiometric equipment but also instrumentation for 'objective' hearing testing such as evoked electric response audiometry (ERA), which is an extremely good tool in evaluation of neurologically normal adult hard-of-hearing patients (Alberti 1970; see Chapter 41). The number of ERA machines available in Canada is definitely limited. In the author's laboratory more than 1500 compensation patients have been evaluated using this technique (Alberti 1974; Alberti, Morgan, and Czuba 1978).

The Provincial Boards have widely differing philosophies about hearing testing methodology. The Ontario Board steadfastly feels the Board should be responsible for fiscal decisions, but that the evaluation of handicap (and thus production of an audiogram) should be undertaken by independent non-Board personnel (in an analogy with the prescribing of drugs, separating the prescriber from the financially involved dispenser), while the British Columbia Board believe that it is the role of the Board not only to decide how much money should be given but also to undertake all tests 'in-house'.

In all Provinces an otologist's (or neuro-otologist's) opinion concerning diagnosis is necessary—but there is disagreement about source of audiograms considered valid for pension purposes, which in part at least stems from a pragmatic attitude about test facilities.

Audiology is a relatively young science in Canada, and specialists in this field are not evenly distributed throughout the country. In Alberta an audiogram produced by any qualified audiologist or otologist is acceptable. In British Columbia only audiograms produced by the Hearing Branch of the Compensation Board in its own central laboratory near Vancouver are acceptable for pension purposes. In Manitoba, because of the low volume, all the compensation work has been contracted to one independent otologist, who has an audiology laboratory in Winnipeg, the largest city of the Province. The same otologist has now started evaluation centres in other parts of the Province. In Newfoundland the Board uses the one audiology laboratory in Saint John's and otologists in other parts of the province. In New Brunswick the Board has provided facilities in a local hospital, which are, however, under the direction of an independent otologist. This is close to the major source of claims—one particular paper manufacturing plant. Claims from other parts of the province are accepted as long as the audiogram accompanying them comes from a specialist and is undertaken 'under the best conditions'. In Northwest Territories any audiogram undertaken by a qualified specialist may be used, while in Nova Scotia only hearing tests undertaken in the Hearing and Speech Clinic in Halifax are valid for pension purposes. This is an extremely high-quality hearing laboratory independent of the Board but financed by the Government, in which the small number of cases can be accommodated.

In Ontario the Board evaluates on the basis of outside reports and audiograms from acceptable ear, nose, and throat consultants. Unfortunately, the majority of the better hearing testing facilities are in the southern part of the province, and the majority of claims so far have come from the North. This has necessitated a considerable amount of unpopular travelling for workers, and a strong desire to be tested close to home, which is in stark contrast to British Columbia where one of the reasons given for central testing is the insistence of workers on testing under the best possible conditions in Vancouver! The Ontario Board will accept evaluations based on audiograms performed by graduate audiologists, most of whom are in the south of the Province.

In all parts of the country claims may be initiated by the worker, his Union, employer, his family doctor, or ENT specialist. In British Columbia this triggers a complete evaluation of the man's occupational and non-occupational noise exposure together with a comprehensive audiological and, if necessary, vestibular investigations at the Hearing Branch of the Board. Although only the Board's audiograms are used for pension calculation purposes, audiograms from all sources, including industrial audiograms, may be used in the apportionment of liability amongst the various employers. The medical/audiological assessment may be appealed by either worker or any employer to a Medical Review Panel. The pattern is similar in the other Provinces except that the medical/audiological evaluation is done by consultants rather than by Board employees.

A recent comparison in Ontario of the audiograms sent in by the initial referring otologist and those produced in a central laboratory demonstrated that peripheral otologists were very poor at picking up the 15–20 per cent of exaggerated hearing loss, which gives considerable weight to the practice of referring cases to a specialized laboratory.

In Quebec, as in Ontario, claimants are referred by the board to independent ENT consultants for evaluation; the board has developed commonsense guidelines covering the information required, audiometry must be undertaken by qualified audiologists. Independent noise surveys of the workplace are required: these are made either by the Environmental Protection Agency or the Natural Resource Ministry. Here also many claimants must travel long distances which generates certain problems. Frequently the claimants fly in small and noisy aeroplanes, and there is a suspicion amongst certain consultants that although the claimants have been away from their occupational source of noise for some time before a final audiogram is undertaken, they are in fact suffering from temporary threshold shift produced by aeroplane flying. Other claimants travel overnight by bus or train and arrive thoroughly tired for a fairly complex psycho-acoustic evaluation, and perhaps some problems arise from this. However, this is more than offset by the more accurate testing undertaken in a central laboratory as the recent survey in Ontario has shown.

In Saskatchewan claimants are evaluated in the Saskatchewan Hearing Aid Plan Clinic, and pensionable disabilities based only on results from that clinic. Thus, there, as in Nova Scotia, work is contracted out to the only government run clinic.

There is a diversity of opinion about the length of time that a claimant must be out of industrial noise before an audiogram can be made which is valid for pension purposes. This ranges from one month—in Alberta—to no waiting period at all in New Brunswick. In British Columbia a period of 14 hours is required; in Manitoba 24 hours; Newfoundland has no established figure; Northwest Territories require 24 hours; the practice of Nova Scotia is not available; Ontario and Saskatchewan require 48 hours, and the Yukon one month. In Ontario the figure used to be six months but when the Act was changed to allow someone to continue working and receive a pension, this was clearly impractical, and indeed Noble has recently (1978) pointed out how little scientific basis there was for such a six-month wait, and even a 48 hour period is somewhat arbitrary.

REHABILITATION

Compensation Boards are also charged with the rehabilitation of industrially injured workers and in the area of hearing loss this largely concerns the provision of hearing aids. An eligible workman can obtain a hearing aid with financial help in part or in whole from the Compensation Board in every Province, although the detailed practice varies.

In British Columbia considerable emphasis is placed on hearing rehabilitation, and eligible workmen are brought to the Board's own audiology unit, having a hearing aid undertaken, a period of orientation and a further rehabilitation if necessary. Aids are bulk purchased and supplied by the Board. In Manitoba hearing aids are provided on the recommendation of an otologist and audiologist, or a hearing aid dealer. In Newfoundland they may be chosen by an otologist or hearing aid technician. In New Brunswick an aid is provided on the recommendation of the examining specialist as it is in the Northwest Territories. In these provinces aids are purchased in the private sector and recompensed fully or in large part; in Nova Scotia aids are provided by the Hearing and Speech Clinic in Halifax. In Ontario the workman may buy his own aid; or may have a hearing aid evaluation undertaken in a local hospital or otologist's office leading to an aid being prescribed. The board will reimburse or pay up to $350 towards the cost of an aid so obtained, although in practice the cost has usually been less. In Quebec aids are purchased privately, and if recommended by an ENT specialist, are reimbursed up to a maximum of $340 for monaural or $680 for binaural aids. In Saskatchewan if an aid is recommended by a qualified audiologist it is usually provided through the Saskatchewan Hearing Aid Plan. If purchased privately, reimbursement will only equal the wholesale bulk price to the provincial plan. Once an aid has been provided, all the boards will also pay for batteries, repairs, and replacements. Binaural aids are extremely unusual benefits.

As the need for a hearing aid frequently leads to the initiation of the hearing loss claim, aids may be provided before a claim is settled or paid for retrospectively once the claim is allowed, as long as they are purchased within one year of the claim being initiated.

Even if a claimant's hearing loss is insufficient to warrant a pension, he may be allowed a hearing aid, as long as the hearing loss is attributable to noise exposure. Thus in Ontario a claim is allowed and the claimant is eligible for a hearing aid with an average four-frequency hearing loss of 25 dB, although no pension is awarded until the hearing loss reaches 35 dB

HEARING CONSERVATION

The provinces differ widely in their interest and legislation concerning hearing conservation. Permissible unprotected noise levels and exposure times vary. In Alberta, an 85 dB eight-hour safe limit has been adopted with a 5 dB doubling and halving, i.e. 90 dB for four hours, 95 dB for two hours, etc. In British Columbia 90 dB is considered safe exposure for eight hours, but 87 for 16 hours within a 24-hour period. It is the only Province to adopt a 3 dB halving and doubling rule. Manitoba follows the lead of Ontario, which currently utilizes a 90 dB eight-hour safe limit with a 5 dB halving, although there is legislation before Parliament to change this to 85 dB with a 5 dB halving and doubling. This rule already exists in Nova Scotia. Quebec has legislated a 90 dBA eight-hour per day cutoff with a 5 dB halving period. In Saskatchewan the only rule appears to be that hearing protection is necessary if sound in the workplace is in excess of 90 dBA, without a time period being mentioned. The lack of court cases and adversary confrontation in law has led to slackness in evaluating total noise exposure and dose. There is a tendency to accept claims if the workman has been exposed to noise in excess of 90 dBA irrespective of the length of exposure. This is in spite of extremely detailed noise measurements available in many cases. None of the provinces consider weekly dosages, nor have any of them come to grips with a longer than eight-hour work period as exist quite frequently in remote construction and drilling sites, where workers may work 12 hour shifts for several days and then have longer periods off.

If noise levels exceed those laid down by law then hearing protection must be provided, and theoretically must be worn, although the policing of this is difficult. The success of a hearing conservation programme depends upon wholehearted support from both management and labour; it requires considerable publicity to persuade workmen that protective devices are worth wearing and not a sign of softness or lack of manhood. Companies have varied enormously in the emphasis they place on hearing conservation procedures: some farsighted engineers brought back V R51 plugs from the Second World War to a big steel plant, which has had the benefit of a successful protection programme for 30 years; other companies are reluctant to start programmes even now! Unquestionably the greatest single incentive has been the rise in claims with its concomitant increase in compensation levies. This, coupled with an increasing awareness and interest in occupational health, has produced some model programmes.

The provinces also vary as to whether screening audiograms are necessary, and in their regulation of their standards. In Alberta the law is quite clear about the frequencies which must be tested, time out of noise, as well as equipment calibration and training of testers. In British Columbia testing may only be done by people trained in the Compensation Board's own hearing branch in the Board method, this is as true of audiologists and otologists as of technicians. Annual screening audiograms are mandatory if workplace noise levels exceed 85 dBA, and they must be completed on a form provided by the Compensation Board which becomes the property of the Compensation Board. They are introducing a method of computerizing the screening audiometric records on a Province-wide basis. The manually filled forms are optically scanned for computer entry; the information is analysed and reports provided both to the Compensation Board and to Industry. In all the other provinces whilst screening audiograms are to be done, none are collected by the Board. The writer suspects that such a scheme would be impractical in provinces with populations the size of Ontario or Quebec.

CONCLUSIONS

Claims for compensation for hearing loss in many parts of Canada have grown rapidly in the past decade, frequently outstripping the facilities required for orderly evaluation. The response to the problem has been part philosophical and part pragmatic. Much research is still needed—currently the Boards of British Columbia and Ontario sponsor extensive projects related to industrial hearing loss. This is reflected in the varying current practices which are constantly evolving. This account outlines the situation in mid-1978; it will undoubtedly be much modified in the next few years.

REFERENCES

ALBERTI, P. W. (1970). New tools for old tricks. *Ann. Otol. Rhinol. Lar.* **79**, 800–7.

—— and MORGAN, P. P. (1974). Occupational hearing loss—an otologist's view of a long-term study. *Laryngoscope, St. Louis* **84**, 1822–34.

—— —— and CZUBA, I. (1978). Speech and pure tone audiometry as a screen for exaggerated hearing loss in industrial claims. *Acta Oto-lar.* **85**, 328–31.

—— —— FRIA, T. J., and LEBLANC, J. C. (1976). Percentage hearing loss: various schema applied to a large population with noise-induced hearing loss. In *Effects of noise on hearing* (ed. D. Henderson, R. P. Hamernick, D. S. Dosangh, and J. H. Mills) pp. 479–98. Raven, New York.

AMERICAN ACADEMY OF OPHTHALMOLOGY AND OTOLARYNGOLOGY COMMITTEE ON CONSERVATION OF HEARING (1959). Guide for the evaluation of hearing impairment. *Trans. Am. Acad. Ophthal. Otolar.* **63**, 236–8.

NOBLE, W. G. (1978). *Assessment of impaired hearing.* Academic Press, New York.
SUTER, A. (1978). The ability of mildly hearing-impaired individuals to discriminate speech in noise. US Environmental Protection Agency. EPA 550/9-78-100.

40 Compensation for occupational hearing loss: the practice in Australia

J. H. MACRAE and R. A. PIESSE

It is obviously preferable to prevent the occurrence of occupational hearing loss rather than compensate for it. Regulations intended to set limitations on the industrial noise exposure of workers, loosely based on the model regulations proposed by the National Health and Medical Research Council of the Australian Department of Health (National Health and Medical Research Council 1974), have been introduced in the Australian States of Queensland and South Australia, are about to be introduced in Victoria, and are in preparation in New South Wales and Western Australia.

In brief, these regulations require employers to ensure that no employee is exposed at any time to a noise level exceeding 115 dB (A), or to a daily noise dose which exceeds 1.0 (equivalent to a continuous noise level of 90 dB(A) for eight hours). More particularly, they require management to carry out noise surveys to determine the extent of the noise problem and the noise exposure hazards of employees, and industries found to be noisy are required to introduce noise reduction and hearing conservation programmes.

Hopefully, the introduction of noise regulations will help in the long run to reduce the incidence of noise induced hearing loss. However, it will never be possible to eliminate occupational hearing loss entirely. In the first place, accidental injuries resulting in hearing loss will continue to occur and, secondly, it would be uneconomical in the foreseeable future to make the regulations so stringent that even individuals highly susceptible to noise induced hearing loss would be protected. There is therefore a permanent requirement for compensation for occupational hearing loss.

WORKERS' COMPENSATION STATUTES

The first workers' compensation statute for an English-speaking country was passed by the United Kingdom Parliament in 1897. In 1902, Western Australia became the first Australian State to enact legislation similar to the United Kingdom statute, followed by Queensland in 1905, New South Wales and Tasmania in 1910, South Australia in 1911, and Victoria in 1914 (Woodhouse and Meares 1974). In Australia, as in the United Kingdom, the introduction of workers' compensation laws was intended to eliminate the uncertainties of obtaining damages for injuries sustained at work by means of common law or employers' liability laws. Prior to the introduction of compensation laws, an employee injured at work had to file a suit against his employer and prove that the injury was due to the employer's negligence. The employer could defeat the claim if he could prove that the employee's injury was due to the ordinary risks of his work, if it was caused by the negligence of a fellow worker, or if the employee contributed in any way to his own injury by his own negligence. The difficulty of proving negligence and these three defences excluded nearly all injured workers from any form of compensation. The social consequences of this state of affairs eventually became intolerable and workers' compensation laws were introduced to rectify the situation.

The workers' compensation laws of Australia, as in the United Kingdom, provide for compensation on a no-fault basis. Under these statutes, an employer is liable to pay compensation when an employee sustains a personal injury arising out of or in the course of his employment or when the employment contributes to the contraction of a disease or to the aggravation, acceleration, or recurrence of a disease. Under all of the legislation there is a general requirement that the onus rests with a claimant to prove his claim to the administering authorities. In the case of an injury, some causal connection must be established to show that it arose out of the employment, but a mere temporal connection is sufficient to show that it arose in the course of employment. In the case of a disease or the aggravation, acceleration, or recurrence of a disease, however, it must be shown that the employment was a contributing factor and this requires a causal connection. Claimants do not have to prove their claims beyond all doubt or by direct evidence, but are required to establish to the satisfaction of the administering authorities that the matters in question in their claims are more likely to be the case than not.

Workers' compensation is provided for by legislation in each State and Territory of Australia and also by the Australian Commonwealth Government. There are in fact ten workers' compensation schemes, administered by ten different authorities, a summary of which is provided in Table 40.1. It

TABLE 40.1 *Workers' compensation legislation in force in Australia (August 1978)*

Statute	Title of Legislation	Administering Authority
New South Wales	Workers' Compensation Act	Workers' Compensation Commission of NSW
Victoria	Workers' Compensation Act	Workers' Compensation Board
Queensland	Workers' Compensation Act	State Government Insurance Office
South Australia	Workmens' Compensation Act	Department of Labour and Industry
Western Australia	Workers' Compensation Act	Workers' Compensation Board
Tasmania	Workers' Compensation Act	Department of Labour and Industry
Aust. Capital Territory	Workmens' Compensation Ordinance	Department of the Capital Territory
Northern Territory	Workmens' Compensation Ordinance	Department of the Northern Territory
Aust. Commonwealth	Compensation (Commonwealth Employees) Act	Office of the Commissioner for Employees' Compensation
Seamen	Seamen's Compensation Act	Department of Social Security

can be seen from this that, in some cases, workers' compensation is administered by Boards, Tribunals, or Commissions. These tribunals have the authority to determine all matters arising under the legislation and, in general, there is no appeal against their decisions, except in questions of law. In the remaining cases, the legislation is administered by government departments, and disputes and appeals are determined by appropriate courts. As a result of the diversity of these schemes, this chapter can only present broad generalizations rather than precisely accurate details and should therefore be regarded as an introductory overview rather than a comprehensive and exhaustive treatise.

COMPENSATION FOR OCCUPATIONAL HEARING LOSS

For the purpose of workers' compensation, two forms of occupational hearing loss are generally distinguished. Firstly, there is the type of hearing loss produced suddenly by a single incident such as an explosion or a blow to the head, which is commonly referred to as deafness arising from personal injury by accident. Secondly, there is the type of hearing loss of gradual onset produced by exposure to high intensities of industrial noise over a long period of time, which is commonly referred to as industrial deafness or noise induced hearing loss, and comes within the category of diseases that are contracted by gradual process.

Since their introduction in the early part of this century, the various statutes have undergone repeated revision and amendment. The history of the development of those sections concerned with occupational hearing loss is complex, differing somewhat in each of the statutes. Lump-sum payments for hearing loss resulting from accidental injury have been included in the legislation since about 1930, but it was not until relatively recently that compensation for industrial deafness, the most commonly occurring form of occupational hearing loss, began to become available to workers. Originally, a worker was entitled to compensation for industrial deafness only if it could be established that his condition totally or partially incapacitated him for work. Since industrial deafness rarely causes incapacity for work, the vast bulk of workers with this condition were therefore excluded from compensation. In fact, it was not until about 1960 that amendments repealing the requirement of incapacity for work began to be introduced into most of the statutes, and this has still not been done in the Acts of Western Australia and Tasmania.

At the present time (1978), all the statutes include schedules or tables of specified injuries for which lump sum compensation is prescribed. Loss of hearing is included in all the schedules but the lump sums prescribed differ greatly, as can be seen from Table 40.2. In all the statutes, hearing loss arising from personal injury by accident is classed as an injury *simpliciter* and is compensated by means of a lump-sum payment of money, as prescribed in the schedule. The circumstances in which a worker who has suffered such an injury may recover compensation vary somewhat from statute to statute,

TABLE 40.2. *Lump-sum compensation for hearing loss in Australian Workers' compensation statutes (August 1978)*

Statute	Total loss of hearing $A	Complete deafness of one ear $A
New South Wales	14 450.00	6850.00
Victoria	15 090.00	4660.00
Queensland	10 020.00	4340.00
South Australia	15 000.00	—
Western Australia	33 649.50	—
Tasmania	12 859.00	5804.00
Aust. Capital Territory	21 177.89	6050.00
Northern Territory	17 500.00	5000.00
Aust. Commonwealth Employees	17 500.00	—
Seamen	17 500.00	5000.00

but most statutes specify that compensation is payable for injuries sustained in the following circumstances: where the injury occurs as a result of or in the course of employment, or is sustained while the worker is travelling between home and work, work and trade school, or home and trade school, or while the worker is attending trade school or where, for compensable conditions, the worker is travelling to receive medical treatment or a medical certificate or compensation. When an employee has suffered an accidental injury involving loss of hearing, he usually has no difficulty in establishing that the hearing loss occurred in the course of his employment by a particular employer and thus his right to compensation and the employer from whom the compensation is due. Industrial deafness, on the other hand, poses more complicated problems.

In order to succeed in making a claim for compensation for industrial deafness, an employee must establish that he suffered a particular degree of hearing loss, that it was as a result of noise exposure, that it arose out of or in the course of his employment, and that it occurred when he was employed by a particular employer or employers. Normally, little difficulty is involved in proving all these things when the worker has sustained a gradual loss of hearing as a result of noise exposure in the employment of one employer only, but, quite commonly, industrial deafness is due to a long history of employment in industry generally with different employers and even in different industries and in this case considerable difficulty is usually encountered.

In order to assist the employee overcome these hurdles, the general trend has been to shift the onus of proof on most of these matters onto the employer, either by the introduction of rules to that effect into the statutes, or where this has not happened, in actual practice by the administering authorities. For example, provided that an employee with a hearing loss was employed for a significant period of time in an industry regarded as likely to cause industrial deafness, the employer has to produce strong evidence if he wishes to establish that the loss was not entirely noise-induced or that it was not entirely caused by the worker's employment. Some statutory assistance has also been given to employees with industrial deafness who have changed employers or industries. In general, the hearing loss is deemed by statute to have been caused by the employer who employed, or had most recently employed, the employee at the time the claim for compensation was made, provided that the working conditions in the employment were likely to give rise to industrial deafness. This employer usually may require contributions from employers who previously employed the worker in noisy conditions, in proportions determined in the individual case by the administering authorities.

Although it is unusual for occupational hearing loss to cause incapacity for work, claims for weekly compensation on the basis of reduced capacity to earn are generally open to workers with damaged hearing. However, with the exception of the scheme in New South Wales where this entitlement is additional to and not in lieu of the entitlement to lump-sum compensation, the receipt of a lump-sum payment cancels the right to weekly payments. A worker who is compensated for occupational hearing loss will also be entitled to hospital and medical benefits, e.g. a hearing aid, in connection with that loss, in addition to other entitlements.

Apart from workers' compensation, a worker may sue his employer for damages at common law if he sustains a personal injury such as hearing loss as a result of negligence or breach of statutory duty by his employer. However, many difficulties confront workers who sue for damages for hearing loss. They must show that they have suffered a hearing loss and establish the cause. If the worker sues for damages for industrial deafness, it may be difficult to establish how much of the hearing loss was caused by noise exposure at work. If the employee has worked for more than one employer, it may be impossible to show how much deafness was caused by each employer. Employers may avoid liability by persuading the court that the measures necessary to reduce the noise would have been unreasonably costly, or that it was not reasonable to expect them to foresee the likelihood of deafness being caused by the noise. Also, the amount of damages may be substantially reduced if the court finds that the worker's own negligence, such as failure to wear ear protection, contributed to the hearing loss and, finally, if the worker's suit is successful, the workers' compensation statutes contain provisions to ensure that the worker does not keep both compensation payments and damages.

THE SETTLEMENT OF COMPENSATION CLAIMS

The way in which claims for compensation for hearing loss are settled differs from scheme to scheme. Each scheme makes use of medical boards and/or medical referees to assist in determining the cause, nature and extent of the harm for which compensation is sought but the role of medical experts is more important in some jurisdictions than in others. In Queensland, for instance, medical boards play a major role in the determination of claims and their findings as to the medical facts of the case are conclusive. In other jurisdictions, medical experts are used less frequently and their findings may be overridden by the administering authorities.

The procedure followed in New South Wales provides one example. When a worker serves a claim for compensation for loss of hearing on an employer in New South Wales, the employer sends the claimant to an otolaryngologist nominated by the employer's insurer. The otolaryngologist may or may not call upon the services of an audiologist in arriving at his assessment of the claimant's hearing loss. If the claimant and the insurer are both satisfied with the otolaryngologist's decisions concerning the nature and extent of the claimant's loss, the claim is finalized by mutual agreement, without being referred to the New South Wales Workers' Compensation Commission. However, if the claimant and the insurer are unable to reach agreement, then either can apply to the Commission for a medical board. Alternatively, or in the event that agreement is not reached as a result of the findings of the medical board, either the claimant or the insurer can lodge an application for determination with the Commission, which functions as a court of record.

Another example, illustrating the differences between schemes, is provided by the way in which claims made by employees of the Australian Commonwealth Government are settled. After serving notice of injury on the employing department, the employee serves a claim for compensation for hearing loss on the Commissioner for Employees' Compensation via a delegate of the Commissioner in the employing department. The delegate has the task of collecting all available relevant information from the claimant and the employing department and forwarding this to the Commissioner and to the National Acoustic Laboratories, where the claimant is tested by an audiologist and examined by a consultant otolaryngologist. The results of the audiological assessment and otolaryngological examination are sent to the Commissioner who then makes a determination concerning payment of compensation to the claimant. If the claimant is not satisfied with the determination, he can request that the matter be referred to a compensation tribunal or, alternatively, make an application to a prescribed court of record in the State in which he is employed, e.g. the New South Wales Workers' Compensation Commission or the South Australian Industrial Court, for a judicial review of the case.

Although none of the statutes requires the use of any particular procedure to arrive at the percentage loss of hearing of claimants, pressure in favour of the use of only one procedure has come from the Otolaryngological Society of Australia (OLSA) and also from the administering authorities who influence which procedure is used by accepting percentage loss assessments based on one procedure rather than another. The recent history of procedures used for compensation purposes can be found in the records of the Annual General Meetings of OLSA. At the 1960 Annual General Meeting, it was decided that no satisfactory method of assessing percentage loss of hearing was available and members were advised to continue using their current methods until further advised. This decision was subsequently objected to on the ground that the prevailing variety of methods led to confusion in the compensation courts and 'in many cases the reputation of the medical witness suffers in the lay mind because the doctors swear to such divergent percentage assessments' (Willis 1962). Accordingly, at the 1963 Annual General Meeting, motions were passed that OLSA should adopt one method for the assessment of percentage loss of hearing and, also, that the Society should adopt the Commonwealth Acoustic Laboratories method of assessing percentage loss of hearing (Murray 1962). This method, modified in 1970 to enable it to be used with hearing threshold levels obtained with audiometers calibrated to ISO reference zero thresholds, was then used widely throughout Australia for compensation purposes until 1975.

In 1974, the National Acoustic Laboratories (formerly called the Commonwealth Acoustic Laboratories) issued a new procedure for evaluating percentage loss of hearing (Appendix 1) (Macrae 1975–6). This was accepted in 1975 by appropriate committees of both the Otolaryngological and Audiological Societies of Australia as the best available procedure for assessing hearing loss on a percentage basis and was adopted in the same year by the Commissioner for Employees' Compensation and, in a slightly modified form, by the Workers' Compensation Committee of New South Wales. It was tested and found acceptable in compensation court cases in Victoria in 1976 and South Australia in 1977 and since then percentage loss assessments obtained with this procedure have been widely accepted by the authorities responsible for the administration of the various workers' compensation statutes.

The Acts of New South Wales, Queensland, South Australia, and Western Australia contain a subsection which requires an adjustment for presbycusis to be carried out. In effect, the subsection asserts that in ascertaining the percentage hearing loss of a worker who is over the age of 50 years, it shall be conclusively presumed that his hearing loss is, to the extent of one-half of a decibel for each complete year in excess of the age of 50 years, to be attributed to presbycusis. At the present time, this has been interpreted by the relevant administering authorities to mean that one-half of a decibel for each year over the age of 50 years should be subtracted from the hearing threshold level at each frequency in each ear before assessing the claimant's percentage loss of hearing. The injustice of this kind of presbycusis adjustment has been pointed out on a number of occasions (e.g Davis 1971; Lebo and Reddell 1972) and the National Acoustic Laboratories have urged that the subsection be repealed.

A subsection of the Compensation (Commonwealth Employees) Act states a principle that is applicable in connection with all the workers' compensation statutes when evaluating the compensable loss of hearing of workers who have both compensable and non-compensable components in their hearing loss. In the case of injury resulting in the loss of hearing by an employee whose hearing is already impaired, compensation is paid for the loss of the workers' residual hearing. If the loss of residual hearing is complete, compensation for total loss of hearing is payable. If a proportion of the residual hearing is lost, that proportion of the amount paid for the total loss of hearing is payable. In this circumstance, the compensable percentage loss of hearing (PLH) is determined by means of the formula

$$\text{Compensable PLH} = \frac{\text{Overall PLH} - \text{Non-compensable PLH}}{100 - \text{Non-compensable PLH}} \times 100$$

On the other hand, if a worker sustains a further hearing loss of a non-compensable nature after having sustained a compensable loss of hearing, the non-compensable component is simply ignored in assessing the compensable percentage loss.

FINANCIAL ASPECTS OF WORKERS' COMPENSATION

In Australia it is generally compulsory for employers to take out policies of insurance covering their workers' compensation liabilities and against common law damages. However, in some States employers meeting certain requirements may act as their own insurers with the approval of the appropriate authorities, and the Australian Commonwealth Government acts as a self-insurer in relation to its own employees. Licences to self-insure are not easy to obtain and are only issued where the size and financial strength of the employer is such that there would be no risk of the employer being unable, at any time, to meet his liabilities.

Some degree of control is generally exercised by the administering authorities in relation to the conduct and solvency of insurers, particularly in relation to the maximum rates of premium that may be charged. Premiums are payable in advance and are calculated according to the employer's estimate of wages. Renewed premiums are adjusted according to the difference between actual wages and the employer's estimate for the previous year. Differential rates are charged for various industries and it is the employer's industry rather than the individual worker's occupation that determines the rate. Premiums paid for workers' compensation insurance are tax deductible and are generally regarded as a direct cost of production to be passed on to the consumer.

The premiums actually paid by employers are affected by the rebate or bonus systems operated by most insurers. These range from informal systems where the employer's claims history is taken into account when quoting the next year's premium, to formal systems where bonuses are declared at the end of each year according to a specific formula based on the insurer's profit and the actual loss ratio of the employer. In each State insurers and self-insurers are required annually to contribute to workers' compensation funds in amounts assessed by the tribunals on the basis of the total premium income of the insurer. The administrative costs of the tribunals and various other expenses are met from these funds. Except in one State, uninsured liability schemes have been set up to ensure that an injured worker is not disadvantaged by his employer's failure to insure. Any amount paid under these schemes is recoverable from the employer. If such recovery cannot be made the amount is collected directly, or indirectly through the workers' compensation funds, from insurers.

Claims for compensation for industrial deafness are at present of minor concern to the Australian insurance industry. This feeling is partly engendered by the comparative ease with which these claims are handled. For the most part, a justifiable claim is made, the claimant's percentage loss of hearing is determined, and the claim is met. This definiteness is a far cry from the complexity and lack of certainty encountered in the settlement of the greater part of workers' compensation claims. More importantly, though, the cost to the industry of claims for industrial deafness is currently only a minute part of the total cost of all claims for workers' compensation. In 1975/6 the cost of industrial deafness claims was approximately $4 million Australia wide, whereas the total amount paid out in settlement of all workers' compensation claims for the same year was $299 million. It is obvious, therefore, that the relative cost of compensation for industrial deafness is at present quite small, being 1.3 per cent of the total. However, it is widely believed throughout the industry that the cost of claims for industrial deafness is going to increase sharply in the future.

Acknowledgements

Sources of information for this chapter included The Conspectus of Workers' Compensation Legislation in Australia, prepared annually by the Australian Department of Social Security and published by the Australian Government Publishing Service, Canberra, and papers by R. O'Keeffe, J. Disney, and B. Bennett included in the Proceedings of the 1978 Annual Conference of the Australian Acoustical Society concerning Occupational Hearing Loss—Conservation and Compensation, to be published by the Australian Acoustical Society, Sydney.

APPENDIX 40.1. PROCEDURE FOR DETERMINING PERCENTAGE LOSS OF HEARING. NATIONAL ACOUSTIC LABORATORIES AUSTRALIAN DEPARTMENT OF HEALTH (31 October 1974)

It is recommended that the following procedure be used to assess the degree of hearing loss of claimants for compensation for loss of hearing under the various Australian Compensation Acts, both Federal and State.

1. Measure the hearing levels (HLs) of the claimant at the audiometric frequencies 500, 1000, 1500, 2000, 3000, and 4000 Hz with an audiometer calibrated to the reference specified in Australian Standard AS-Z43 Part 2, Reference Zero for the Calibration of Pure Tone Audiometers. This reference is commonly known as ISO-1964 or simply ISO.

2. Determine the better and worse ear at each of these frequencies. At a particular frequency, the better ear is the ear with the smaller HL. The better ear at one frequency may be the worse at another.

3. Using the HLs of the better and worse ears, read the percent loss of hearing (PLH) at each frequency from the appropriate table (Table 40.A1 (a–f)) and add these six values of PLH together to obtain the overall (binaural) PLH.

Example

Frequency	Hearing levels		Better ear	Worse ear	PLH
	Right ear	Left ear			
500	40	10	10	40	1.7
1000	45	25	25	45	4.2
1500	50	40	40	50	7.0
2000	55	55	55	55	7.9
3000	60	70	60	70	6.6
4000	65	85	65	85	7.2
				Overall PLH =	34.6%

4. It is recommended that monaural evaluation of hearing loss not be carried out for compensation purposes. However, monaural evaluation is possible with these tables. The HL-worse ear dimension of the tables is ignored, and the monaural PLH is read from the top diagonal set of values, using the HL-better ear scale only.

Example

Frequency	HLs-RT ear	PLH
500	30	2.6
1000	40	7.2
1500	50	9.0
2000	60	9.1
3000	70	7.7
4000	80	8.9
	Monaural PLH =	44.5%

TABLE 40.A1(a). *Values of percentage loss of hearing corresponding to given hearing levels in the better and worse ears at 500 Hz*

HL — Worse Ear	HL — Better ear															
	≤15	20	25	30	35	40	45	50	55	60	65	70	75	80	85	90	≥95
≤15	0																
20	0.3	0.7															
25	0.6	1.1	1.5														
30	0.9	1.5	2.0	2.6													
35	1.3	1.9	2.5	3.3	4.1												
40	1.7	2.3	3.0	3.9	4.9	5.8											
45	2.0	2.7	3.3	4.3	5.4	6.5	7.4										
50	2.2	2.9	3.6	4.6	5.8	7.0	8.1	9.0									
55	2.5	3.2	3.9	4.9	6.1	7.3	8.6	9.7	10.6								
60	2.7	3.4	4.1	5.1	6.3	7.6	8.9	10.1	11.2	12.2							
65	2.9	3.6	4.3	5.3	6.5	7.8	9.1	10.4	11.7	12.8	13.7						
70	3.1	3.8	4.5	5.5	6.7	8.0	9.3	10.6	11.9	13.2	14.4	15.3					
75	3.2	3.9	4.6	5.6	6.8	8.1	9.4	10.7	12.1	13.4	14.7	15.9	16.7				
80	3.3	4.0	4.7	5.7	6.9	8.2	9.5	10.8	12.1	13.5	14.8	16.1	17.2	17.9			
85	3.3	4.0	4.7	5.7	6.9	8.2	9.5	10.8	12.1	13.5	14.8	16.2	17.4	18.3	18.9		
90	3.3	4.0	4.7	5.7	6.9	8.2	9.5	10.8	12.2	13.5	14.8	16.2	17.4	18.4	19.1	19.5	
≥95	3.3	4.0	4.7	5.7	6.9	8.2	9.5	10.8	12.2	13.5	14.8	16.2	17.4	18.4	19.2	19.7	20.0

TABLE 40.A1(b). *Values of percentage loss of hearing corresponding to given hearing levels in the better and worse ears at 1000 Hz*

HL — Worse Ear	HL — Better ear															
	≤15	20	25	30	35	40	45	50	55	60	65	70	75	80	85	90	≥95
≤15	0																
20	0.4	0.9															
25	0.7	1.3	1.9														
30	1.2	1.9	2.5	3.3													
35	1.6	2.4	3.2	4.1	5.2												
40	2.1	2.9	3.7	4.9	6.1	7.2											
45	2.5	3.3	4.2	5.4	6.8	8.1	9.2										
50	2.8	3.7	4.5	5.8	7.3	8.7	10.1	11.2									
55	3.1	4.0	4.8	6.1	7.6	9.2	10.7	12.1	13.2								
60	3.4	4.3	5.1	6.4	7.9	9.5	11.1	12.6	14.1	15.2							
65	3.6	4.5	5.4	6.6	8.2	9.8	11.4	13.0	14.6	16.0	17.2						
70	3.9	4.7	5.6	6.9	8.4	10.0	11.6	13.3	14.9	16.5	18.0	19.1					
75	4.0	4.9	5.8	7.0	8.5	10.1	11.8	13.4	15.1	16.7	18.4	19.8	20.9				
80	4.1	5.0	5.8	7.1	8.6	10.2	11.8	13.5	15.2	16.8	18.5	20.1	21.5	22.4			
85	4.1	5.0	5.9	7.1	8.6	10.2	11.9	13.5	15.2	16.9	18.5	20.2	21.7	22.9	23.6		
90	4.1	5.0	5.9	7.1	8.6	10.2	11.9	13.5	15.2	16.9	18.6	20.2	21.8	23.0	23.9	24.4	
≥95	4.1	5.0	5.9	7.1	8.6	10.2	11.9	13.5	15.2	16.9	18.6	20.3	21.8	23.0	24.0	24.7	25.0

TABLE 40.A1(c). *Values of percentage loss of hearing corresponding to given hearing levels in the better and worse ears at 1500 Hz*

							HL — Better ear									
	≤15	20	25	30	35	40	45	50	55	60	65	70	75	80	85	90	≥95
≤15	0																
20	0.3	0.7															
25	0.6	1.1	1.5														
30	0.9	1.5	2.0	2.6													
35	1.3	1.9	2.5	3.3	4.1												
40	1.7	2.3	3.0	3.9	4.9	5.8											
45	2.0	2.7	3.3	4.3	5.4	6.5	7.4										
50	2.2	2.9	3.6	4.6	5.8	7.0	8.1	9.0									
55	2.5	3.2	3.9	4.9	6.1	7.3	8.6	9.7	10.6								
60	2.7	3.4	4.1	5.1	6.3	7.6	8.9	10.1	11.2	12.2							
65	2.9	3.6	4.3	5.3	6.5	7.8	9.1	10.4	11.7	12.8	13.7						
70	3.1	3.8	4.5	5.5	6.7	8.0	9.3	10.6	11.9	13.2	14.4	15.3					
75	3.2	3.9	4.6	5.6	6.8	8.1	9.4	10.7	12.1	13.4	14.7	15.9	16.7				
80	3.3	4.0	4.7	5.7	6.9	8.2	9.5	10.8	12.1	13.5	14.8	16.1	17.2	17.9			
85	3.3	4.0	4.7	5.7	6.9	8.2	9.5	10.8	12.1	13.5	14.8	16.2	17.4	18.3	18.9		
90	3.3	4.0	4.7	5.7	6.9	8.2	9.5	10.8	12.2	13.5	14.8	16.2	17.4	18.4	19.1	19.5	
≥95	3.3	4.0	4.7	5.7	6.9	8.2	9.5	10.8	12.2	13.5	14.8	16.2	17.4	18.4	19.2	19.7	20.0

HL — Worse Ear

TABLE 40.A1(d). *Values of percentage loss of hearing corresponding to given hearing levels in the better and worse ears at 2000 Hz*

							HL — Better ear									
	≤15	20	25	30	35	40	45	50	55	60	65	70	75	80	85	90	≥95
≤15	0																
20	0.2	0.5															
25	0.4	0.8	1.1														
30	0.7	1.1	1.5	2.0													
35	1.0	1.5	1.9	2.5	3.1												
40	1.2	1.8	2.2	2.9	3.7	4.3											
45	1.5	2.0	2.5	3.2	4.1	4.9	5.5										
50	1.7	2.2	2.7	3.5	4.4	5.3	6.1	6.7									
55	1.9	2.4	2.9	3.7	4.6	5.5	6.4	7.3	7.9								
60	2.0	2.6	3.1	3.8	4.7	5.7	6.7	7.6	8.4	9.1							
65	2.2	2.7	3.2	4.0	4.9	5.9	6.8	7.8	8.8	9.6	10.3						
70	2.3	2.8	3.4	4.1	5.0	6.0	7.0	8.0	8.9	9.9	10.8	11.5					
75	2.4	2.9	3.5	4.2	5.1	6.1	7.1	8.1	9.1	10.0	11.0	11.9	12.5				
80	2.5	3.0	3.5	4.2	5.2	6.1	7.1	8.1	9.1	10.1	11.1	12.1	12.9	13.4			
85	2.5	3.0	3.5	4.3	5.2	6.1	7.1	8.1	9.1	10.1	11.1	12.1	13.0	13.7	14.1		
90	2.5	3.0	3.5	4.3	5.2	6.1	7.1	8.1	9.1	10.1	11.1	12.2	13.1	13.8	14.4	14.7	
≥95	2.5	3.0	3.5	4.3	5.2	6.1	7.1	8.1	9.1	10.1	11.1	12.2	13.1	13.8	14.4	14.8	15.0

HL — Worse Ear

TABLE 40.A1(e). *Values of percentage loss of hearing corresponding to given hearing levels in the better and worse ears at 3000 Hz*

		≤15	20	25	30	35	40	45	HL — Better ear 50	55	60	65	70	75	80	85	90	≥95
	≤15	0																
	20	0.1	0.2															
	25	0.3	0.5	0.7														
	30	0.5	0.7	1.0	1.3													
	35	0.7	1.0	1.3	1.7	2.1												
HL — Worse Ear	40	0.8	1.2	1.5	1.9	2.4	2.9											
	45	1.0	1.3	1.7	2.2	2.7	3.2	3.7										
	50	1.1	1.5	1.8	2.3	2.9	3.5	4.0	4.5									
	55	1.2	1.6	1.9	2.4	3.0	3.7	4.3	4.8	5.3								
	60	1.4	1.7	2.1	2.6	3.2	3.8	4.4	5.1	5.6	6.1							
	65	1.5	1.8	2.2	2.7	3.3	3.9	4.6	5.2	5.8	6.4	6.9						
	70	1.6	1.9	2.3	2.7	3.4	4.0	4.7	5.3	6.0	6.6	7.2	7.7					
	75	1.6	2.0	2.3	2.8	3.4	4.1	4.7	5.4	6.0	6.7	7.3	7.9	8.4				
	80	1.6	2.0	2.3	2.8	3.4	4.1	4.7	5.4	6.1	6.7	7.4	8.1	8.6	9.0			
	85	1.7	2.0	2.3	2.8	3.5	4.1	4.7	5.4	6.1	6.7	7.4	8.1	8.7	9.1	9.4		
	90	1.7	2.0	2.3	2.8	3.5	4.1	4.8	5.4	6.1	6.7	7.4	8.1	8.7	9.2	9.6	9.8	
	≥95	1.7	2.0	2.3	2.8	3.5	4.1	4.8	5.4	6.1	6.7	7.4	8.1	8.7	9.2	9.6	9.9	10.0

TABLE 40.A1(f). *Values of percentage loss of hearing corresponding to given hearing levels in the better and worse ears at 4000 Hz*

		≤20	25	30	35	40	45	HL — Better ear 50	55	60	65	70	75	80	85	90	≥95
	≤20	0															
	25	0.1	0.4														
	30	0.3	0.6	0.8													
	35	0.5	0.8	1.0	1.4												
HL — Worse Ear	40	0.6	1.0	1.3	1.7	2.2											
	45	0.8	1.2	1.5	2.0	2.6	3.1										
	50	1.0	1.3	1.7	2.2	2.8	3.4	3.9									
	55	1.1	1.5	1.8	2.4	3.0	3.7	4.3	4.8								
	60	1.2	1.6	2.0	2.5	3.2	3.9	4.6	5.2	5.7							
	65	1.3	1.7	2.1	2.6	3.3	4.0	4.7	5.4	6.0	6.5						
	70	1.4	1.8	2.2	2.7	3.4	4.1	4.8	5.6	6.3	6.9	7.4					
	75	1.5	1.9	2.3	2.8	3.5	4.2	4.9	5.6	6.4	7.1	7.7	8.2				
	80	1.5	1.9	2.3	2.8	3.5	4.2	4.9	5.7	6.4	7.1	7.9	8.5	8.9			
	85	1.5	1.9	2.3	2.8	3.5	4.2	4.9	5.7	6.4	7.2	7.9	8.6	9.0	9.4		
	90	1.5	1.9	2.3	2.8	3.5	4.2	4.9	5.7	6.4	7.2	7.9	8.6	9.1	9.5	9.7	
	≥95	1.6	1.9	2.3	2.8	3.5	4.2	4.9	5.7	6.4	7.2	7.9	8.6	9.1	9.6	9.8	10.0

REFERENCES

DAVIS, H. (1971). A historical introduction. In *Occupational hearing loss* (ed. D. W. Robinson). Academic Press, New York.
LEBO, C. P. and REDDELL, R. C. (1972). The presbycusis component in occupational hearing loss. *Laryngoscope, St. Louis* **82**, 1399.
MACRAE, J. H. (1975–6). A procedure for classifying degree of hearing loss. *J. oto-lar. Soc. Aust.* **4**, 26.
MURRAY, N. E. (1962). Hearing impairment and compensation. *J. oto-lar. Soc. Aust.* **1**, 135.
NATIONAL HEALTH AND MEDICAL RESEARCH COUNCIL, AUSTRALIAN DEPARTMENT OF HEALTH (1974). Model regulations for hearing conservation. Australian Government Publishing Service, Canberra.
WILLIS, R. (1962). Editorial. *J. oto-lar. Soc. Aust.* **1**, 83.
WOODHOUSE, A. O. and MEARES, C. L. D. (1974). *Compensation and rehabilitation in Australia.* Australian Government Publishing Service, Canberra.

41 Non-organic hearing loss in adults

P. W. ALBERTI

Non-organic hearing loss in adults (NOHL) is currently a relatively common finding, chiefly because of wars and the vast increase in compensational industrial hearing loss. The expression is used for a large number of conditions in which hearing test results do not reflect the true hearing status. There are many causes, which range from inattentiveness and lack of comprehension of the test procedure, through deliberate concealment or exaggeration of a hearing loss, to pure psychiatric disease. The varying aetiology is reflected in the multitude of synonyms applied to the condition. The expression 'non-organic hearing loss' is used as a generic term in the European English-speaking literature, while in the United States the term 'pseudohypacusis' is currently in favour; some others are malingering, hysterical deafness, psychogenic deafness, feigned hearing loss, sinistrosis, pseudo-organic deafness, and functional hearing loss. These and other expressions are well reviewed by Martin (1978). There has been much debate in the literature about the relative differences between true hysterical hearing loss, which is entirely subconscious, and pure malingering, which is consciously motivated for gain, but in the writer's opinion too much has been made of this. The relationship of NOHL to psychological disorders has been the subject of an enormous literature which will not be discussed in detail. The reader is referred to the Round Table on Psychogenic Deafness (1962), a series of papers by Chaiklin and Ventry (1965 a, b; Ventry and Chaiklin 1965 a, b; Ventry, Trier, and Chaiklin 1965; Beagley and Knight (1968); Beagley (1973); and Sohmer, Feinmesser, Baurberer and Edelstein (1977).

This chapter deals mainly with the clinical problems of detection and accurate quantification of NOHL. Quantification has become important because of the large sums of money involved in compensation and pension payments; it has become practical on a large scale with the development of electrophysiological tests for hearing.

HISTORY

Hanley and Tiffany (1954) were able to describe over 40 tests for auditory malingering. The original tests for non-organic hearing loss in adults were developed in Europe in the late nineteenth century, because the constant series of wars in which Germany and Austria were involved gave rise to their fair share of NOHL later. The pensioning of service-related hearing loss by the United States after the Second World War made it essential to develop effective methods of audiometry for NOHL.

Politzer (1894) described many of the clinical features and indicated that feigned dullness of hearing is more common than feigned total deafness; he described a battery of tests which had been devised in the nineteenth century to detect NOHL. Some of the tests were so complex that he warned that the tester was as likely to become confused by them as the subject. He emphasized that clinical acumen is the single most important feature in the identification of NOHL. Politzer's account was so good that it was quoted almost verbatim in a fairly lengthy section by Fowler in 1939, who in addition proposed the use of the lie detector to identify feigned hearing loss, thus antedating the development of an effective form of electrodermal audiometry by almost a decade. Fowler also gave a good description of the audiometric Stenger test and stated that 'the most difficult are those with moderate or even severe deafness who, . . . may attempt malingering to add to their disability'. He thus encapsulated the clinical problem which remains today.

In the years immediately following 1945 there was much literature about the psychotherapeutic aspects of NOHL, including diagnosis and treatment by pentothal narcosis. This was well reviewed by Robin (1952).

INCIDENCE

The incidence of NOHL in adults depends very much on the population under test. It is low if the major role of the facility is diagnostic site-of-lesion audiometry, high if the major role is pension, compensation or medicolegal assessment. Hearing losses may be concealed or exaggerated. The majority of the literature deals with exaggeration, but in certain circumstances the converse is more common. The writer has seen men with familial high-frequency hearing losses attempting to simulate normal hearing in order to join the armed forces, and middle-aged miners out of work as their mines closed, simulating normal hearing in an attempt to gain employment in another mine which was hiring labour. The most blatant example was a normal-hearing person being substituted for the job applicant at the time of the hearing test!

The overwhelming majority of cases are those in which the hearing loss is exaggerated and in appropriate populations the incidence currently is reported at between 20 and 25 per cent of all patients being tested. This is true of our own experience with compensation claims (Alberti, Morgan, and LeBlanc 1974) and similar figures are reported from the American Veterans' Administration (VA) (Johnson, Work, and McCoy 1956; Ventry and Chaiklin 1965b). However, in a given population the actual incidence may vary with the mechanism of compensation awards, and the reported incidence with the acumen of the clinician. The sums of money and numbers of people involved are large. For example Gaynor (1974) comments that the VA in the United States in 1970 alone, paid over $52 000 000 as compensation for hearing loss. Currently, in Sweden, 24 000 workers receive about 85 million Swedish kronor in annual compensation for noise-induced hearing loss from the government (Axelsson, Axelsson, and Jonsson 1978). The large sums of money involved make the detection and accurate quantification of NOHL imperative.

DETECTION OF NOHL

Clinical acumen

The single most important factor in the identification of NOHL is an alert, suspicious clinician—both at the time of otological evaluation and during the audiological tests, and it should be remembered that the overwhelming majority of adults with NOHL have an underlying organic hearing loss which is being exaggerated.

The clinical history will frequently alert the clinician to the possibility of NOHL. It should be considered wherever the result of an evaluation is directly turned into payment, whether this be in terms of a monthly pension award for occupational hearing loss, or a medicolegal financial settlement following injury.

The typical adult with NOHL, in our experience, is claiming compensation for occupational hearing loss. There are some legal claims from motor vehicle accidents, although the latter are more likely to involve balance problems.

The patient may have less education than the average claimant, and often has had a recent change in occupation which has lowered his income. In our experience he is frequently being tested in a language which is not his native one and very careful instruction can have a major effect on the accuracy of the hearing test.

The attitude of the patient throughout the history and examination can be revealing. The patient exaggerating his hearing loss frequently exaggerates his listening techniques. If he wears a hearing aid it is worn aggressively and is much adjusted, otherwise a hand may be cupped over the ear associated with much head turning. The patient may sit forward in the chair and is often an ostentatious lip-reader. He may ask for much to be repeated, although in the circumstances of a face-to-face encounter such a request should be unnecessary for all but the very hard of hearing patient.

There are many tricks developed to outwit the exaggerating claimant. If when talking one covers one's mouth or turns one's back the patient may go on hearing what is said. Once the interview is over some general conversation about a recent sporting event at a normal conversational level with one's back turned to the patient often produces an appropriate response, as may some quietly spoken but inflammatory comment about the patient's prospect of success in the claim that is being made. Clinicians develop their own armamentarium of similar manoeuvers, including a battery of tuning-fork tests and responses to confirm the presence of NOHL, but which are outside the scope of this account (see Chapter 14).

Unquestionably the place where NOHL is most likely to be detected is during the audiometric evaluation. The importance of clinical suspicion on the part of the tester *cannot be over-emphasized*. This section will deal only with people who exaggerate a hearing loss. The very small percentage of those claiming to have better hearing than they actually have will not be dealt with, except to say that the techniques for quantification described later are equally appropriate to them.

There are many reasons for inexact hearing thresholds, including unfamiliarity with the test procedure, both by patient and by an inexperienced tester, and a lack of understanding of instructions. The patient who believes he must be absolutely certain that he hears a test tone before responding, will give elevated thresholds. It is easy to forget that patients are being asked to participate in quite complex psychoacoustic measurements in alien and sometimes intimidating surroundings. In addition, in some parts of Europe and in many parts of North America, patients must travel long distances to reach regional centres, and after an all night bus or train ride may be too tired to respond appropriately to tests.

Routine hearing tests

INTRODUCTION

The clinician undertaking the hearing test must be alert to the possibility of NOHL. Without this further tests will not be undertaken and many cases may be missed. We have repeatedly found that the detection rate of new staff is low and that it takes some time for them to accept that NOHL does exist. Hearing testing facilities are usually concerned with accurate site of lesion testing. By contrast, the target in evaluation of NOHL is an accurate quantification of the hearing level. For most diagnostic purposes a range of 10 dB about any given point is not critical, whereas if a pension is determined by the decibel hearing loss an error of 10 dB may prove very costly either to the claimant or to the paying authority. The audiological emphasis is different and must be learned.

One of the most important features in detecting NOHL is discrepancy between tests—the patient who hears speech well but admits to hearing no pure-tones, or who has a soft voice and yet an apparently profound bilateral sensorineural hearing loss, or stapedius reflex thresholds below the voluntary pure-tone thresholds. The tester should be vigilant and if internal discrepancies like this are detected, should proceed to special tests.

THE TEST BATTERY

It is often beneficial to start the test with impedance testing, instructing the patient to sit still because the machine is going to tell us about his hearing without need for any response from him. This has an impressive and salutory effect on responses to further hearing tests, particularly if the impedance bridge is connected to a highly visible write-out device.

Observation of the patient's reactions during the test procedure may give the first clue to the presence of NOHL. The patient should be seated so that the examiner can watch his face and preferably be asked to respond to stimuli by means of finger rather than a push button signal because the flickering, tentative movements of a finger demonstrate many shades of meaning which may be missed with the on/off responses of a light. There are differences in reaction time between someone stimulating a hearing loss and someone responding normally, which a good clinician can detect and use to identify NOHL. The number of false responses between signals, particularly if an unexpected delay is inserted between tone presentations, may give a clue; the subject with NOHL makes many fewer false-positive responses than a normal subject. Two characteristic responses in NOHL are a delay in responding, i.e. a much longer than usual reaction time with the tone having to be on longer than usual to obtain a response, and the responses which are given to progressively greater increments of intensity as the threshold is searched. The subject may respond initially at a given level, and fail to respond 10 dB below, but on the next occasion that the original level is bracketed will not respond until 5 or 10 dB higher. This may persist so that a threshold which was originally suspected is ultimately admitted, some 30 dB higher. In addition, responses in a normal (non-NOHL) patient are usually well established and brisk 10 dB above threshold—the NOHL subject remains hesitant throughout the test (Wood, Goshorn, and Peters 1977). Many of these points have been well described by Green (1978) when he writes of UFOs (useful finger observations) and the sightings that can be made from them such as 'malingerfingers'.

In patients with unilateral hearing loss it is worthwhile in the first instance performing tests without masking. The absence of a shadow curve in a claimed total hearing loss is a strong suggestion that NOHL is present. Also, the subject may deny hearing in one ear, but turn his head as the signal is switched from ear to ear.

Many subjects are quite adept at maintaining their particular hearing level as the admitted 'threshold' and they can reproduce their inappropriate results with considerable reliability. The mechanism whereby this is done may be related to fixing a particular loudness level to which they respond, or by introducing internal masking. This may be done by the subject humming constantly to himself during the test (Gaynor 1974). The maximum effects are produced at frequencies below 4 kHz and may produce a shift of 40 dB at 250 and 500 Hz gradually dropping to 20 dB at 4 kHz. This can be discovered by the tester using a monitoring microphone.

SPEECH AUDIOMETRY

Incorrect but meaningful patient responses during speech audiometry, particularly with spondaic words, e.g. 'cowgirl' for 'cowboy', 'hot air' for 'airplane', 'north-east' for 'north-west', strongly suggest the presence of NOHL, as do half-word responses, e.g. 'cow', 'air', 'north'. Here, too, the response latencies may be very long. A further very useful guide is a discrepancy between speech reception thresholds and pure-tone thresholds. Fletcher (1929) pointed out years ago that the pure-tone average (PTA) in the speech frequencies 500, 1000, and 2000 agreed well with the speech reception threshold (SRT) as long as the pure-tone audiogram was relatively flat. If it is sloped the SRT agrees with the PTA of the better two frequencies. Carhart (1952) was first to suggest that the discrepancy between these two might be used to identify non-organic hearing loss; Ventry and Chaiklin (1965a) stated that this technique identified 70 per cent of patient with confirmed pseudohypacusis. In our own experience (Alberti, Morgan, and Czuba 1978) we found that out of a population of 600 compensation claimants, 120 of whom had a confirmed NOHL, 62 per cent were correctly identified by an SRT–PTA difference of greater than 10 dB. If we considered only those where the PTA and SRT were more than 10 dB apart, 85 per cent were exaggerating. The weakness of the test is that a significant proportion of those who exaggerate pure-tone thresholds do not show this SRT–PTA difference, because they appear to be able to exaggerate their SRTs as well as pure-tones. The value of speech audiometry in the detection of NOHL has been emphasized by Coles and Priede (1971) who also give results with speech discrimination tests in NOHL (Priede and Coles 1976).

SHAPE OF PURE-TONE AUDIOGRAM
It has been suggested at various times that the pure-tone audiogram has a characteristic shape in NOHL. It seems to be generally accepted at present that it is likely to follow an equal loudness contour because that is the most readily simulated. The shape therefore varies with the true underlying ear pathology. Since at the present time the majority of cases of NOHL in adults coexist with high-frequency noise-induced hearing loss, either from military or civil noise, the most usual shape is of a sloping audiogram worse in the high frequencies, but flatter than usual at the lower frequencies. We have made considerable use of this as a screening test. In a large series of patients we found that in those with poor low-frequency hearing (40 dB or worse at 500 Hz), one-third were exaggerating their threshold loss and that they comprised 85 per cent of the total NOHL group. In patients with presumed occupational hearing loss, poor low-frequency hearing either means an unreliable threshold or the presence of other ear disease, and in any event is an indication for more detailed evaluation (Klockhoff *et al.* 1974; Alberti *et al.* 1978).

Frequently the bone conduction loss is not exaggerated as much as the air conduction, suggesting a conductive loss. A normal tympanogram and normal acoustic reflexes make a true conductive hearing loss extremely unlikely and suggest NOHL.

ACOUSTIC REFLEX THRESHOLDS
We routinely perform tympanometry and obtain acoustic reflex thresholds (ARTs) as part of the hearing test battery. The latter are frequently useful in identifying the presence of NOHL, although not in quantifying it (see below). ARTs are always greater than pure-tone thresholds, and even in an ear with a significant cochlear loss, are usually at least 20 dB higher than the

pure-tone threshold. Any patient in whom the pure-tone reflex thresholds are within 20 dB of the pure-tone threshold is probably giving inaccurate pure-tone threshold responses; any patient in whom the pure-tone reflex threshold is equal to or apparently more sensitive than the pure-tone threshold is certainly giving inaccurate responses (Alberti 1970; Thomsen 1955).

SISI TEST

The results of the SISI test may suggest the presence of NOHL (Kumpf 1975). This test, which is a statistical application of the difference limen, usually gives high scores in the presence of a cochlear hearing loss. In the presence of a simulated sensorineural hearing loss the results are usually between zero and 25 per cent, which either suggest a central lesion (unlikely), or NOHL. Naturally, if there is a coexistent cochlear loss, the SISI score will be high.

TONE DECAY

Patients with NOHL may exhibit excessive tone decay. If this is present bilaterally there is a very great chance that it is due to NOHL rather than to any organic lesion.

Differential diagnosis

While many of the above findings are common in NOHL, they may also exist in other conditions and the diagnosis may be difficult. One of the commoner confounding factors in our clinic has been collapsing ear canals. Here, the placement of the headphone deforms the ear canals so that they are closed, giving rise to a greater air conduction (AC) loss than is really the case, and an apparent conductive pathology. However, the presence of a normal tympanogram and ARTs suggest this is unlikely. Inspection of the ear canals may show a narrow entrance and the air conduction tests should be repeated with a small plastic tube in the ear canal. This may produce a dramatic improvement in AC thresholds. True fluctuating hearing loss may also represent a problem as apparent AC threshold discrepancies appear from test to test. One of the more difficult distinctions is with a true retrocochlear hearing loss where the signs may be very similar, including increased response latencies, undue stumbling over speech tests, discrepancies between SRT and PTT, normal SISI, type 5 Békésy, etc. If there is any doubt in the tester's mind, advanced audiological, radiological, and neurological investigations should be performed.

Special tests to detect NOHL

Once suspicion has been raised, the number of tests available both to identify and quantify NOHL is enormous. The particular tests used in any one clinic depend on the experience of the testers and the available equipment. Thus those who gained great experience in the evaluation of NOHL in the American VA system in the 1950s and 60s used Békésy and electrodermal response audiometry extensively and place considerable credence on them. These tests were less commonly used in Europe where electric response audiometry (ERA), initially late vertex responses, latterly electrocochleographic (ECochG) and brain-stem evoked potentials (BSERA) has been widely adopted; thus in these areas ERA has found favour.

Unquestionably, tester familiarity with a technique leads to more accurate results. Tests must be used routinely, so that testers can be familiar with responses and interpretation of results, and unless there is considerable familiarity with any test—whether it be ERA, EDA, Békésy audiometry, etc.—the interpretation made and quantification produced is unlikely to be reliable.

Although there are many tests described which may identify and perhaps quantify NOHL, there are very few studies which evaluate their predictive value. What is the probability of NOHL being the cause of a type 5 Békésy audiogram? More important, what proportion of patients with NOHL do not show type 5 response? Unfortunately the literature gives little indication of either the sensitivity or the specificity of the many tests described, and the investigator is left with an embarrassing plethora of techniques without knowing which give the best value in terms of sensitivity, selectivity, time, cost, etc.

HARRIS'S TEST

Kerr and his colleagues (Kerr, Gillespie, and Easton 1975) have recently re-introduced a very simple test to detect NOHL (Harris 1958). Thresholds of hearing are established separately by ascending and descending means. Audiograms are performed starting at approximately 90 dB HL, frequency-by-frequency, reducing the intensity by 10 dB per step until no sound is heard; the threshold is then elevated by 5 dB steps until a sound is just heard. This is plotted as the descending threshold. The same frequency is again tested, this time rising from 0 dB until an ascending threshold is achieved. In the normal person the descending thresholds are marginally better than ascending thresholds. In the malingerer the descending thresholds are 25–30 dB less sensitive than the ascending thresholds.

BÉKÉSY AUDIOMETRY

There is a wealth of literature concerning the use of Békésy audiometry, including many reports of its value in identifying simulated hearing loss. Jerger and Herer (1961) noted that patients with NOHL frequently gave better hearing thresholds to continuous tone sweep frequency tracings than for pulsed tones, a configuration they called a type 5 Békésy audiogram. It is occasionally found in central hearing problems, but is overwhelmingly more common in NOHL. Resnick and Burke (1962) showed that this was true also when a fixed frequency was used.

Many modifications have been made to routine Békésy audiometry in efforts to identify patients with NOHL, including lengthening of the off-time between cycles and diminishing the length of the pulse tone. Pulsed

Békésy audiometry is normally carried out with 200 ms tones separated by 200 ms of silence. Hattler (1970) introduced the LOT (lengthened off-time) test in which the on time remained 200 ms but the off-time between tones was increased to 800 ms. He found that the difference between continuous and pulse tones in NOHL became even more marked when this was done. He claimed that this increases the indentification rate of NOHL to 95 per cent from the 40 per cent found with routine Békésy audiometry. Unfortunately the number of type 5 responses decreases with subject experience both in the standard and LOT Békésy tests (Martin and Monroe 1975).

When presentation times are short an intensity/duration relationship exists in pure-tone threshold measurements. This has been made use of in 'brief-tone' audiometry where thresholds to pure-tones of progressively shorter durations are measured. The thresholds are tracked by means of Békésy self-recording audiometry. This type of audiometry has had a considerable vogue in central hearing testing. It has also been applied to the test battery for identification of NOHL, particularly by Dean, Wright, and Valerio (1976), although they cautioned that an existing organic hearing loss (as may occur at higher frequencies with noise-induced losses) may invalidate the test.

THE LOMBARD TEST

The Lombard phenomenon has been well known for many years. A person speaking raises the voice above the level of background noise subconsciously. This phenomenon is exploited in a test for severe unilateral hearing loss and for profound bilateral hearing loss. The subject claiming a unilateral hearing loss is given a passage to read aloud. After a sentence or two a Barany noise box is applied to (or paper rubbed over) the good ear. If the good ear is the only hearing ear then the sound applied is enough for the patient's voice to rise well above the previous level, whereas if the other ear is hearing relatively normally there will be no change in intensity of the passage being read.

The Lombard test may also be undertaken using an audiometer. Under headphones the patient is asked to read a passage into a microphone and to continue reading whilst sounds are presented. In the case of unilateral loss a white noise stimulus is applied to the good ear at high intensity, and the reading voice will be raised, which can be monitored on the VU meter. If a severe bilateral hearing loss is claimed then white noise presented at a level below the noise threshold should not affect the hearing level. The patient is asked to read and the noise presentation gradually raised until a level is reached where the reading voice is elevated. If this is below the admitted voluntary thresholds then NOHL is present.

The test is not foolproof for subjects can learn to maintain constant voice levels against varying levels of background noise.

TEST USED TO DETECT NOHL

The above tests are useful in establishing the presence of NOHL. However, this is only the start of the testing dilemma. It is usually important to *quantify* the hearing level, both for financial and for therapeutic reasons, e.g. appropriate hearing aid fitting. There are fewer tests which can be used to quantify accurately the hearing thresholds in NOHL and the commonest technique is still to 'beat up' the audiogram, i.e. explain again what is required of the patient and then painstakingly re-apply the technique. To know where to stop is difficult but made easier by some of the tests described in this section. Some form of ERA is, in the author's hands, by far the most useful tool.

The Stenger test

This test has been used for years to establish the validity of unilateral hearing losses. The principle upon which the test is based is that if identical sounds are presented to the two ears then the subject will only appear to hear it in the ear which the sound is louder. The test can be undertaken with two identical tuning forks placed at varying distances from the ears (Chapter 14) but is more commonly performed with an audiometer (Chapter 15). If a tone of 10 dB above threshold at any frequency is presented to the good ear and a similar tone presented to the ear in which a hearing loss is claimed, the patient's response will depend upon the relative loudness of the sounds. If the sound in the poor ear is presented at or below its actual threshold then the patient will lateralize the sound to the good ear. If the tone is presented at a greater perceived loudness to the poor ear than the good ear, then the sound will appear to be in the poor ear and disappear from the good ear. The patient who is giving reliable thresholds will identify the sound as being heard in the worse ear, while the patient with NOHL, knowing that this cannot be admitted, will deny hearing a sound at all. This response is called a positive Stenger.

The technique can be modified to establish hearing thresholds which are made by determining the intensity levels at which the sound presented to the poor ear interferes with the sound heard in the good ear. A tone of 10 dB above threshold at the frequency under test is presented to the good ear simultaneously with tones of increasing intensity in the poor ear. Initially the sound is heard in the good ear but as the intensity is increased in the poor ear the sound is ultimately heard in that ear. The point at which this takes place, at which the patient denies hearing any sound, is said to be within 20 dB of the threshold of the ear in question. The test may also be conducted using speech material.

There is some controversy in the literature about the sensitivity of the Stenger test. Chaiklin and Ventry (1965) felt that there has to be a considerable difference between the ears or a considerable non-organic component before the test is of value. More recently Kinstler and his colleagues (Kinstler, Phelan, and Lavender 1972) concluded that the Stenger, both for pure-tones and for speech, predicted hearing loss of the functional type with a high degree of accuracy. They correctly identified 25 of 31 subjects. A technique for combining the Stenger with self-recording Békésy audiometry has been evaluated, applied and found to be effective in the VA (Watson and Voots 1965), although the test is complex and has not been widely adopted.

Delayed auditory feedback (DAF)

SPEECH DAF

Normal speech production is self-monitored by intensity, pitch, and rhythm. Anything that interferes with self-monitoring disrupts the normal pattern of speech. This is made use of in the delayed auditory feedback test. If speech is recorded and played back to the speaker after a short delay, the sound of the delayed speech may interfere with continuing speech production. The test is undertaken using a tape recorder with separate record and playback heads. The speaker's voice is recorded on one head and played back into headphones from a playback head. The delay consists of the time taken for the tape to pass from the recording head to the playback head, and is dependent upon the speed of the tape recording and the distance between the heads. With most commercial recorders it is possible to achieve delays of between 100 and 200 ms. It is usually possible to switch the feedback from the playback to the recording head at will. Delayed speech heard by the subject will usually result in a raised voice and some stuttering, as the subject attempts to speak above the speech and has his own self-monitoring interfered with. This can be used as a method of identifying NOHL, for if the changes in speech are produced by intensities below the admitted thresholds, then a non-organic hearing loss almost certainly is present. Refinements of the test include tape recording of speech during presentation and analysis of rate of reading and absolute intensity changes in the voice. Unfortunately not all subjects show the phenomenon, and with practice, more can learn to suppress it. In addition, subjects not fluent in the test language rarely establish sufficient rhythm of speech to allow evaluation of the test.

PURE-TONE DAF

An adaptation of this test to pure tones is said to provide threshold information. Instead of speaking into a microphone the subject is asked to tap a morse key at an established rhythm, e.g. de-de-de-dah pause de-de-de-dah. The key is used as an interrupter switch for the audiometer, the tones from which are listened to on a headphone via a tape recorder rigged as for DAF speech. If the sound is heard by the subject an introduction of the delay will alter the rhythm of tapping or break it down completely. The intensity of the tone heard can be adjusted and a threshold of interference established. This can be repeated at any number of frequencies and an 'audiogram' achieved. The morse key must be covered so that the patient does not establish visual monitoring of the tapping pattern. The test is not universally applicable, for some patients do not learn the rhythm of tapping, others do not have adequate manual dexterity, and the relationship between the interference level and the true threshold varies from subject to subject.

Various claims have been made for the reliability and accuracy of this test since its introduction by Chase in 1959 (Chase, Harvey, Standfast, Rapin, and Sutton 1959; Ruhm and Cooper 1962, 1964). According to Ruhm and Cooper (1964) changes may occur within 5 dB of the true threshold, although others report they may not be detectable until 30 dB above threshold (Alberti 1970; Martin 1978). The test is therefore useful in a qualitative way (Beagley 1973) although of doubtful value for accurate threshold estimation (Alberti 1970).

Doerfler–Stewart test

This test achieved considerable prominence in the United States, particularly in the VA programme, to detect binaural non-organic hearing loss. Basically it compares responses to speech versus noise, and does so at different levels of intensity of speech and noise, drawing from this a series of conclusions about the patient's hearing levels by means of establishing speech reception thresholds, noise interference levels, and noise detection thresholds. The test is complex and whilst still applied in certain clinics in the United States, should be considered of historical value. It is well reviewed by Hopkinson (1978).

Threshold estimation from acoustic reflex measurement

Acoustic reflex thresholds (ARTs) to pure-tones and noise are easy to elicit in people with normal middle-ear function, and are tempting as a basis for the development of objective hearing tests. The use of ARTs in the identification of NOHL has already been described. Niemeyer and Sesterhenn (1974) introduced a technique for hearing threshold estimation based on the difference in ARTs for pure-tones and broad-band noise. They found that in a normal person the threshold for broad-band noise is lower (more sensitive) than for pure-tones, but that in the presence of a cochlear hearing loss the threshold for broad-band noise becomes elevated more rapidly than that for pure-tone stimuli. They therefore based a formula for estimation of pure-tone thresholds on the difference in reflex thresholds for pure-tone and broad-band noise stimuli. The results were initially verified by Jerger and his colleagues (Jerger, Burney, Mauldin, and Crump 1974) although they altered the methodology somewhat. In addition the use of high-pass and low-pass filtered noise has enabled some degree of slope prediction to be attempted.

Other authors have enthusiastically adopted the technique. Miller and her colleagues (Miller, Davies, and Gibson 1976) suggest that it will predict hearing thresholds to within −15 +25 dB in 90 per cent of cases. This is hardly a degree of accuracy on which one would wish to award a pension. Similarly Van Wagoner and Goodwine (1977) have adopted the SPAR test (sensitivity prediction by acoustic reflex) and recommended it particularly in adult medicolegal cases. They used a technique similar to Jerger's and found that they were able to classify patients into hearing loss groupings of normal, mild, moderate, and severe loss, with an overall 72 per cent accuracy, and predict the slope with 60 per cent accuracy. The test was most accurate for predicting normal hearing and least accurate for predicting severe hearing losses. Van Wagoner goes as far as stating 'In the currently available clinical test battery for non-organic hearing loss we observed that no single test matches SPAR for its accuracy in predicting the extent of loss, its objective nature, its ease of administration and interpretation and often its cost of implementation'. The test is easy to administer but requires individual biological calibration in each laboratory and its accuracy is, in this writer's opinion, very low.

Others have questioned the rationale of the Niemeyer–Sesterhenn method and have attempted to use the white-noise threshold on its own as a method of predicting hearing loss (Johnsen, Osterhammel, Terkildsen, Osterhammel, and Huis in'TVelt 1976). However, in our hands this method has not proved to be sufficiently accurate for reliable prediction.

Sesterhenn and Breuninger (1977) described a pre-activation of the stapedius reflex threshold by a second tone of quite different frequency (usually at 8 kHz). The hearing threshold at the frequencies 0.5 to 4 kHz is deduced from the amount the pure-tone ART at these frequencies is lowered by the presence of the pre-activating tone. The authors make many caveats for the technique, which will probably have limited application.

Margolis and Fox (1977) comment on many of these problems and give thoughtful analysis of the different techniques employed. A recent major paper by Jerger and his colleagues (Jerger, Hayes, Anthony, and Mauldin 1978) reviews the current status of hearing-level prediction from ARTs. They believe that the two major uncontrollable factors in this test battery are change in reflex thresholds with patient age, for according to them the reflex threshold for pure-tones is lowered as people become older, although that for noise does not vary. Secondly minor middle-ear disorders can grossly elevate thresholds. They write that the effect of the sensorineural hearing loss on acoustic reflexes is complex and varies with audiometric shape and the degree of the loss. They feel the best approach to prediction may be to use the bandwidth effect, i.e. white-noise–pure-tone threshold differences, to detect a loss, but to use absolute reflex thresholds, especially to broad-band noise, to predict the degree of loss. In a large study of compensation claimants the test was, in our hands, too inaccurate to be of any quantitative value (Ityde, Alberti, Morgan, Symons, and Cummings 1980).

The subject is tantalizing and the technique clearly has value in gross categorization of hearing levels in young children, but it does not appear to have the degree of accuracy required to play a major role in the quantification of adult NOHL.

Electrodermal audiometry—psychogalvanic skin response testing

This test has a long history and was probably used to test hearing as early as 1918 (Albrecht 1918). The test was developed and brought into clinical use shortly after the Second World War by Bordley, Hardy, and Richter (1948) and consisted of the application of Pavlovian conditioning to audiometric technology. Skin resistance to current flow may vary from a variety of reasons including the presence of a noxious stimulus. Whether the change in resistance is due to sweating, or changes in blood flow to the skin is irrelevant. The changes in skin resistance can be measured by a galvanometer. The patient is conditioned by simultaneous presentation of sound and unpleasant electric shocks which result in skin resistance changing. When the patient is conditioned by a few shocks, a sound alone will produce a change of skin resistance. The change in skin resistance is measured by attaching electrodes to two fingers—preferably not adjacent to each other—and passing a small current so that the skin acts as a resistance in the circuit. The circuit is connected to a galvanometer which indicates changes in skin resistance which occur whenever a sound is heard, if conditioning has been effective.

The test had considerable vogue in the VA and as late as 1978 was still the technique of choice of certain authors (Engelberg 1978). The test is however unpleasant for the patient, relatively difficult to interpret, and subject to a variety of artifactual responses. The condition of the skin is important and the test may be affected by medication which the patient is taking. Recent regulations concerning connection of biomedical equipment to a patient has led to the banning of shock stimuli in the USA, although some investigators are turning to other stimuli such as air jets in the palpebral fissure. In the writer's opinion at the present time the test has been completely superseded by ERA.

Electric response audiometry

Currently there are three well-accepted methods of investigating the auditory system by means of electric response audiometry. The first to be introduced was the recording of late vertex potentials (cortical ERA), the second electrocochleography, and more recently brain-stem electric response audiometry. The vertex responses are the largest but are nevertheless difficult to separate from on-going brain-wave activity, and thus did not come into prominence until averaging devices were available. Improvement in amplifiers, transducers, and averagers have enabled ECochG and BSERA to be used for clinical testing of the auditory system. As far as NOHL in adults is concerned, it is probably unnecessary to use an invasive technique and thus ECochG has only a minor role, if any, to play.

Very recently, there has been a great deal of research into the use of brain-stem evoked potentials, particularly the so-called wave V, in threshold measurement. The technique is non-invasive, and although the responses are minute, their ability to withstand stimulus repetition rates of more than 20 per second results in an averaging time comparable to that of the late vertex response.

These potentials have deservedly achieved widespread use in testing babies and young children, important advantages over the late potentials being their relative stability and resistance to sedation and anaesthesia. For the adult patient with NOHL, the benefits of brain-stem audiometry are not yet clear. Firstly the classical ERA method is almost always successful in these patients—a strong contrast to testing children. Furthermore, the necessity of minimizing electromyogenic interference, the relative lack of frequency specificity, and the previously reported poor definition of response for stimulus frequencies at or below 1 kHz are disadvantages. More recent experience, however, gives grounds for greater optimism in this respect, but further work on these problems is required before the role of brain-stem audiometry in NOHL can be accurately assessed.

At present it is probably true to state that the most accurate and rapid threshold determinations are made with the averaged late-vertex response, although the amount of work being undertaken on BSERA is so great that they probably will have a role to play in adults, as well as in young children.

Goldstein and Price (1966) were probably the first to report the use of evoked response audiometry in the detection of NOHL, but two papers in 1968 established its role. Beagley and Knight (1968) reported the use of ERA in 21 cases of suspected non-organic hearing loss as part of a test battery, thereby setting the pattern for the correct use of this technique. In the same year McCandless and Lentz (1968) demonstrated that in their hands in normal hearing adults there is no significant difference between hearing thresholds arrived at by ERA or conventional techniques. They suggested that patients with NOHL fall into three groups: (i) those who have real organic hearing loss but initially were inaccurate—they were frequently anxious and gave many false-positive results but who after repeated testing stabilized. (ii) Those who were initially obviously unreliable but were relatively easy to condition into providing accurate responses. (iii) Those consistently unreliable, who gave very elevated voluntary thresholds, but whose thresholds by ERA averaged 50 dB better. Alberti (1970) also demonstrated that in his hands the threshold responses obtained by evoked response audiometry and conventional means were similar, and in a series of normal subjects with hearing losses, but whose conventional test results were known to be reliable, felt that the 90 per cent confidence interval for the test at the frequencies 0.5, 1, and 2 kHz was 10 dB or better.

Not all workers are as enthusiastic. For example, Rose and his colleagues (Rose, Keating, Hedgecock, Miller, and Schreurs 1972) found in 50 adults in whom both conventional and ERA audiometry were undertaken using a PAR 140 machine at two frequencies, 0.5 and 2 kHz, that there was a less than 70 per cent agreement within 10 dB. However, results from the same clinic (Cody 1973; Cody and Townsend 1973) indicated that vertex-response thresholds as determined in patients with a functional loss of hearing correlate accurately with their true organic hearing thresholds.

Unquestionably the accuracy of ERA is strongly dependent upon proper technique and experience in judgement of the responses. In the presence of aberrant EEG activity, or of difficulty in electrode placement, or of a very restless patient, the responses may be inadequate or difficult to interpret. The absence of a widely accepted objective method for scoring results means that the estimation of thresholds is subjective and requires considerable experience and skill. It is much less accurate in children, but in neurologically normal adults it is now accepted as one of the best tests available. In our laboratory, where more than 1500 adult patients have been tested with ERA, more than 500 with NOHL, the estimation errors are acceptably small.

More recently, Pratt and Sohmer (1978) compared hearing thresholds determined by behavioural responses and various electrical responses in the same subject. They conclude the electrical response measures, especially auditory nerve and brain-stem responses, are reliable indicators of hearing threshold. They have found that the brain-stem responses were more reliable than the cortical evoked responses, the former being reliable to within 6 dB (± 6 dB), and the latter to 12 dB (± 7 dB). However, the cortical responses were evoked by clicks rather than pure-tones, considerably reducing the utility of the test for accurate quantification at individual frequencies.

ERA has not yet been universally accepted in North America as a technique for the quantification of NOHL—a recent article on functional hearing level (Engelberg 1978) fails to mention the technique at all, and Martin (1978) in a comprehensive chapter is also not completely enthusiastic. However, there is an increasing body of world literature to support the use of this test in NOHL (Bochenek, Sulkowska, Filkowska *et al.* 1974; Flack Knothe, and Hofmann 1974; Heron 1974; Buechel 1977).

Beagley (1973) has given a thoughtful review of his experience with 77 cases of NOHL and comments that 'the ERA threshold has proven of great value in making out a prima facie case of NOHL'. He then states that the diagnosis should be confirmed by other techniques, which is also the practice in our clinic.

We have found that ERA can be performed about as quickly as a full Békésy test battery and has the advantage of producing threshold estimates. It is the technique of choice in our hands, as long as it is coupled with revalidation by means of conventional pure-tone testing. Our major reason for adopting this technique was that it significantly reduced the time taken to establish a threshold estimate, an important factor in a busy clinic. This is largely because of its ability to provide a threshold to 'shoot' at. We attempt never to rely on the results of one test alone. We use discrepancies in routine tests to suggest the need for ERA and if it shows different results from conventional tests then the conventional tests are repeated until there is congruity between the results of at least two tests, either ERA and SRT or ERA and conventional pure-tone tests, or preferably all three. Occasionally the ERA responses are poor for technical reasons and this must be recognized. Then other identification techniques are used and the audiologist 'beats up' the pure-tones until satisfied nothing more can be done. The philosophy that more than one type of test result is required to establish a valid threshold is important and should be adapted to all areas of NOHL estimation.

SUGGESTED PROTOCOL

Hearing testing for NOHL requires some different skills and emphasis than site of lesion testing. Any clinic undertaking this work should have available pure-tone and speech audiometry, impedance audiometry, and ERA. Other techniques such as DAF are useful but not essential. There should be a systematic programme of evaluation of all the techniques used, so that the testers know the degree of reliance to be placed on any test. Tester familiarity with complex equipment and techniques is essential; any technique is liable to produce unreliable results if not used regularly. We use ERA several times daily so that each tester is completely at ease with the technique. A suggedsted test protocol is as follows:

1. Impedance testing as described above, providing visible evidence for the patient of a test result which does not require his co-operation.
2. Speech audiometry, so that the SRTs may be established. Speech discrimination testing is done at the same time. The type of responses given to the speech tests may well alert the tester to the potential presence of NOHL. If this is so, the patient is then re-instructed.
3. Pure-tone audiometry, by conventional means, testing both air and bone conduction.
4. If there is a unilateral hearing loss the Stenger test is performed for pure-tones, and if the tester believes the results so far have been reliable it is expedient at this stage to perform whatever further advanced puretone tests are undertaken for site of lesion testing, such as tone decay and ABLB.
5. In those patients who are likely to gain from the result of the hearing test, e.g. industrial or medicolegal claims, ERA should, ideally, be undertaken routinely. As this may not be possible, some selection is necessary. It should be performed in all patients in whom the tester, for any reason whatsoever, believes the results may be unreliable, and whenever discrepancies have come to light in the routine test battery, as for example puretone/SRT differences greater than 10 dB. In addition it is prudent to perform ERA on a random sample of patients, so that skills are maintained. The occasional finding of an unsuspected case of NOHL has a salutory effect. We strongly urge that the ERA be performed and evaluated by a different tester than the one who has performed the routine test battery; this helps to eliminate a number of tester biases.
6. If, when the ERA and conventional test results are compared, there is a discrepancy of 10 dB or greater at any two frequencies, or if there is still unexplained discrepancy between other tests in the battery, NOHL is

diagnosed and a major effort made to reconcile the differences in order to achieve a true hearing threshold.
7. The patient should always be allowed a gracious way out, and is re-instructed using terms such as 'We believe you may have misunderstood our instructions, we want you to tell us when you suspect you hear the faintest sound. Do not wait until you are quite certain that you hear a sound' etc. The conventional pure-tone audiogram is then repeated and usually produces much better results. It should be emphasized that NOHL in adults usually exists on top of an organic hearing loss, and the amount of exaggeration is usually in the order of 15–20 dB. There are occasional examples of huge discrepancies, but they make up less than 15 per cent of all NOHL cases. The majority of patients respond well to recounselling and the discrepancies are nullified. However, in some cases repeated testing and demonstration of discrepancies is necessary.

The writer is not prepared to give a legal opinion on the basis of one test result alone, and if there is a discrepancy between ERA and PTT we work with the patient until at least two test results coincide, preferably ERA and PTT although occasionally it is necessary to rely on validation of the ERA by the SRT score. The very occasional subject is extremely sophisticated, belligerent, or intoxicated, so that testing is almost impossible. The man who constantly moves throughout the ERA test, or who has managed to establish NOHL for SRT and PTT and in whom the ERA responses are not clear, may be extremely difficult to test. We will usually request that the patient return for further testing sessions, perhaps using a different tester and introducing some of the other techniques described.

Perhaps the most difficult of all subjects is the one with a genuine discrepancy in hearing thresholds between the two ears, which is however being exaggerated. The significance of unequal thresholds in NOHL has recently been commented upon (Alberti, Symons, and Hyde 1979), and the examiner must be ever alert to the possible presence of other ear disease; the claimant for compensation is self-selecting himself as someone with a hearing problem: he is not necessarily providing a diagnosis. It must be remembered that other ear disease has at least as high an incidence in noise-exposed subjects as in the population at large. It is easy to miss a retrocochlear lesion because of the similarity of the responses in NOHL and some central disorders, and one must remember to perform the full battery of site-of-lesion tests in addition to tests for NOHL. It should be remembered that shadow curves are as possible with ERA as with routine techniques and appropriate masking must be used. If necessary ERA can be performed for bone conducted stimuli.

In the writer's opinion the majority of other tests described should be abandoned in favour of ERA, if the prime purpose is detection and quantification of NOHL. They are less efficient than ERA and when patient and tester time is at a premium do not warrant the effort expended on them because the results can be obtained more rapidly and readily in other ways. The clinician should, however, remain alert to the signs suggesting NOHL in tests which he uses for other reasons. If Békésy audiometry is routinely used for site of lesion testing, then its use may indeed reveal a type V audiogram in someone undergoing site-of-lesion tests. However, the suspected presence of NOHL is not an indication to undertake a Bekesy audiogram if ERA is available, because it does not quantify the lesion and adds unnecessary time to the test protocol.

With the current epidemic of compensation claims for noise-induced hearing loss in the western world, the number of cases of NOHL will inexorably rise. Clinicians must remain alert to the possibility of its occurrence and be prepared to perform the appropriate test battery to quantify it. If appropriate equipment such as ERA is unavailable, or if the number of cases tested is low, then the clinician should be prepared to refer the patient to centres which have adequate experience with the problem, in which case they need rely only on tests for the *detection* of NOHL. In our hands (Alberti *et al.* 1978) PTT–SRT discrepancies and unexpected pure-tone thresholds are reliable indicators. Despite the plethora of tests available for the detection of NOHL, an alert, suspicious clinician is still the most effective agent for identifying this type of hearing loss.

REFERENCES

ALBERTI, P. W. (1970). New tools for old tricks. *Ann. Otol. Rhinol. Lar.* **79**, 800.

—— MORGAN, P. P., and CZUBA, I. (1978). Speech and puretone audiometry as a screen for exaggerated hearing loss in industrial claims. *Acta oto-lar.* **85**, 328.

—— —— and LeBLANC, J. C. (1974). Occupational hearing loss: an otologist's view of a long-term study. *Laryngoscope, St. Louis* **84**, 1822.

—— SYMONS, F., and HYDE, M. L. (1979). Occupational hearing loss. The significance of asymmetrical hearing thresholds. *Acta oto-lar.* **87**, 723.

ALBRECHT, W. (1918). Die Trennung der neicht organischen von der organischen Horstorung mite Hilfe des psychogalvanischen Reflexes. *Arch. Ohr-Nas-Kehlkheilk.* **101**, 1.

Audiology (1962). Round table on psychogenic hearing loss and stimulation. *Audiology* **1**, 112.

AXELSSON, K., AXELSSON, A., and JONSSON, A. (1978). Aspects on personal noise protection. *Scand. Audiol.* **7**, 247.

BEAGLEY, H. A. (1973). The role of electrophysiological tests in the diagnosis of non-organic hearing loss. *Audiology* **12**, 470.

—— and KNIGHT, J. J. (1968). The evaluation of suspected non-organic hearing loss. *J. Lar. Otol.* **82**, 693.

BOCHENEK, W., SULKOWSKA, W., FILKOWSKA, D. *et al.* (1974). Impedance and Electrophysiologic audiometry in the diagnosis of occupational hearing loss. *Med. Pracy.* **24**, 381.

BORDLEY, J. E., HARDY, W. G., and RICHTER, C. P. (1948). Audiometry with the use of galvanic skin resistance response. *Bull. Johns Hopkins Hosp.* **82**, 569.

BUECHEL, E. (1977). The possibilities of electric response audiometry in medical/legal assessment? *Lar. Rhinol. Otol. Grenzgeb.* **56**, 177.

CARHART, R. (1952). Speech audiometry in clinical evaluation. *Acta oto-lar.* **41**, 18.

CHAIKLIN, J. B. and VENTRY, I. M. (1962). Round Table on psychogenic deafness. *Int. Audiol.* **1**, 112.
—— —— (1965a). Patient errors during spondee and pure-tone threshold measurements. *J. audit. Res.* **5**, 219.
—— —— (1965b). The efficiency of audiometric measures used to identify functional hearing loss. *J. audit. Res.* **5**, 196.
CHASE, R. A., HARVEY, S., STANDFAST, S., RAPIN, I., and SUTTON, S. (1959). Comparison of the effects of delayed auditory feedback on speech and key tapping. *Science, N.Y.* **129**, 903.
CODY, D. T. R. (1973). Cortical evoked responses in neuro-otological diagnosis. *Archs Otolar.* **97**, 96.
—— and TOWNSEND, G. L. (1973). Some physiologic aspects of the average—vertex response in humans. *Audiology* **12**, 1.
COLES, R. R. A. and PRIEDE, V. M. (1971). Nonorganic overlay in noise-induced hearing loss. *Proc. R. Soc. Med.* **64**, 194.
DEAN, L. A., WRIGHT, H. N., and VALERIO, M. W. (1976). Brief-tone audiometry in pseudohypacusis. *Archs Otol.* **102**, 621.
ENGLEBERG, M. W. (1978). Functional hearing level. *Otol. Clins N. Am.* **11**, 741.
FLACH, M., KNOTHE, J., and HOFFMAN, G. (1974). Objective audiometry (evoked response audiometry) and otological. fitness assessment. *Mchr. Ohrenheilk.* **108**, 388.
FLETCHER, H. (1929). *Speech and hearing.* Van Nostrand, New York.
FOWLER, E. P. (1939). Tests for hearing. In *Looseleaf Medicine of the Ear* (ed. E. P. Fowler), p. 374. Nelson, New York.
GAYNOR, E. B. (1974). Humming and non-organic hearing loss. *Archs. Otolar.* **100**, 199.
GREEN, D. S. (1978). On air conduction testing. In *A handbook of clinical audiology*, 2nd edn (ed. J. Katz). Williams and Wilkins, Baltimore.
GOLDSTEIN, R. and PRICE, L. L. (1966). Clinical use of EEA with an average response computer: a case report. *J. Speech Hear. Dis.* **31**, 75.
HANLEY, C. and TIFFANY, W. R. (1954). Auditory malingering and psychogenic deafness. *Archs Otolar.* **60**, 197.
HARRIS, D. A. (1958). A rapid and simple technique for the detection of non-organic hearing loss. *Archs Otolar.* **68**, 758.
HATTLER, K. W. (1970). Lengthened off-time: a self-recording screening device for non-organicity. *J. Speech Hear. Dis.* **35**, 113.
HERON, T. G. (1974). Evoked response audiometry and hearing impairment in adults. *Proc. Mine med. Offrs' Ass.* **54**, 9.
HOPKINSON, N. T. (1978). Speech tests for pseudohypacusis. In *A handbook of clinical audiology*, 2nd edn (ed. J. Katz). Williams and Wilkins, Baltimore.
HYDE, M. L., ALBERTI, P. W., MORGAN, P. P., SYMONS, F., and CUMMINGS, F. (1980). Puretone threshold estimation from acoustic reflex thresholds—a myth? *Acta oto-lar.* **89**, 345.
JERGER, J., BURNEY P., MAULDIN, L., and CRUMP, B. (1974). Predicting hearing loss from the acoustic reflex. *J. Speech Hear. Dis.* **18**, 11.
—— HAYES, B., ANTHONY, L., and MAULDIN, L. (1978). Factors influencing prediction of hearing level from the acoustic reflex. *Monogr. contemp. Audiol.* **1**. 1.
—— and HEARER, G. (1961). An unexpected dividend in Békésy audiometry. *J. Speech Hear. Dis.* **26**, 390.
JOHNSEN, J. D., OSTERHAMMEL, D., TERKILDSEN, K., OSTERHAMMEL, P., and HUIS IN' T VELT, F. (1976). The white noise middle ear muscle reflex

threshold in patients with sensorineural hearing impairment. *Scand. Audiol.* **5**, 131.
JOHNSON, K. O., WORK, W. P., and MCCOY, G. (1956). Functional deafness. *Ann. Otol.* **65**, 154.
KERR, A. G., GILLESPIE, W. J., and EASTON, J. M. (1975). Deafness, a simple test for malingering. *Br. J. Audiol.* **9**, 24.
KINSTLER, D. B., PHELAN, J. G., and LAVENDER, R. W. (1972). The Stenger and speech Stenger tests in functional hearing loss. *Audiology* **11**, 187.
KLOCKHOFF, I., DRETTNER, B., and SVEDBERG, A. (1974). Computerized classification of the results of screening audiometry in groups of persons exposed to noise. *Audiology* **13**, 326.
KUMPF, W. (1975). SISI test und aggravation von schwerhorigkeit. *Lar. Rhinol. Otol. Grenzgeb.* **54**, 372.
MCCANDLESS, G. A. and LENTZ, W. E. (1968). Evoked response (EEG) audiometry in non-organic hearing loss. *Archs Otolar.* **87**, 123.
MARGOLIS, R. H. and FOX, C. M. (1977). A comparison of three methods for predicting hearing loss from acoustic reflex thresholds. *J. Speech Hear. Res.* **20**, 241.
MARTIN, F. D. and MONROE, D. A. (1975). The effects of sophistication on type 5 Békésy patterns in simulated hearing loss. *J. Speech Hear Dis.* **40**, 508.
MARTIN, F. N. (1978). Evaluation of pseudohypacusis. In *A handbook of clinical audiology*, 2nd edn (ed. J. Katz). Williams and Wilkins, Baltimore.
MILLER, R., DAVIES, C. B., and GIBSON, W. P. R. (1976). Using the acoustic reflex to predict the puretone threshold. *Br. J. Audiol.* **10**, 51.
NIEMEYER, W. and SESTERHENN, G. (1974). Calculating the hearing threshold from the stapedius reflex threshold for different sound stimuli. *Audiology* **13**, 421.
POLITZER, A. (1894). *A textbook of diseases of the ear and adjacent organs* (translated from 3rd German edition by O. Dodd; ed. Sir William Dalby) p. 681. Lee Brothers, Philadelphia.
PRATT, H. and SOHMER, H. (1978). Comparison of hearing threshold determined by auditory pathway, electrical responses and behavioural responses. *Audiology* **17**, 285.
PRIEDE, V. M. and COLES, R. R. A. (1976). Speech discrimination tests in investigation of sensorineural hearing loss. *J. Lar. Otol.* **90**, 1081.
RESNICK, D. M. and BURKE, K. S. (1962). Békésy audiometry in non-organic auditory problems. *Archs Otolar.* **76**, 38.
ROBIN, I. G. (1952). In *Diseases of the ear nose and throat*, 2nd edn (ed. W. C. Scott-Brown) p. 318. Butterworth, London.
ROSE, D. E., KEATING, L. W., HEDGECOCK, L. D., MILLER, K. E., and SCHREURS, K. K. (1972). Comparison of evoked response audiometry and routine clinical audiometry. *Audiology* **11**, 238.
RUHM, H. B. and COOPER, W. A. Jr (1962). Low sensation level effects of puretone delayed auditory feedback. *J. Speech Hear. Res.* **5**, 185.
—— —— (1964). Delayed feedback audiometry. *J. Speech Hear. Dis.* **29**, 448.
SESTERHENN, G. and BREUNINGER, H. (1977). Determination of hearing threshold for single frequencies from the acoustic reflex. *Audiology* **16**, 201.
SOHMER, H., FEINMESSER, M., BAURBERER, T. L. and EDELSTEIN, E. (1977). Cochlear, brainstem and cortical evoked responses in non-organic hearing loss. *Ann. Otol. Rhinol. Lar.* **86**, 227.
THOMSEN, K. A. (1955). Case of psychogenic deafness as demonstrated by measuring impedance. *Acta oto-lar.* **45**, 82.

VAN WAGONER, R. S. and GOODWINE, S. (1977). Clinical impression of acoustic reflex measures in an adult population. *Archs Otolar.* **103**, 582.
VENTRY, I. M. and CHAIKLIN, J. B. (1965a). Evaluation of pure-tone audiogram configurations used in identifying adults with functional hearing loss. *J. Audit. Res.* **5**, 212.
—— —— (1965b). Multidiscipline study of functional hearing loss. *J. audit. Res.* **5**, 179.
—— TRIER, T., and CHAIKLIN, J. B. (1965). Factors relating to persistence in resolution for functional hearing loss. *J. audit. Res.* **5**, 231.
WATSON, J. E. and VOOTS, R. J. (1965). Clinical application of the Reger modification of the Stenger test. *Int. Audiol.* **4**, 149.
WOOD, T. J., GOSHORN, E. L., and PETERS, R. W. (1977). Auditory reaction times in functional and non-functional hearing loss. *J. Speech Hear. Res.* **20**, 177.

42 Forensic audiology*

R. HINCHCLIFFE

INTRODUCTION

As David and Brierley (1968) point out, each political society in the world has its own Law. In fact, it frequently happens that several Laws co-exist within the same state. Moreover, law is not static; it is in a state of flux, of evolution. The development of the Law is shaped by logic, history, custom, and utility, as well as the accepted standards of right conduct (Cardozo 1921).

In view of this dependence on political, cultural, and historical factors, the law relevant to audiology will vary from country to country. This chapter will be concerned primarily with English law. Technically, as David and Brierley point out, the area of application of English law is limited to England and Wales. English law is neither the law of the United Kingdom nor that of Great Britain because Northern Ireland, Scotland, the Channel Islands and the Isle of Man are not ruled by 'English law'. However, because of historical ties this English law has applicability in various degrees to countries other than England.

The many facets of this English law which have a bearing on otolaryngological practice and research (Hinchcliffe and Hinchcliffe 1976) are also applicable to audiology. In this chapter it will be appropriate to restate some of these principles and mention changes in the law which have taken place since 1976.

GENERAL CONSIDERATIONS

There are two sources of law, i.e. case law and Statute (code) law.

British case law comprises two systems of law, i.e. Common Law and Equity. Equity was a peculiar development of the Middle Ages which sought to modify the rigidity of the Common Law by proceeding on flexible principles of 'good conscience'. Common Law comprises the ancient unwritten law of the country. It developed tentatively and casually, based upon the decisions of judges in preceding cases. The Common Law doctrine of abiding by precedent is known as *stare decisis* (short for *stare decisis et non quieta movere*). However, the only thing in a judge's decision binding as an authority upon a subsequent judge is the principle upon which the case was decided (*Osborne to Rowlett*). This principle on which a case is decided is known as the *ratio decidendi*.

---

* A Table of Statutes and a Table of Cases are given on pages 957 and 958.

However, Dias (1970) contends that the rigidity of *stare decisis* is largely mythical and judges have considerable latitude in evading unwelcome authorities. In the first place, a judge may lower the level of generality of a precedent when stating its facts and, in so doing, distinguish one case from another. Thus judges have much discretion in the handling of precedents. Moreover, as Stuttard (1969) points out, there is no test which can be applied to show which part of a previous case constituted the *ratio decidendi*. Anything which is not part of the *ratio decidendi* and which is not part of the facts of a case is referred to as *obiter dicta* (things said by the way). Consequently the Common Law has the capacity to develop and to progress. As Lord Evershed said, the ancient rules of the English Common Law have the characteristic that in general they can never be said to be final and limited by definition, but have the capacity of adaptation in accordance with the changing circumstances of succeeding ages (*Haley v. London Electricity Board*).

Tort

The law of *torts* was a creation of the Common Law and it was evolved from the principle of providing a remedy for an unjustifiable injury done by one person to another. A tort is a civil wrong. As pointed out by Lord Denning, the province of tort is to allocate responsibility for injurious conduct. In the context of this chapter, the three most important torts are Nuisance, Negligence, and Trespass to Person.

A *nuisance* has been defined as 'an inconvenience materially interfering with the ordinary comfort, physically, of human existence, not merely according to elegant or dainty modes of living, but according to plain and sober and simple notions among the English people' (*Walter v. Selfe*). A nuisance is thus an unlawful interference with a person's use or enjoyment of land, or of some right over or in connection with it.

Negligence is a failure to provide against reasonably foreseeable hazards. Indeed the concepts of foreseeability is an essential element in all cases of nuisance and negligence (Privy Council in the Wagon Mound Case (*Overseas Tankship (U.K.) Limited v. Miller Steamship Co. Limited*, Wagon Mound No. 2)—so called because it refers to the ship S.S. *Wagon Mound*. However, as Munkman (1962) points out, the concept of foreseeability has been shown up as vague, capricious, and subjective when applied to anything much more complex than bows and arrows or horses and carts. Some learned judges are able to foresee very little; others, by taking a complex succession of events step by step, are able to foresee almost anything. Moreover, the same Court can reach opposite results on two cases based on the same happening. In the Wagon Mound case, different plaintiffs took action on the same occurrence. The lower court in one case held that a particular event was not reasonably foreseeable, whilst, in the second case, another lower court held that the same event might have been foreseeable.

In British courts, the concept of 'foreseeability' is usually interpreted in the sense given to it by Lord Oaksey in the case of *Bolton v. Stone* (the plaintiff was injured by a cricket ball hit over a fence on to a road. It was held that the cricket club was not liable as the possibility of injury was so slight). The reasonable man does not take precautions against everything which he can foresee, but only against those things which he can foresee are reasonably likely to happen.

In an action for negligence, the plaintiff must prove that the defendant was under a duty of care to him, that there was a breach of such duty, and that, as a direct consequence, the plaintiff suffered damage. Thus, the essential requisites have been given as the 'four Ds': 'Duty of care, Dereliction of Duty, Damage, Directness'.

In practice, there is usually no doubt about the existence of the duty of care and it is then assumed to exist. However, in the case of *Donoghue v. Stevenson*, Lord Atkin formulated the general concept that 'you must take reasonable care to avoid acts or omissions which you can reasonably foresee will be likely to injure your neighbour'. He then defined 'neighbours' as 'persons so closely and directly affected by my act that I ought reasonably to have them in contemplation as being so affected when I am directing my mind to the acts or omissions which are called in question'. Thus there will be a 'duty' situation wherever the relationship of the parties is such that the likelihood that the plaintiff would be affected by the defendant's conduct ought reasonably to have been contemplated by the defendant.

Defences available in an action for negligence are, apart from denying the alleged negligence, that: (i) it was an inevitable accident (mishap); (ii) the negligence was that of someone else; (iii) the risk was assumed by the plaintiff (*volenti non fit injuria*); and (iv) there was contributory negligence by the plaintiff.

It is a defence to an action in tort that the defendant neither intended to injure the plaintiff nor could have avoided doing so by the use of a reasonable care.

Until 1945, contributory negligence was a complete defence to an action in tort. However, in that year, the Law Reform (Contributory Negligence) Act was enacted. Section 1 of that Act states that 'Where any person suffers damage as the result partly of his own fault and partly the fault of any other person, a claim in respect of that damage shall not be defeated by reason of the fault of the person suffering the damage, but the damages recoverable in respect thereof shall be reduced to such an extent as the court thinks just and equitable having regard to the claimant's share in the responsibility for the damage'. In two decisions in 1971, 5 per cent and 20 per cent were deducted from damages awarded as the result of road accidents in which the plaintiff was not wearing a seat belt. Associated with the concept of contributory negligence is the doctrine of 'hypothetical causation'. About 15 years ago a steel erector was killed by a fall from a tower. Although on the day in question no safety belts were available, it was held, from the evidence given, that the deceased would not have worn one. The plaintiff's act of omission may therefore constitute a *novus actus interveniens*.

Trespass to the person is any direct, intentional interference with an individual without lawful justification. Trespass to person encompasses both *assault* (the threat or attempt to use force against another person) and *battery* (the actual application of force). Unlike the law of negligence, the plaintiff need not prove that the defendant was negligent or had a duty of care to him. He need only prove that the act was harmful to him. He must, however, establish an intention. Where the battery does not amount to a serious crime, a defence of *volenti* can be maintained, as in the law of negligence.

Statute Law

Statute Law is enacted by legislation in a legislature which, in Britain, is Parliament. The unprecedented development of legislation in the nineteenth century owed much to the concepts and reforming zeal of Bentham (1789) who has subsequently been considered as one of the greatest analytical jurists of all time (Friedmann 1949). In his Theory of Legislation, Bentham defined the main function of law as being to provide subsistence, to aim at abundance, to encourage equality, and to maintain security. From these concepts there emerge the increasing social legislation which reached its peak in the middle of the twentieth century.

As Dias (1970) points out, there is now universal recognition that deliberate law making is indispensable to the efficient regulation of the modern state. The most important consequence of judicial acceptance of the supremacy of Parliament is the doctrine that no court can challenge the validity of an Act. As J. Ungoed-Thomas (1968) said 'What the statute itself enacts cannot be unlawful, because what the statute says and provides is itself the law, and the highest form of law that is known in this country. It is the law which prevails over every other form of law' (*Cheney v. Conn*). This contrasts with the position in some other countries where a higher court can declare statutes as 'unconstitutional' and therefore inoperative. However, with Britain joining the European Economic Community, the doctrine of unlimited supremacy of Parliament may have to be modified. This may well be the only legal safeguard for the possibility, envisaged by Dicey (1905), that Parliament could, if it wished, enact a law ordering all blue-eyed babies to be killed.

In respect of Acts of Parliament, the role of judges is limited to interpreting them. For this purpose, there are three rules, i.e. the Literal Rule, the Golden Rule, and the Mischief Rule. The Literal Rule states that the words in an Act are to be interpreted in their natural, ordinary, and plain meaning. Where such a literal interpretation would be absurd or ambiguous, the Golden Rule states that the statute should be interpreted such that it makes good sense. The mischief Rule may also be applied to an otherwise ambiguous statute. This rule states that one should look to discover what 'mischief' an act was intended to remedy. It thus follows that decisions based upon an application of an Act and its interpretation by the courts are all important; the actual provision of the Act is less important.

Statute Law may impose certain limitations on the Common Law. In particular, the Limitation Act 1939 stated that actions founded on tort shall not be brought after the expiration of a certain duration (six years) from the date on which the cause of action accrued. The Law Reform (Limitation of Actions) Act 1954 reduced this period to three years in connection with actions for damages for negligence, nuisance, or breach of statutory duty where personal injury was concerned. The time commences on the date on which the cause of action accrues. Thus, until 1963, an injustice might have arisen in a case where an injury was inflicted in a way that could become discoverable only after a lapse of time. Such a manner is, of course, characteristic of many occupational disorders, noise-induced hearing loss *par excellence*. This injustice was removed by the Limitation Act 1963. This Act enables the plaintiff to bring a claim even though the three year limit is past, provided that he neither knew about the injury, nor ought to have known about it, and provided that he brings the claim within one year.

MEASURES TO PROVIDE EDUCATIONAL, MEDICAL, AND SOCIAL SECURITY

Hearing-impaired individuals benefit from the general social legislation. It is convenient to discuss this under the headings: Education, Health, Rehabilitation, and Financial Security.

Education

As Boyle (1960) pointed out, education of the hearing-impaired became a statutory duty in 1893. Each school authority was charged with the duty of providing education for deaf children in its area, and the age range for compulsory school attendance of such children was fixed from 7–16 years. In 1937, the lower limit was dropped to 5 years of age. The Education Act 1944 provided for the education of hearing-impaired children from the age of 2 years. Moreover, Section 34 of that Act said that local educational authorities had a duty to ascertain which children in their areas required special educational treatment. After a child has attained the age of 2 years a notice may be served upon the parents to submit the child for examination by a competent medical officer of the appropriate area.

As Henderson (1960) indicated, it has been government policy for a number of years (Ministry of Education 1954) that no handicapped child should be sent to a special school when it can be educated satisfactorily in an ordinary one. Where a special school is necessary, a day school is preferable.

Health

The modern state is seen to have a duty in providing health services that all of its citizens can use, irrespective of whether or not they can afford to purchase them (Abel-Smith 1976). The British NHS (National Health Service) is just one of these.

The National Health Service Act (1946) provided for the establishment of a comprehensive health service which encompassed every aspect of medical care and covered everybody everywhere in the country. The NHS came into operation on 5 July 1948. *Inter alia*, it covers the investigation and management of disorders of hearing.

Although the NHS entailed radical administrative changes, it constituted an evolutionary rather than a revolutionary measure. As Milne and Chaplin (1969) point out, the purpose of the Act was 'not so much to create any completely new service as to secure a strengthening and expansion and a more rational and integrated organisation of an already existing wide range of personal health services and to make them freely available to all in need of them'. The adoption of a national health service was foreshadowed by the Second World War Beveridge Plan for Social Security.

The socialistic swing after the Second World War provided the necessary political climate for a national health service plan to be implemented. The absence of either any large number of denominational hospitals or of any large health insurance scheme, such as the American Blue Cross, facilitated the implementation. Thus, viewed in this geographical and historical perspective, doubts may arise that the British Health Service could be exported, lock, stock, and barrel, to any other country. Indeed, as Abel-Smith (1976) points out, developing countries, for example, are almost by definition short of the resources which contribute to economic and social development—highly educated man-power, entrepreneurial skill for running large enterprises, and sums available for investment. As Godber (1975) pointed out in a foreword to the Maxwell Report, the technical quality of services given under the best circumstances at selected centres in the developed countries probably does not vary a great deal. Those able to use such centres will do equally well in any country. The outcome for the whole people, however, depends on the extent to which such services are available to all who need them. Comprehensive care may be achieved either through a nationally organized service or through a system—usually based at least partly on insurance—of assistance in obtaining a service for payment, without unification of the administration. The wide variations in the proportion of the GNP (Gross National Product) expended on health must raise the question of efficiency in deployment. Britain devotes a smaller proportion of its GNP to health than do many other countries but the Maxwell Report (1975) indicates that as good a result is obtained from this funding as is obtained with greater fundings in other countries. Indeed, Cochrane (1976) considers that the NHS remains the most cost-effective service in the world.

The NHS provides a series of hearing aids, termed the Medresco hearing aids, for subjects with impaired hearing. Although body-worn hearing aids only were introduced initially, current issues are predominantly of the ear level type. About 82 000 hearing aids are issued each year by the NHS. The estimated number of users of NHS hearing aids is about 600 000. To cope with this workload, there are only about 30 audiological scientists and 850 medical staff (all grades).

The NHS has also indirectly been responsible for the establishment of a new medical specialty, Audiological Medicine, and an associated scientific cadre, Audiological Science. The practice of these specialties is restricted to the diagnosis, care, and management of patients with disorders of hearing.

Unfortunately, the NHS is now beset with problems of accountability (Klein 1976), allocation of resources (British Medical Association 1971), finance, and morale (Royal College of Surgeons 1976).

There are undoubted geographic variations in audiological health care. For example, in one particular year, three areas (with a total population of 104 000) issued a total of 5 hearing aids, whereas another area (with a population of 176 000) issued 48 aids; this indicates a relative incidence of about 6 : 1; geographic differences in the prevalence of hearing impairment in Britain are not greater than 2 : 1 (Gregory 1964). It has been suggested that an *Inverse Care Law* operates, i.e. primary physicians in the areas with most illness and deaths tend to have larger lists and less hospital support (Hart 1971).

With a view to remedying these various problems, it has been suggested that, in respect of NHS expenditure, there should be a system of administrative audit akin to medical audit to reinforce the present system of Parliamentary accountability (Klein 1976). Resources allocation and priorities have been the subjects of special study by the DHSS (Department of Health and Social Security). The Royal Commission on the National Health Service, under the Chairmanship of Sir Alec Merrison, was set up in 1976 'to consider in the interests both of the patients and of those who work in the NHS the best use and management of the financial and man power resources of the NHS'.

The problems of resource allocation sometimes referred to as opportunity costs, were the subject of a recent report by the DHSS's (1967a) Resource Allocation Working Party (RAWP). RAWP's basic unquestionable premise was that resources should be allocated according to need. The report suggested that, after considering the populations involved, a more equitable distribution of money amongst the various geographical regions of the NHS should take into account need in the form of relative morbidity rates. Although many illnesses that use resources are not usually fatal, and many fatal conditions are not preceded by costly illnesses, standardized mortality ratios (SMRs), which are readily available, correlate well with morbidity measures. Consequently, SMRs for each region should be introduced into the population weightings. But how far should one extend this weighting system? Men in the professional groups (social class I) have better mortality records than almost all other groups for all diseases, whilst labourers and unskilled workers (social class V) have a poorer record in every category (DHSS 1976). Moreover, the children of manual workers still have poorer hearing than those of non-manual workers (Richardson, Peckham, and Goldstein 1976). Should there therefore be a corresponding weighting in the allocation of resources in respect of socio-economic class? Finally, there are geographical variations in respect of the costs in providing resources.

The question of how to choose priorities is a difficult one; the principles and criteria have recently been discussed by Gray (1979). The future development of the Government's Health and Personal Social Services have been discussed in the DHSS's (1976b) Priorities Document. It was the first time an effort had been made to establish rational and systematic priorities throughout the health and personal social services. Such an effort, the document concedes, is long overdue but it is given even greater urgency by the economic limitations outlined in the Government's White Paper on Public Expenditure up to 1979/80, the period with which the document is also concerned. The White Paper on Public expenditure has shown that, despite the standstill in public expenditure as a whole from 1976/77 to 1979/80, the Government realized the need for a continuing, though reduced, growth in the health and personal social services during this period. This growth is designed to take account of demographic changes, especially the rising number of elderly people, and the increasing sophistication and, therefore, the cost, of medical care.

The DHSS says in the Priorities Document that it has been accepted that service provision for the deaf and hard-of-hearing should be given some priority. The main objectives are to improve the standards in audiology departments and hearing-aid centres by expansion of staff and facilities, including facilities for follow-up and rehabilitation of patients provided with hearing aids. One specific objective concerns the present behind-the-ear hearing-aid programme which is due to be completed by 1979/80, by which time the annual central expenditure on the programme is expected to have increased from about £5 000 000 to over £8 000 000. In the same document, the DHSS says that there is a need to develop social service provisions for the deaf, including the establishment of residential accommodation for those who are both blind and deaf. The document also says that preventive measures to identify the risk of permanent handicaps in the new-born and the young (for example, screening services to detect hearing impairments in young children) are vitally important if the incidence of handicap is to be reduced.

The Report of the Royal Commission on the National Health Service (1979) recommended, *inter alia*, that health departments should be more critically involved in the development of new specialities, e.g. audiological medicine.

Finally one should add that the NHS will need to be monitored perhaps more closely and more scientifically than at present. Doll (1974) has pointed out three ways in which this can be done, i.e. (a) medical outcome, (b) social acceptability, and (c) economic efficiency. To these one may add (d) measurement of job satisfaction in regard to all skill groups and (e) measurement of industrial harmony (Hinchcliffe 1977).

Rehabilitation

Recent years have seen legislation introduced to cover the social aspects of rehabilitation which were not covered by the National Health Services Act.

The Disabled Persons (Employment) Act 1944 provided for facilities to enable disabled persons to secure employment. The Act incorporated recommendations of the Inter-departmental Committee of the Rehabilitation and Resettlement of the Disabled (Tomlinson Committee). The Act defined a disabled person as one who, on account of injury, disease, or congenital deformity, is substantially handicapped in obtaining or keeping employment but who is capable of full-time employment. Every disabled person could apply for inclusion in the Register of Disabled Persons. Application for registration, which was open to any adult, had to be made to the nearest Disablement Resettlement Officer (DRO). A disabled person would be registered for a period of 1–10 years depending on the severity of his disability. The DRO is often quite helpful in obtaining employment for a person with profound hearing impairment. 3 per cent of the personnel employed by firms with 20 or more employees should be disabled persons. Exception from this requirement may be obtained from the DRO.

Having the right job in the first place is most important and the DRO should know where all the jobs and all the open-minded employers are to be found. He is generally the centre of the triumvirate, teacher, DRO, and WOD (Welfare Officer for the Deaf) who join in conference to launch the adolescent on his new life. It is to the DRO that the youngster will turn again, either directly or through his interpreter, if things go wrong or he wants a change (*Hearing* 1971a).

The Disabled Persons (Employment) Act 1958 incorporated recommendations made by the Piercy Committee which enquired into services for the rehabilitation, training, and resettlement of disabled persons.

The Chronically Sick and Disabled Persons Act 1970 imposes a statutory duty upon Local Authorities to ascertain the number of disabled people in their areas. As a result, over $\frac{3}{4}$ million people were so listed in 1975.

The Act requires the Local Authorities Social Services Departments, when they are satisfied that it is necessary, to meet the needs of handicapped persons by providing, or assisting in obtaining, the following services: (a) practical assistance in the home; (b) library, radio, television, or similar leisure facilities in the home; (c) leisure and travelling facilities outside the home and assistance in taking advantage of educational facilities; (d) support in lessening the personal and social consequences of illness and disability to individuals and their families; (e) assistance in carrying out adaptations to their homes or provision of additional facilities to secure greater safety, comfort, and convenience; (f) facilitating the taking of vacations; (g) meals at home and away from home; and (h) a telephone and any special equipment necessary for use of the instrument.

There are thus a number of ways in which the hearing handicapped person could benefit under the Act. Unfortunately, the Act suffers in being permissive rather than mandatory legislation. There is indeed considerable variation in the amount of money spent by Local Authorities in implementing the Act. At least one Local Authority has provided a private hearing aid for a person (young mother with a progressive senorineural hearing loss) who had inadequate help from a Medresco hearing aid and who did not qualify under the Employment and Training Act.

The Employment and Training Act 1973 led to the establishment of the Employment Service Agency (ESA) in October 1974 and the Training Services Agency (TSA) in April 1974. The ESA which is now part of the Manpower Services Commission, administers local employment offices and the chain of 26 Employment Rehabilitation Centres. These centres provide retraining for particular jobs in industry. Under the Act vocational training is provided for the disabled who are in need of such help. The Government also supports, or liaises with, rehabilitation units run by voluntary organizations. An example of one of these is the Royal National Institute for the Deaf's Unit at Court Grange (*Hearing* 1971b). This unit was established in 1962 for youths aged between 16 and 24 years who were showing signs of emotional instability and required specialized help in readjusting. The objective was to endeavour to provide the will to lead a full, happy, and industrious life. It was accepted that it was necessary to acquire competence in a trade and a proper attitude to be able to work with dignity and satisfaction. Instruction is given in bricklaying, carpentry, farming, gardening, painting, and decorating. There are close links between the ESA and other services, especially medical, for the disabled. Thus there are arrangements for the DROs, who are now responsible to the Agency, to obtain appropriate medical advice when counselling disabled persons.

The Employment Protection Act 1975 provides for greater job security. An employee suspended from work on medical grounds is entitled to 26 weeks' full pay unless offered suitable alternative employment.

Financial security

A system of financial security, termed personal social security was instituted alongside the NHS. This system costs more than £2×10^9 per annum. It provides for disablement, injury, invalidity, maternity, sickness and widow benefits, retirement pensions, and death grants.

The principle of public responsibility for the relief of poverty was accepted in Britain as early as the sixteenth century. It was embodied for England and Wales in the Poor Law Act 1601 (a similar Act was passed by the Scottish Parliament in 1579) which required the parishes to provide from local taxation for the sick, the needy, and the homeless (Central Office of Information 1970).

The National Insurance Act 1911 was the first statutory scheme of social insurance in Britain. It introduced compulsory insurance against unemployment for workers in certain industries and against medical costs and loss of earnings through sickness for lower paid workers. The Act embodied a principle which was new to public provision although it was characterized by the mutual assistance schemes of the 'friendly societies' and the trade unions to which some workmen belonged. This principle was the payment of benefits as of right in return for contributions instead of there being a test of need. Adequate funds to secure the benefits was ensured by the inclusion of employers and the Government as contributors in addition to the insured workmen.

The National Insurance Act 1946 embodied recommendations of Beveridge's (1942) Report on Social Insurance and Allied Services. A comprehensive system of insurance against loss of income due to interruption of earnings was implemented. The National Insurance Act 1965 consolidated the 1946 Act and subsequent amending legislation. Everyone is now required to participate in the National Insurance Scheme. Earnings-related short-term benefits were introduced by the National Insurance Act 1966. Invalidity benefits for the chronic sick were introduced by the National Insurance Act 1971.

A system of insurance against industrial accidents or occupational disease was provided by the National Insurance (Industrial Injuries) Act 1946. This Act superseded the Workmen's Compensation Acts 1925–45. The 1946 Act and subsequent amending legislation was consolidated in the National Insurance (Industrial Injuries) Act 1965. This Act also redefined disabilities or diseases entitling a person to compensation. Moreover, occupational noise-induced hearing loss was now covered.

The Ministry of Social Security Act 1966 provided for the establishment of the Supplementary Benefits Commission. This Commission administers a scheme of supplementary benefits. These benefits are cash payments made as of right to individuals whose income falls below a minimum level that has been laid down by Parliament. For the purposes of the 1966 Act a man is liable to maintain his wife and children, and a woman, her husband and children.

The Child Benefit Act 1971 provided for a single payment to replace family allowances and income tax allowances for dependent children.

MEASURES TO PROTECT AGAINST NOISE

In the United Kingdom, the generation and the effects of noise are controlled both by Common Law and by Statute.

That part of the Common Law known as tort deals with both the annoyance aspects of noise and the hearing-damaging aspect. The particular sections of the Law of Tort governing the annoyance and the damaging effect of noise are the Law of Nuisance and the Law of Negligence respectively.

Law relating to noise annoyance

COMMON LAW

That air-borne noise alone may constitute a nuisance was established in 1867 in the case of *Crump v. Lambert*, and structure-borne noise in the case of *Hoare & Company v. McAlpine* in 1923.

In contrast to the statute law on noise, it is no defence for the defendant to show that he has taken all reasonable steps and care to prevent the noise (*Rushmer v. Polsue and Alfieri Limited*). The judgement of Warrington, J. in this case was expressly approved by the House of Lords on appeal. With respect to this case, Lord Loreburn stated that 'It would be no answer to say that the steam hammer is of the most modern improved pattern and is reasonably worked'. This principle was upheld in the more recent case of *Halsey v. Esso Petroleum Co. Limited*. The plaintiff was granted both damages for loss caused by acid smuts from the defendants' depot and injunctions to restrain the making of noise at night and the emission of pungent smells at any time. The action was also of note because the plaintiff brought noise level measurements to court in evidence.

A landlord may be liable if he has authorized the creation of a nuisance expressly or by implication. Thus a landlord has been held liable for his tenant's blasting operations because he had let the property for that specific purpose (*Harris v. James*).

Gunfire, especially when malicious, can be a cause for nuisance. A fox farmer was granted an injunction restraining his neighbour from firing guns so as to frighten the foxes during the breeding season (*Hollywood Silver Fox Farm v. Emmett*).

Structure-borne sound (vibration) may also result in a successful action for nuisance. A particular case was in connection with pile-driving operations which set up vibrations that damaged the plaintiff's buildings (*Barette v. Franki Compressed Pile Co. of Canada*).

Noises other than those due to gunfire or machinery can also constitute a nuisance. In the case of *Tinkler v. Aylesbury Dairy Co. Limited*, it was held that noise resulting from moving milk churns when being loaded interfered with the personal comfort of the nearby residents and thereby constituted a common-law nuisance. Noise from carts and shouts from their drivers during night-time, so that they made the plaintiff unable to sleep, also constituted a common-law nuisance (*Bartlett v. Marshall*). Noisy animals can also constitute a common-law nuisance, e.g. cockerels crowing (*Leeman v. Montagu*). More recently, in the case of *Harrison v. Metropolitan Police*, the plaintiff obtained an injunction with respect to the howling and barking of dogs kept in a police station compound. These noises had disturbed his sleep and made it difficult for him to work in his study even when he wore earplugs and had installed both double glazing in the bedroom and internal shutters.

Malice may be a factor in an action for noise nuisance. In the case of *Christie v. Davey*, a music teacher was granted an injunction restraining a neighbour from knocking on the party wall and otherwise creating a noise to interfere with professional teaching.

However, temporary noise, e.g. that due to the demolition of a building, may not, if the operation is reasonably conducted and all proper reasonable steps taken to ensure that no undue inconvenience is caused to neighbours, form a basis for a successful action for nuisance at common law (*Andreae v. Selfridge*). Nevertheless, a teacher in New Zealand was successful in claiming damages in the New Zealand Supreme Court because nearby construction noise forced him to shout and this caused him to develop a tumour on the vocal folds (*The Times* 1969).

At common law, prescriptive right is a defence in an action for nuisance.

This arises after twenty years but the time begins only when the act in fact becomes a nuisance. Thus it was held that the defendant had no prescriptive right in a case where he had used the machinery for more than twenty years but the vibrations caused by it became a nuisance only when the plaintiff, a physician, put up a consulting room at the end of his garden near the noise (*Sturges v. Bridgman*). This decision thus also upheld the principle, established in the case of *Bliss v. Hall*, that it is no defence to show that the plaintiff came to the nuisance.

STATUTE LAW

Prior to the Noise Abatement Act 1960, noise control was vested in Local Authorities under provisions set out in, and effected principally by, by-laws made under the Local Government Act 1933.

The Noise Abatement Act has now been superseded by the Control of Pollution Act 1974. Part III of the Act deals with noise. The first section (Sec. 57) of this part imposes a duty on every Local Authority to have its area periodically inspected to detect noise nuisances and for the purpose of establishing noise-abatement zones.

Where a Local Authority is satisfied that noise amounting to a nuisance exists, or is likely to occur or recur, Sec. 58 requires the Authority to serve a notice requiring the abatement of the nuisance or prohibiting or restricting its occurrence or recurrence. The notice must specify the time, or times, within which the requirements of the notice are to be complied with. Under Sec. 58 (5) it shall be a defence to prove that the best practical means have been used for preventing, or for counteracting the effects of, the noise. Sec. 72 (2) defines 'practicable' as 'reasonably practicable having regard among other things to local conditions and circumstances, to the current state of technical knowledge and to the financial implications'.

Sec. 59 (1) says that a Magistrates' Court may act under this section on a complaint made by the occupier of any premises if he is aggrieved by noise amounting to a nuisance.

Secs. 60 and 61 effect control of noise on construction sites. In connection with intended work, Sec. 60 (2) enables the appropriate Authority to serve a notice specifying the plant or machinery that is, or is not, to be used, specify the hours during which the work may be conducted and specify the level of noise which may be generated.

Sec. 62 governs noise in the streets. A loudspeaker may not be operated for any purpose between 2100 h and 0800 h, and for commercial advertising at any time.

Sec. 63 provides for the establishment of noise abatement zones. Sec. 64 requires Local Authorities to keep a *Noise Level Register*. This records noise level measurements made of noise emanating from premises within such a zone. Sec. 66 provides for a 'Noise Reduction Notice' to be served on persons responsible for exceeding permitted levels within the zone.

Sec. 68 provides for the fitting of silencers to machinery.

Sec. 73 (1) says, *inter alia*, that 'noise' includes vibration.

Sec. 74 provides a maximum penalty of £200 for first offences and £400 for subsequent offences, together with a fine of £50 for each day that the offence continues after the conviction.

There are also a number of other anti-noise provisions embodied in miscellaneous Acts. Sec. 28 of the Town Police Clauses Act 1847 prohibits the wantonly disturbing of residents by knocking on the door or ringing the door bell. Sec. 55 of the Metropolitan Police Act 1839 provides that 'no person other than persons acting in obedience to lawful authority shall discharge any cannon or other firearm of greater calibre than a common fowling piece within three hundred yards of any dwelling house . . .'. Sec. 1 of the Metropolitan Police Act 1864 provides that 'any householders within the Metropolitan Police District, personally or by his servant, or by any police constable, may require any street musician or street singer to depart from the neighbourhood of the house of such householder on account of the illness or on account of the interruption of the ordinary occupation or pursuits of any inmate of such house, or for other reasonable or sufficient cause; and every person, who shall sound or play upon any musical instrument or shall sing in any thoroughfare or public place near any such house, after being so required to depart, shall be liable to a penalty not more than forty shillings. . .'.

Law relating to noise-induced hearing loss

This is a topic of such importance that it merits separate mention (Chapters 36–40).

MEASURES TO PROTECT AGAINST UNWANTED EFFECTS OF DRUGS

The Law of Negligence may afford protection for the patient against the adverse effects of therapeutic substances or procedures. The doctor, the hospital, or the pharmaceutical manufacturer could be liable. Injury sustained as a result of being given a drug could be considered as an aspect of products liability. Decisions in a given case would be based on *Donoghue (or M'Alister) v. Stevenson* which has been referred to earlier. The Plaintiff in that case had drunk ginger beer from an opaque bottle which was subsequently found to contain a decomposed snail. The Plaintiff who became ill, was unable to sue under the Law of Contract because another person had purchased the bottle. The Law of Contract may also not be applicable for other reasons. For example, in *Pfizer v. Ministry of Health*, the House of Lords ruled that the supply of drugs under the NHS scheme was not a contract, even when a prescription charge had been levied. The patient has a statutory right to demand the drug; the hospital has the statutory obligation to supply it.

The case of *Watson v. Buckley* showed that a Plaintiff may sue (successfully) the distributors of an unsafe pharmaceutical product, in that case a hair dye.

Much of the legal interest in the adverse effect of drugs centres on thalidomide, α-(N-phthalimido) glutarimide. This was a psychotropic drug which was discovered in 1954, first marketed in Germany in 1956 and, in the United Kingdom in 1958. An ataxic polyneuritis was soon observed as an adverse effect. Wiedemann (1961) reported congenital abnormalities in cases where the mothers had taken the drug in the early stages of pregnancy. In the same year, the drug was withdrawn from the market. During the 5-year period that it was on the market, thalidomide probably produced 10 000 defective children, about 400 in the United Kingdom. The congenital abnormality was characterized by phocomelia, microtia, and, frequently, defective hearing. Legal proceedings began in 1962 but the case was never fully litigated. Instead, there were a series of settlements, beginning in 1968 and ending 10 years later (*The Times* 1978). Nevertheless, as Teff and Munro (1976) point out, the thalidomide catastrophe has had many repercussions and a profound influence on the Law. It provoked an extensive assessment by the Law Commission on the Problem of Liability for Antenatal Injury. This culminated in the *Report on Injuries to Unborn Children* 1974. Based upon the Law Commission's recommendations, the Congenital Disabilities (Civil Liability) Act 1976 provided for the unborn child to sue for negligence. At the time of the thalidomide catastrophe, doubts were expressed as to whether or not a right of action existed with regard to ante-natal injury. This was exemplified by a decision in 1884 in the United States in which it was held that a child was part of its mother and had no independent legal personality (*Dietrich v. Northampton*). However, Mr Justice Hinchcliffe held that the mother had a right of action and was entitled to damages for 'grievous shock at seeing her child born deformed'.

The likelihood of a thalidomide claim to have succeeded also hinged, as it does in occupational noise-induced hearing loss cases, on the general state of medical and scientific knowledge at the time in question. The time in question was between 1956 and 1958 when the drug was being developed. The likelihood of success of a claim would also hinge on whether or not the pharmaceutical company could be held to have discharged their duty of care. At the time in question, teratogenicity tests were not part of standard screening procedures for new drugs. Risks which ought reasonably to have been known must be interpreted in the light of medical knowledge and experience prevailing at the time (*Roe v. Ministry of Health*).

As Teff and Munro (1976) point out, public reaction to the thalidomide tragedy created an atmosphere in which both the medical profession and the pharmaceutical industry were prepared to accept controls. The result was the Medicines Act 1968. This Act provided for the legal control of various aspects of the advertising, manufacture, labelling, distribution, and use of medicines.

The 1968 Act provided for the establishment of the Medicines Commission. Licences for new product and certificates to subject these to clinical trials must be obtained from the Commission's Committee on Safety of Medicines. The Committee also monitors adverse reactions to drugs already in use. As a result the hazards of practolol, 4-(2-hydroxy-3-

isopropylaminopropoxy) acetanilide, were detected and their frequency assessed. The drug, which is a beta-adrenergic blocker, was used for the treatment of angina pectoris, cardiac dysrhythmias, and hypertension. It produces an oculo-mucocutaneous disorder (Felix, Ive, and Dahl 1974) which is sometimes associated with tinnitus and/or impairment of hearing (Wright 1975). The hearing disorder is sensorineural but various audiometric patterns occur, including one that is similar to that of noise-induced hearing loss (McNab Jones, Hammond, Wright, and Ballantyne 1977).

MEASURES TO PROTECT AGAINST HEALTH SERVICES AND THEIR PERSONNEL

Common law

NEGLIGENCE

Health Services and their personnel are liable for acts of negligence. In the Court of Appeal Lord Denning has said that the hospital authorities are responsible for all of their staff (*Roe v. Ministry of Health*). However, a clinician is not liable because some other doctor might have shown greater skill and knowledge. In actions for negligence in respect of medical practice, the law is applied almost entirely on the expert evidence of medical witnesses—evidence from competent practitioners that, in the same circumstances, they would have done, or would not have done, what the Defendant did.

It is normal for the Plaintiff to establish that the Defendant's negligence had caused him injury. However, the onus is on the Defendant if the principle of *res ipsa loquitur* operates. For example, a patient went into hospital with two stiff fingers (due to Dupuytren's contracture) and came out with four. In reversing the decision of the trial court, Lord Denning held it to be a case of *res ipsa loquitur* (*Cassidy v. Minister of Health*). Two conditions are required before this doctrine will apply. First, the event which caused the damage must have rested within the control of the Defendant. Secondly, the mere occurrence of the event itself implies that the Defendant has been negligent. One would also presume that this doctrine would be applied to cases of permanent complete facial palsy following a stapedectomy. Recently, a Plaintiff underwent this operation and the stapes was replaced with a politef piston. The only unusual feature encountered at operation was a greater than usual amount of posterior meatal wall which had to be drilled before the stapes and foramen ovale were exposed. The patient developed a complete ipsilateral facial palsy 48 hours after the operation. A subsequent exploration showed that facial nerve had been damaged in the horizontal portion of a facial nerve canal, at which site there was a dehiscence. The claim for damages was settled for £10 000 (Annual Report and Accounts 1978).

In respect of the *directness* of the causation, actions for medical negligence may allow for a 'chain of causation'. Thus failure in the treatment of the infected finger of a pregnant woman was held to be the cause of a voice disorder. The chain of causation here was via a septicaemia and subsequent damage to the cranial nerves.

In respect of medical practice, Lord Denning has said that a doctor was not to be held negligent simply because something went wrong. He was liable only when he fell below the standard of care of a *reasonably competent* practitioner *in his field* so much that his conduct might be deserving of censure or be inexcusable (*Cole v. Hucks*). However, this holds only when the mishap cannot be avoided by any such precaution as a reasonable man may be expected to take. Risks are inherent in most medical and surgical procedures but a practitioner must not take 'an unwarranted and unnecessary risk'. The 'broken needle' cases best illustrate the law relating to medical mishaps. When the needle of a hypodermic syringe breaks off during a diagnostic or therapeutic procedure, the Plaintiff must produce evidence of negligence as such. The evidence may be that the needle was not the appropriate one for the particular injection or that it was inserted wrongly.

There is now a mounting number of negligence cases of audiological interest. Of particular concern are those associated with clearing the ear of cerumen and the use of ototoxic drugs.

A perforated ear drum following aural syringing in a 50-year-old man resulted in otorrhoea which in turn resulted in inability to go swimming or take a shower which resulted in an expensive holiday to the Canary Islands being ruined. The doctor who syringed the ear recorded that 'unfortunately, the nozzle of the syringed slipped during the procedure and the external auditory canal was lacerated'. The case was settled out of Court for £4222. This sum covered a 'profound sensorineural hearing loss' on the affected side as well as surgical fees for a myringoplasty and legal fees (Annual Report and Accounts 1978).

In another case of a perforated ear drum following syringing, the Plaintiff was reported to have suffered a 'permanent 40-dB hearing loss and tinnitus' (*James v. SKF (UK)*).

In a third case of ear-drum perforation following syringing, subsequent treatment (repeated myringoplasties) by a Consultant was considered to have made things worse rather than better. 'There was a 50 per cent hearing loss in the affected ear with vestibular function significantly diminished.' The claim was settled after negotiation by payment and damages of £8000 and costs of £810 (Annual Report and Account 1979).

However, not all claims in respect of ear-drum perforations due to syringing have been successful. An 18-year-old youth attended for a medical examination at a Recruiting Centre. Impacted wax in both ears required syringing. The youth denied any previous ear trouble. Syringing was successful in clearing the wax from one ear but 'the third and last effort to eliminate the wax (from the other ear) proved so painful that the doctor desisted, instilled more oil into the ear and told the young man to return a week later. . . . the boy reported at the examination centre a week later with a piece of lint over his ear on which there was some brownish-yellow discharge. . . . had had some bleeding from the ear during the evening the day when it had been syringed. . . . On examination, the ear was found to be cleared of debris and there was a small perforation in the tympanum.' 'The papers were submitted to two experienced otologists, both of whom were of the opinion that it is impossible to perforate a healthy ear drum by syringing.' In view of this evidence, the Judge gave Judgment for the doctor with costs (Taylor 1971).

An Australian case mentioned by Lockhart (1980) is cited as an example of the duty of a doctor to use competent assistants. The Plaintiff, who had been surfing, attended hospital complaining of 'a thundering noise in the ear'. After examination of the Plaintiff's ear in the casualty department, a resident doctor asked a student nurse to provide the Plaintiff with some glycerol and phenol ear drops. The nurse misunderstood and the Plaintiff was given what was essentially pure phenol. As a result 'a part of his ear drum was destroyed, and his hearing was permanently impaired'. The Judge said that 'the real cause of the error was the giving of instructions in terms which were not as specific as they should have been to a pupil nurse who was not competent to take them. The doctor should not have given her instructions, or he should, before giving her the instructions, have satisfied himself that she was competent to take them and knew what was intended' (*Henson v. The Board of Management of the Perth Hospital and Another*).

A woman who had been admitted to hospital suffering from boils was prescribed a course of streptomycin. The day after the last injection, symptoms of damage to the vestiblocochlear nerve developed and the Plaintiff was left with the loss of her sense of balance. The claim for negligence was based upon the fact that a total of 30 injections had been ordered by the house surgeon but 34 injections had been given. The Judge considered that it was the last injection which had caused the damage. The Defendants were therefore liable. (*Smith v. Brighton and Lewes Hospital Management Committee*).

Mistakes must be differentiated from mishaps. As a general rule in the Law of Torts, a mistake is no defence. However, the law has taken a different view in respect of medical mistakes. A mistake in diagnosis has been construed as an 'error of judgment' (see Fig. 42.1).

Thus, in an action for damages brought by a widow in respect of the misdiagnosis of her late husband's chest pain, the judge ruled that the case was one of mistake and not of negligence because the doctor had examined the case carefully for an hour. However, failing to make a correct diagnosis must be differentiated from failure to examine a patient adequately. The latter may amount to negligence. Failure to use a stethoscope in a Casualty Department to diagnose fractured ribs in an intoxicated injured patient has been held to be negligent. Failure to request a radiological examination in possible bony disorders or injuries would probably be held to be negligent. But, surprisingly, failure to employ an endoscope which would have diagnosed a rare condition may not amount to negligence. If a doctor does not

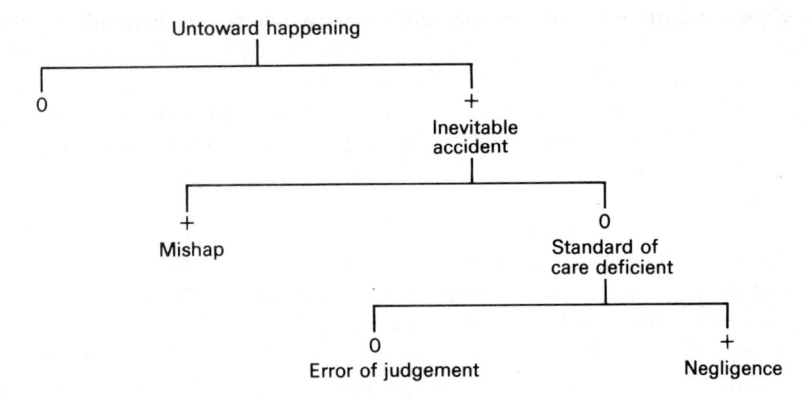

```
                    Untoward happening
        ┌──────────────────┴──────────────────┐
        0                                     +
                                         Inevitable
                                          accident
                          ┌──────────────────┴──────────────────┐
                          +                                     0
                        Mishap                            Standard of
                                                         care deficient
                                          ┌──────────────────┴──────────────────┐
                                          0                                     +
                                   Error of judgement                        Negligence
```

Fig. 42.1. The nature of medicolegal error.

feel competent to diagnose a particular case, he may be held negligent for failing to refer the case to the appropriate specialist. Although, in cases concerning surgical treatment, the question of negligence hinges on what other competent practitioners would, or would not, have done, so often the principle of *res ipsa loquitur (vide supra)* is applied. This principle would hold where the wrong operation was performed or the wrong side was operated on. Lord Goddard held that the principle applied in 'swab cases' also (*Mahon v. Osborn*).

In a recent Court of Appeal decision, Lord Denning said that 'if medical men were to be found liable whenever they did not effect a cure—or whenever anything untoward happens—it would do a great disservice not only to the profession itself but to society at large. Heed should be taken of what had happened in the United States. There "medical malpractice" cases were very worrying, especially as they were tried by juries who had sympathy for the patient and none for the doctor—who was insured—and damages were colossal. Experienced practitioners refused to treat patients for fear of being accused of negligence. In the interest of all we must avoid such consequences. The courts must say firmly that, in a professional man, an error of judgment was not negligent' (*Whitehouse v. Jordan and Another*) 1979. However, the case went to the House of Lords where disagreement was expressed with this statement. Their Lordships nevertheless upheld the Court of Appeal's decision in reversing the trial Judge's finding. In concurring with Lord Wilberforce, Lord Fraser stated that Lord Denning must have meant to say that an error of judgment 'is not *necessarily* negligent'. Another Law Lord, Lord Edmund-Davies, concluded by saying 'doctors and surgeons fell into no special legal category, and, to avoid any future disputation of a similar kind, His Lordship would have it accepted that the true doctrine was enunciated—and by no means for the first time—by Mr Justice McNair in *Bolam v. Friern Hospital Management Committee* in words applied by the Privy Council in *Chin Keow v. Government of Malaysia*: "When you get a situation which involves the use of some special skill or competence, then the test as to whether there has been negligence or not is not the test of the man on the top of a Clapham omnibus, because he has not got this special skill. The test is the standard of the ordinary skilled man exercising and professing that special skill." If a surgeon failed to measure up to that standard in any respect ("clinical judgment" or otherwise) he had been negligent and should be so judged.' (*Whitehouse v. Jordan and Another, 1980.*)

The institution of an experimental therapeutic procedure can be particularly hazardous—legally for the doctor as well as medically for the patient. The law governing the institution of new (experimental) treatments of patients was established over 300 years ago (*Slater v. Baker and Stapleton*). In this case, the Plaintiff sued the then Head Surgeon (Mr Baker) of St Bartholomew's Hospital. Mr Baker had re-fractured the Plaintiff's healed leg so that it could go through the 'operation of extension using a heavy steel invention with fearsome teeth'. On appeal, the Chief Baron held that, 'although the Defendants in general may be as skilful in their respective professions as any two gentlemen in England, yet the Court cannot help saying that, in this particular case, they have acted ignorantly and unskilfully contrary to the known rules and usage of surgeons'. The law applicable to actions for negligence in respect of new therapeutic procedures was systematized in a Scottish case (*Hunter v. Hanley*) by Lord President Clyde in 1955. Three facts must be established. First that there does exist a normal, usual practice. Secondly, that the Defendant had not adopted that practice. Thirdly, that the course of management adopted was one that no professional man of ordinary skill would have taken if he had been acting with ordinary care.

A defence of *volenti non fit injuria* in medical cases of actions for negligence can only be made if *consent*—informed consent, has been freely given. Any medical or surgical procedure, including the simplest diagnostic examination which is conducted without the patient's consent (expressed or implied) is a trespass to person (see later). For minor diagnostic and therapeutic procedures, consent is usually implied. It is argued that, when a patient presents himself seeking treatment, he has clearly implied his consent to a physical examination and, at least, some minor therapeutic procedure. Sitting down in the examination chair or lying down on a couch may be taken as tacit consent. In other cases, written consent should be obtained. If an emergency operation is necessary to save a patient's life and consent cannot be obtained, the principle of 'agency of necessity' is invoked.

In a recent claim for damages arising out of an unsuccessful stapedectomy, the Plaintiff claimed that he had not carefully read the consent form and was under the impression that it signified authority only for a general anaesthetic and an examination. The Plaintiff was employed as a claims manager by an insurance company where careful scrutiny of forms and their small print is all important. Not surprisingly, therefore, the Judge completely rejected the Plaintiff's evidence.

In some experimental therapeutic procedures, actions for negligence have hinged not on whether or not an unusual course of action was adopted but on whether or not *informed consent* had been really given. In a case in the United Kingdom, where a facial paralysis developed after an operation involving the insertion of an electronic device in the para-aural tissues to treat deafness, the Judge held that there was inadequate warning of all the risks involved. However, in *non-experimental* therapeutic procedures, the courts will admit to the necessity for 'therapeutic misrepresentation'. In an action for negligence arising from damage to the recurrent laryngeal nerve during a thyroidectomy, the trial judge said 'on the evening before the operation, the surgeon told the plaintiff that there was no risk to her voice, when he knew that there was some slight risk, but he did that for her own good because it was of vital importance that she should not worry. He told a lie, but he did it because in the circumstances it was justifiable. The law does not condemn the doctor when he only does what a wise doctor so placed would do... And none of the doctors called as witnesses have suggested that the surgeon was wrong' (*Hatcher v. Black*).

The Medical Protection Society offer the following recommendations to doctors for a successful defence in negligence cases:

1 Keep clear and accurate records.
2 Report early to the Society any incident which might give rise to a possible claim, setting out full details of the incident while it is fresh in the memory and giving the names and addresses of anyone else who witnessed the incident.
3 Seek the advice of the Society before replying to a letter of complaint which might lead to an allegation of negligence or breach of terms of service or an accusation of professional misconduct.
4 Reply promptly to letters from the Society or its solicitors requesting comments or instructions.
5 Keep the Society informed of any change of address, so that letters do not go astray. If a principal witness goes overseas without leaving a forwarding address and cannot be traced when a trial is imminent, the Defence is embarrassed (Annual Report and Accounts 1978).

TRESPASS TO PERSON

It is not a battery to make a medical examination of a patient who consents to it. But a battery does take place if a person is examined against his/her own will (*Latter v. Braddell and Sutcliffe*). However, Lord Justice Winn's Committee on Personal Injuries Litigation concluded (Cmnd. 3691, 1968, para. 312) that it 'entertained no doubt that every claimant for personal injuries must be bound to submit himself to medical examination of a reasonable character which is reasonably required, subject, of course, to proper safeguards and to the claimant's right to object to any particular doctor'. Nevertheless, Mr Justice Lawson condemned the procedure whereby a person could be compelled to submit to a medical examination by indirectly staying proceedings as not being conducive to respect for the administration of justice (*Baugh v. Delta Walter Fittings*). Mr Justice

Lawson pointed out that a requirement to submit to a medical examination could be justified only where Parliament had specifically authorized it. Compulsory medical examinations are required by various statutes, e.g. of school children under the Education Act 1944. Even then, the examination can only be done after the requisite notice has been served on the parent.

Recently, the Court of Appeal held that 'if a Defendant in a personal injuries case made a reasonable request for the Plaintiff to be medically examined by a doctor whom the Defendant had chosen then the Plaintiff should accede to such a request unless he had reasonable ground for objecting to that particular doctor and was prepared to disclose his reason to the Court' (*Starr v. National Coal Board*). In giving Judgment in this case, Scarman L. J. said that 'the Defendant is not to be regarded as making an unreasonable request merely because he wishes to have the Plaintiff examined by a doctor unacceptable to the Plaintiff . . . it can only be the interests of justice that could require one or other of the parties to have to accept an infringement of a fundamental human right cherished by the common law. The Plaintiff can only be compelled, albeit indirectly, to an infringement of his personal liberty if justice requires it. Similarly, the Defendant can only be compelled to forego the Expert Witness of his choice if justice requires it'.

A recent forensic audiological case concerned attempts to impose constraints on the nature and extent of the medical examination to be conducted by an Expert Witness. The Plaintiff alleged that he was suffering from impaired hearing as a result of exposure to an occupational noise hazard. He had a partial hearing loss on one side, a total hearing loss on the other side, and he also suffered from tinnitus and recurrent episodes of vertigo. The Defendant's Expert Witness proposed to conduct a medical examination that would have included zonography of the internal acoustic meatuses, caloric tests and transtympanic electrocochleography. The patient refused to submit to the examinations and the Defendant applied to stay the proceedings. The application first came before a Registrar who was also furnished with an Affidavit sworn by the Expert Witness for the Plaintiff. The Affidavit stated, *inter alia*, that the radiological examination would 'involve considerable radiation dosage to the brain and eyes' . . . 'My experience is that the caloric test is frightening to some patients, causes giddiness to most, nausea to many and vomiting to a few.' Transtympanic electrocochleography 'is somewhat unpleasant and frightening for many patients. It is not without danger; very occasionally it has punctured the inner ear membranes and damaged the ear; or caused infection.' The Registrar accepted these statements and concluded that it would not be appropriate to grant a stay as asked by the Defendant. However, he did say, in referring to the X-ray examination, 'it seems to me that this is an infringement of his (the Plaintiff's) liberty which, if it were the only test proposed, and subject to it not involving the Plaintiff in more than the safe dosage limit of X-rays, the Plaintiff could be obliged to accept.'

The Defendant appealed and the case was heard by Mr Justice Webster on the 22 July 1980. The Judge refused to choose between the conflicting evidence produced by two Expert Witnesses. 'For the reasons for the decisions I have already reached it has not been necessary for me to determine any factual conflict between the evidence of the Plaintiffs and the Defendants. All it is for me to determine is a reasonableness of the Defendant's request as reasonably seen by them and the reasonableness of the Plaintiff's objection as seen by him, and then to compare the weight of the reasonableness of the request with the reasonableness of the objection. For that purpose it does not seem to me (at any rate, in this case) to be necessary to involve such conflicts as there are between the various deponents, and I accordingly dismiss that application' (*Prescott v. Bulldog Tools Limited*).*

It is within the discretion of a judge to admit the evidence derived from a specimen of blood that has been unlawfully obtained (*R. v. Trump*).

Surgical operations which are technically successful may amount to a trespass if consent has not been obtained. Thus, during an operation on an ear, a surgeon in the United States found that the other ear was more extensively diseased. He therefore operated on both ears. Although he did so skilfully and successfully, the Court, on appeal, found for the Plaintiff.

In a recent English case (*Chatterton v. Gerson and Another*), the Plaintiff claimed that consent to a therapeutic procedure, which was associated with complications, was vitiated by a lack of explanation of what the procedure entailed and what were its implications. Consequently, the Plaintiff had given *no real* consent. The procedure was therefore a trespass to her person that was a battery. There was no claim that the doctor had been negligent. The Judge said that the duty of a doctor was to explain what he intended to do, and its implications, in the way that a careful and responsible doctor in similar circumstances would have done. His Lordship was satisfied that the doctor had told the Plaintiff what the procedure (an intrathecal phenol injection for pain relief) was all about. The Plaintiff's consent was not vitiated by any lack of information. The Judge also said that it would be very much against the interests of justice if actions which were really based on a failure by the doctor to perform his duty adequately to inform were pleaded in trespass. The action therefore failed.

Statute law

There is one statute that has been designed with the exclusive purpose of protecting hearing-impaired people. This is the Hearing Aid Council Act 1968. For the purpose of the Act, a body termed the Hearing Aid Council was set up. The Council has the function of securing adequate standards of competence and conduct among persons engaged in dispensing hearing aids. It also advises on methods for improving training facilities for hearing aid dispensers. Section 1 (3) requires the Council to draw up both standards of competence and codes of practice for dispensers. Section 1 (6) provides for the Council to receive complaints from members of the public and to investigate such complaints. Section 2 requires the Council to establish a

* See note added in proof on page 960.

register of dispensers of hearing aids. A person may be registered if, prior to the commencement of the Act, he had acted as a dispenser of hearing aids for a period of at least six months in the two years prior to the Act, or he satisfies the standards of competence laid down by the Council. The Council was also empowered by Section 5 (1) to set up a committee termed the Investigating Committee to investigate disciplinary cases. The function of the Investigating Committee was to decide whether a disciplinary case (a case being investigated) ought to be referred to the Disciplinary Committee. If a person is judged by the Disciplinary Committee to have been guilty of serious misconduct in connection with the dispensing of hearing aids, the Committee may direct his name to be erased from the register.

Section 14 of the Act defined a 'dispenser of hearing aids' as 'an individual who conducts or seeks to conduct oral negotiations with a view to effecting the supply of a hearing aid, whether by him or another, to or for the use of a person with impaired hearing'. A 'hearing aid' was defined as 'an instrument intended for use by a person suffering from impaired hearing to assist that person to hear better but does not include any instrument or device designed for use by connecting conductors of electricity to equipment or apparatus provided for the purpose of affording means of telephonic communication'.

LAW RELATING TO EVIDENCE

As Martin (1979) points out, an expert, when giving evidence must state the reasons for his opinions, how they were reached and by what criteria his conclusions can be tested. It is for the Court to determine whether or not it wishes to accept his opinion, or which of conflicting opinions, if any, it prefers. The Court is not bound to accept any opinion, even if undisputed.

The standard of proof in civil cases is that of the balance of probabilities (*Cooper v. Slade*).

Confidential information communicated to medical practitioners is not protected by privilege (*Garner v. Garner*). However, a witness may refuse to produce a document or give evidence until ordered by the Court to do so. In any claim for damages for personal injury, the Court has the power under Sections 31 and 32 of the Administration of Justice Act 1970 to order the disclosure and production of documents. Section 31 relates to legal proceedings which are contemplated. Section 32 relates to legal proceedings which have been commenced. It entitles either party to the action to apply for an order for the production of relevant documents in the possession of a third person who is not a party to the action. Documents which may be the subject of an order under either Section include medical correspondence, records, reports, and X-rays. As a result of three decisions in the Court of Appeal in the early 1970s, it had become the practice in applications under both Sections 31 and 32 for medical records to be disclosed only to a Medical Expert nominated by the applicant, and not to the applicant himself or to his solicitors. In the case of *McIvor v. Southern Health and Social Services Board*, a hospital submitted that the consequences of not confining production of hospital records to the medical advisers of the applicant would in some cases be so dire that Parliament must have intended to confer on the courts a power so to do. The hospital's appeal to the House of Lords was dismissed. The House of Lords held that the Act meant what it said. However, the medical protection societies strongly advise their members to consult with them before complying with any request for the disclosure of records. It does not follow that every application from solicitors for the disclosure of records in the possession of a doctor must automatically be complied with, for the applicant has to satisfy the Court on affidavit that there are grounds for making an order (Annual Report and Accounts 1978).

The ownership of medical records, including X-ray films, is discussed by Speller (1974). Ordinarily, medical records belong to the hospital authority. But should a radiologist's or other report be made in respect of a private patient by virtue of a private arrangement with the patient or, as likely as not, with the consultant on his behalf, then, even though the radiologist or other specialist concerned is on the staff of the hospital, the hospital is not the owner of the record. What the patient pays for is not a photograph but the expert reading by the radiologist of the film and for his opinion on what he believes to be the facts disclosed, that reading and opinion being communicated to the medical practitioner by whom the patient was referred for his guidance. If, as is customary, the report is accompanied by a print of the film, that does not alter the argument provided the radiologist is regarded—as he properly must be—as the expert giving an opinion. It would not seem that there would be any grounds on which such a patient could claim possession of an X-ray photograph taken but, presumably, as well as in the case of part-paying and general-ward patients, the photographs and radiologist's reports will be available for the use of medical practitioners at other hospitals where the patient may later be treated.

In a recent test case, it was held that an expert medical report is meant for the impartial assistance of the court and not simply to buttress one party's case. A doctor is right in refusing to amend a report at the behest of the solicitor requesting it (Medicolegal 1979). Concern has indeed been expressed in recent times regarding the manner in which expert evidence comes to be organised by lawyers. Comments have been made both in the Court of Appeal and in the House of Lords. In a House of Lords Judgment, Lord Wilberforce has said that 'while some degree of consultation between experts and legal advisers was entirely proper it was necessary that expert evidence presented to the Court should be, and should be seen to be, the independent product of the expert, uninfluenced as to form or content by the exigencies of litigation. To the extent that it was not, the evidence was likely to be not only incorrect but self-defeating.' (*Whitehouse v. Jordan and Another 1980*).

There is a curious notion amongst some medical men that they must, as well as presenting their expert evidence, also dwell on the rights and wrongs of a legal case. As Martin (1979) points out, a witness, however distinguished, cannot assume the mantle of a judge; he does not relieve the court of its responsibility for the judicial decision. Lord President Cooper has clearly distinguished between the separate roles of the expert and of the court (*David v. Edinburgh Magistrates*).

CONCLUSIONS

It is clear that there is a plethora of enactments and a considerable body of the Common Law which governs the practice of Audiological Medicine. With the notable exception of the Hearing Aid Council Act 1968, however, the relevant case law and statute law is not specific to Audiology. Moreover, as indicated by the incorporation of the provisions of the Noise Abatement Act 1960 into the Control of Pollution Act 1974, there is a tendency to provide non-specific legislation.

APPENDIX 42.1 TABLE OF STATUTES

1601 Poor Law Act
1839 Metropolitan Police Act
1847 Town Police Clauses Act
1864 Metropolitan Police Act
1911 National Insurance Act
1933 Local Government Act
1939 Limitation Act
1944 Disabled Persons (Employment) Act
1944 Education Act
1945 Law Reform (Contributory Negligence) Act
1946 National Health Service Act
1946 National Insurance (Industrial Injuries) Act
1954 Law Reform (Limitation of Action) Act
1958 Disabled Persons (Employment) Act
1960 Noise Abatement Act
1963 Limitation Act
1965 National Insurance (Industrial Injuries) Act
1966 Ministry of Social Security Act
1968 Hearing Aid Council Act
1968 Medicines Act
1970 Administration of Justice Act
1970 Chronically Sick and Disabled Persons Act
1971 Child Benefit Act
1971 National Insurance Act
1973 Employment Training Act
1974 Control of Pollution Act
1975 Employment Protection Act
1976 Congenital Disabilities (Civil Liability) Act

APPENDIX 42.2. TABLE OF CASES

Andreae v. Selfridge (1937). 3 All E.R. 255
Barette v. Franki Compressed Pile Co. Canada (1955). 2 D.L.R. 665
Bartlett v. Marshall (1896). 60 J.P. 104

Baugh v. Delta Water Fittings (1971). *The Times* Law Report, 13 May
Bliss v. Hall (1838). 4 Bing. (N.C.) 183
Bolam v. Friern Hospital Management Committee (1957). 1 W.L.R. 582, 586
Bolton v. Stone (1951). 1 All E.R. 1078 (H.L.); A.C. 850
Cassidy v. Minister of Health (1951). 2 K.B. 343
Chatterton v. Gerson and Another (1980). *The Times* Law Report, 6 February
Cheney v. Conn (1968). 1 All E.R. 779
Chin Keow v. Government of Malaysia (1967). 1 W.L.R. 813
Christie v. Davey (1893). 1 Ch. 316
Cole v. Hucks (1968). *The Times*, 9 May
Cooper v. Slade (1858). 1 H.L.C. 746
Crump v. Lambert (1867). L.R. 3 Eq. 409
David v. Edinburgh Magistrates (1953). S.C. 34
Dietrich v. Northampton (1884). 138 Mass. 14
Donoghue (or M'Alister) v. Stevenson (1932). A.C. 562
Garner v. Garner (1920). 26 T.L.R. 196
Haley v. London Electricity Board (1965). A.C. 778
Halsey v. Esso Petroleum Co. (1961). 2 All E.R. 145
Harris v. James (1876). 45 L.J.Q.B. 545
Harrison v. Metropolitan Police (1972). *The Times*, 28 March, p. 4
Hatcher v. Black (1954). T.L.R.
Henson v. The Board of Management of the Perth Hospital and Another (1938). 41 W.A.L.R. 15
Hoare & Co. v. McAlpine (1923). 1 Ch. 167
Hollywood Silver Fox Farms v. Emmett (1936). 1 All E.R. 825
Hunter v. Hanley (1955). S.L.T. 213
James v. SKF (UK) (1977?) Unreported
Latter v. Braddell and Sutcliffe (1881). 44 L.T. 368
Leeman v. Montagu (1936). 2 All E.R. 1677
McIvor v. Southern Health and Social Services Board (1978). 2 All E.R. 625
Mahon v. Osborn (1939). 1 All E.R. 535
Osborne v. Rowlett (1880). 13 Ch.D. 774, at p. 785
Overseas Tankship (UK) Ltd v. Miller Steamship Co. Pty. Ltd, Wagon Mound (No. 2) (1967); 1 A.C. 617 (P.C.); (1966). 2 All E.R. 709
Pfizer v. Ministry of Health (1965). 2 W.L.R. 387
Prescott v. Bulldog Tools (1980). Unreported
R. v. Trump (1979). *The Times*, Law Report, 28 December
Roe v. Minister of Health (1954). 2 Q.B. 66
Rushmer v. Polsue and Alfieri Ltd (1906). 1 Ch. 234
Slater v. Baker and Stapleton (1767). K.B. 2 Wils. 359
Starr v. National Coal Board (1977). 1 W.L.R. 63
Sturges v. Bridgman (1879). 11 Ch.D. 852
Tinkler v. Aylesbury Dairy Co. (1888). 5 T.L.R. 52
Walter v. Selfe (1851). 4 DeG and Sm 315
Watson v. Buckley, Osborne, Garrett & Co. Ltd, and Wyrovoys Products Ltd (1940). 1 All E.R. 174
Whitehouse v. Jordan and Another (1979). *The Times* Law Report, 5 December
Whitehouse v. Jordan and Another (1980). *The Times* Law Report, 17 December

REFERENCES

ABEL-SMITH, B. (1976). *Value for money in health services*. Heinemann, London.
ANNUAL REPORT AND ACCOUNTS (1978). The Medical Protection Society Limited, London.
ANNUAL REPORT AND ACCOUNTS (1979). The Medical Protection Society Limited, London.
BENTHAM, J. (1789). *Introduction to the principles of morals and legislation*. Payne, London.
BEVERIDGE, W. (1942). Social Insurance and Allied Services. A Report to His Majesty's Paymaster-General. HMSO, London.
BOYLE, E. (1960). In *Modern educational treatment of deafness* (ed. A. W. G. Ewing). Manchester University Press.
BRITISH MEDICAL ASSOCIATION (1971). Gaps in medical care. Report by the Board of Science and Education, British Medical Association. *Br. med. J. Suppl.* ii, 71.
CARDOZO, B. N. (1921). *The nature of the judicial process*. Yale University Press, New Haven, Conn.
CENTRAL OFFICE OF INFORMATION (1970). Social Security in Britain. Central office of Information Reference Pamphlet. HMSO, London.
COMMITTEE ON PERSONAL INJURIES LITIGATION (Winn Committee) (1968). Report Cmnd. 3691. HMSO, London.
DAVID, R. and BRIERLEY, J. E. C. (1968). *Major legal systems in the world today*. Stevens, London.
DEPARTMENT OF HEALTH AND SOCIAL SECURITY (1976a). Priorities for Health and Personal Social Services in England. A Consultative Document. HMSO, London.
—— (1976b). Sharing Resources for Health in England. Report of the Resource Allocation Working Party. HMSO, London.
DIAS, R. W. M. (1970). *Jurisprudence*. Butterworth, London.
DICEY, A. V. (1905). *Lectures on the relation between law and public opinion in the 19th century*. Macmillan, London.
DOLL, R. (1974). To measure NHS progress. Fabian Occasional Paper 8. Fabian Society, London.
FELIX, R. H., IVE, F. A., and DAHL, M. G. C. (1974). Cutaneous and ocular reactions to practolol. *Br. med. J.* iv, 321–4.
FRIEDMANN, W. (1949). *Legal theory*. Stevens, London.
GODBER, G. (1975). Foreword. In *Health care: the growing dilemma*, 2nd edn (ed. R. Maxwell). McKinsey, New York.
GRAY, J. A. M. (1979). Choosing priorities. *J. med. Ethics* 5, 73–50.
GREGORY, P. Deafness and Public Responsibility. Occasional Papers on Social Administration, No. 7. Bell, London.
HART, J. J. (1971). Inverse care law. *Lancet* i, 405–12.
Hearing (1971a). D-R-O's Editorial. *Hearing* 26, 323.
—— (1971b). West Country D-R-O's at Court Grange. *Hearing* 26, 324–7.
HENDERSON, P. (1960). Handicapped children. Their treatment and special education in England and Wales. In *The modern educational treatment of deafness* (ed. A. W. G. Ewing). Manchester University Press.
HINCHCLIFFE, D. and HINCHCLIFFE, R. (1976). Administrative, ethical and legal aspects. In *Scientific foundations of otolaryngology* (ed. R. Hinchcliffe and D. F. N. Harrison). Heinemann, London.
HINCHCLIFFE, R. (1977). Socialized medicine in the UK. In *Medico-Socio-*

Economic Issues in ORL in Six Countries (ed. J.-I. Suzuki). Proc. Special Plenary Session on Socio-Economic Problems in Oto-Rhinolaryngological Practice. XI World Congress of Otorhinolaryngology, Buenos Aires, 13–19 March 1977.
KLEIN, R. (1976). Accountability in the NHS: whose head on the block? *Br. med. J.* **ii**, 1211–12.
LOCKHART, M. R. (1980) Chapter 8. In *Medical Practice* (ed. J. Leahy Taylor). John Wright, Bristol.
MCNAB JONES, R. F., HAMMOND, V. T., WRIGHT, D., and BALLANTYNE, J. C. (1977). Practolol and deafness. *J. Lar.* **91**, 963–73.
MARTIN, C. R. A. (1979). *Law relating to medical practice.* Pitman Medical, Tunbridge Wells.
MAXWELL, R. (1975). *Health care: the growing dilemma*, 2nd edn. McKinsey, New York.
MEDICOLEGAL (1979). Medical reports not to the lawyers' liking. *Br. med. J.* **ii**, 1376.
MILNE, J. F. and CHAPLIN, N. W. (1969). *Modern hospital management.* Institute of Hospital Administrators, London.
MINISTRY OF EDUCATION (1954). Circular 276, 25 June.
MUNKMAN, J. (1962). *Employer's liability.* Butterworth, London.
RICHARDSON, K., PECKHAM, C. S., and GOLDSTEIN, H. (1976). Hearing levels of children tested at 7 and 11 years: a national study. *Br. J. Audiol.* **10**, 117–21.
ROYAL COLLEGE OF SURGEONS OF ENGLAND (1976). Evidence of the Royal College of Surgeons of England to the Royal Commission on the National Health Service, Pt. 1.
ROYAL COMMISSION ON THE NHS (Merrison Commission) (1979). A service for patients. HMSO, London.
SPELLER, S. R. (1974). *Law relating to hospitals and kindred institutions.* Lewis, London.
STUTTARD, A. R. D. (1969). *English Law notebook.* Butterworth, London.
TAYLOR, J. L. (1971). *The doctor and negligence*, p. 110. Pitman Medical, Tunbridge Wells.
—— (1980). *Medical Malpractice.* John Wright, Bristol.
TEFF, H. and MUNROE, C. R. (1976). *Thalidomide: the legal aftermath.* Saxon House, Farnborough, Hants.
The Times (1969). 4 September, page 6.
—— (1978). 4 August, page 1.
WIEDEMANN, H. R. (1961). Hinweis auf eine derzeitige Häufung hypo- und aplasticher Fehlbildungen des Gliedmassen. *Med. Welt* **37**, 1863–6.
WRIGHT, P. (1975). Untoward effects associated with Practolol administration: oculomucocutaneous syndrome. *Br. med. J.* **i**, 595–8.

NOTE ADDED IN PROOF

In a more recent decision in 1981, Mr Justice Mais ordered an action to be stayed unless the Plaintiffs submitted to caloric testing and polytomography. Liberty to apply for ECochG was also provided for (*Bird v. Cadbury Schweppes Overseas Ltd; Pearson v. Cadbury Schweppes Overseas Ltd*).

43 Some psychosocial aspects of deafness

JOHN C. DENMARK

Many people have little understanding of the psychosocial implications of deafness. There are a number of reasons for this, one of the most important being the fact that the word 'deafness' is used as a blanket term covering a variety of different conditions.

The results of hearing loss depend upon many variables but the most important are the degree of loss and the age of onset. For example the problems of the child who is born profoundly deaf are of an entirely different order from those of a person who loses all his hearing in adult life. The child that is born deaf has a sensory deficit which interferes with all aspects of his development, while the person who is deafened in adult life suffers a sensory deprivation which may affect his whole life-style and call for many readjustments. Deafness which is present from early life before the acquisition of language and speech (prelingual deafness), and deafness which is acquired after this stage (postlingual deafness), have entirely different implications.

PRELINGUAL PROFOUND DEAFNESS

CHILDHOOD HEARING LOSS

This may be congenital or acquired at any later age, and can vary in degree from minimal unilateral impairment to bilateral total loss. Any attempt to be definitive about the degree of deafness is, however, complicated by the fact that a deaf child may have little useful hearing without a hearing aid and yet be able to hear reasonably well with one. Some workers would label such a child 'profoundly deaf' while others, correctly in the author's view, would describe such a child as 'partially hearing'.

The term prelingual profound deafness should be confined to hearing impairment which is profound, which cannot be alleviated to any useful degree by hearing aids, and which is either congenital or acquired in early life before the development of language and speech. Prelingually profoundly deaf children should be differentiated from those who have sufficient residual hearing to enable them to discriminate speech with or without hearing aids and also from those children who become deaf postlingually, i.e. after speech and language have developed.

The prelingually profoundly deaf child

The basic problem of prelingually profoundly deaf children is that they cannot acquire speech and language normally. About the end of the first year of life the normal child begins to imitate speech. To do so he has both to hear the speech of others and to monitor his own voice. He soon begins to associate words with people and with objects, and so begins the process of internalization of language. Slowly at first, but then with increasing rapidity, he achieves a command of language, and by the age of four years the normal hearing child has already grasped most of the fundamental grammatical and syntactical complexities of his native tongue. Later, with further intellectual development and with education, he learns to read and write—he learns to understand and express in another form the language he has acquired through hearing.

For the child who is profoundly deaf from birth or early age the development of speech and the acquisition of verbal language are both formidable tasks. The fact that he cannot hear means that he is unable to imitate the speech of others or monitor his own voice. The prelingually deaf child has to acquire verbal language through another sensory channel—through vision—by lipreading or by the written word. Lipreading, however, is extremely difficult because of its inexactitude, for some of the sounds of speech are not accompanied by movements of the mouth or lips, while their movements are in many cases the same for different words. A more important aspect is that lipreading presupposes a knowledge of verbal language, which, in the case of the young prelingually profoundly deaf child, is absent. Consequently the deaf child has to acquire verbal language through the written word. This presents a further difficulty for the ability to read and write requires a certain degree of intellectual development, so that even normally hearing children with good language development are not capable of literacy in their early years. The deaf child has a long preverbal stage for he only begins to acquire the rudiments of language much later than his hearing peers, and even then he progresses very slowly.

Manual methods of communication, i.e. fingerspelling and sign language are used universally by prelingually profoundly deaf adults. Fingerspelling consists of spelling out each word, letter by letter, by using different configurations of the fingers of one or both hands to represent the different letters of the alphabet (Fig. 43.1). Manual sign languages of deaf people involve the use of the hands and arms to convey the meanings of words and concepts. Sign languages differ to some extent from country to country and are different in structure from the native spoken language (Fig. 43.2). Some deaf people who use manual communication methods have an excellent command of verbal language, while others are seriously retarded linguistically. The former will usually employ a combination of fingerspelling and sign language, while those with poor language will use only sign language and gesture.

For centuries controversy has existed whether or not manual methods of communication should be employed to overcome the communication problems of deaf children. The arguments are really concerned with sign language, for young children are not literate and cannot, therefore, fingerspell. Some workers, the so called 'pure oralists', mainly teachers of the deaf, believe that deaf children should concentrate upon speech, lipreading, the

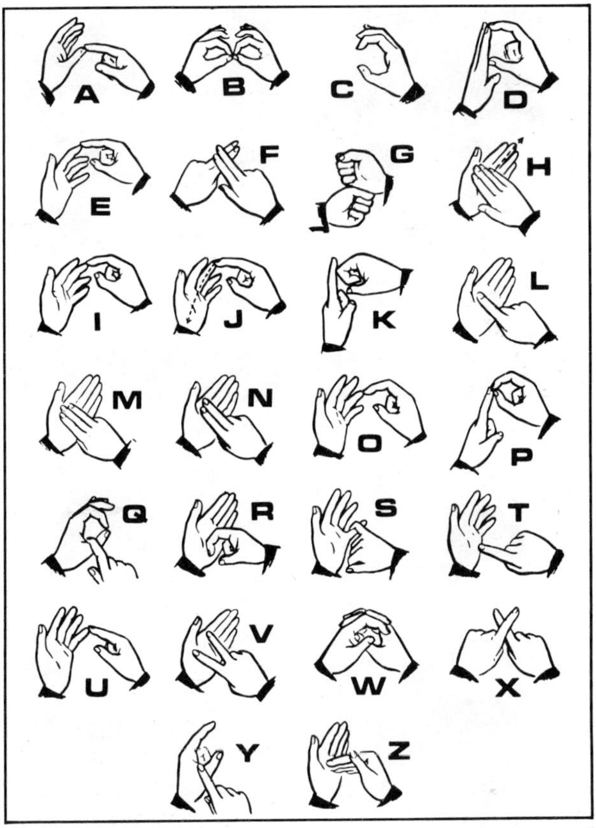

Fig. 43.1. The manual alphabet.

written word, and any useful residual hearing. They do not allow the use of sign language, arguing that deaf children will use it because it is the easiest method, and so will not be motivated to develop speech and lipreading skills. There is, however, no evidence to support this. Indeed all the evidence tends to support the opposite view that combined oral and manual methods should be employed with all deaf children from the earliest years—years when a meaningful form of communication is so vitally important for future intellectual, social, and emotional development (Denmark 1973).

The hearing aid has undoubtedly been of immeasurable benefit to hearing impaired children and many who would otherwise have had to be treated as profoundly deaf have been enabled to be treated as partially hearing. Nevertheless, its advent appears to have led to the development of a myth that *all* deaf children have useful residual hearing and can, therefore, learn to speak. This is not the case: but the perpetuation of this myth has undoubtedly been a major factor in delaying the introduction of manual methods of communication into schools for the deaf. Changes are now

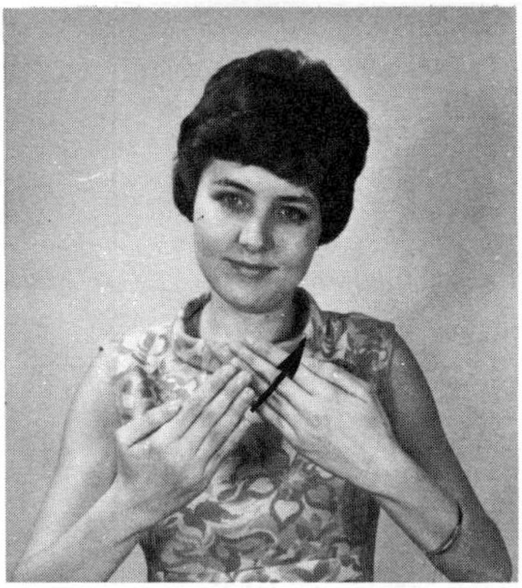

NEW 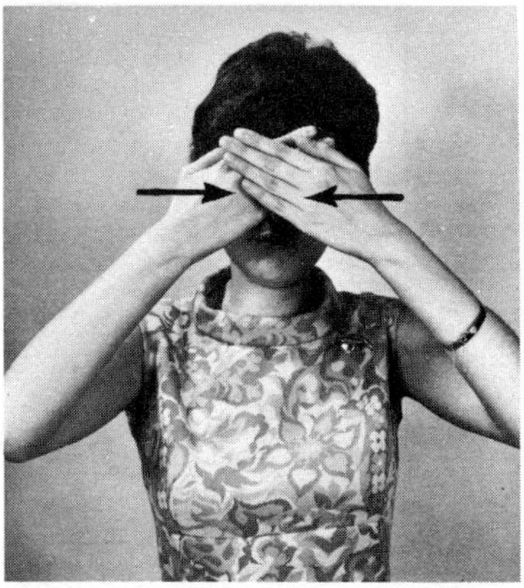 NIGHT

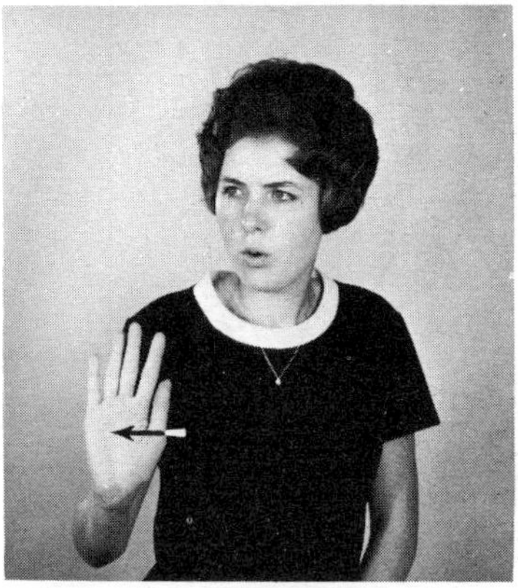

NO 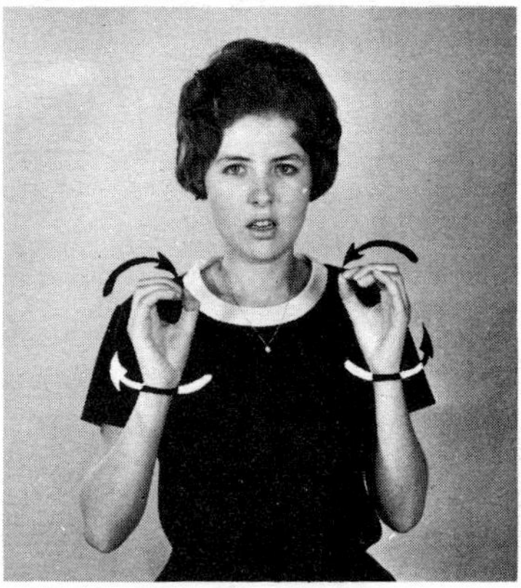 NOTHING

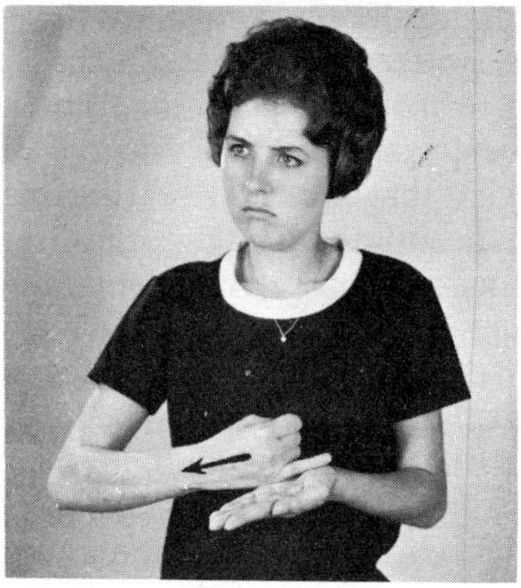

OBJECT (to) 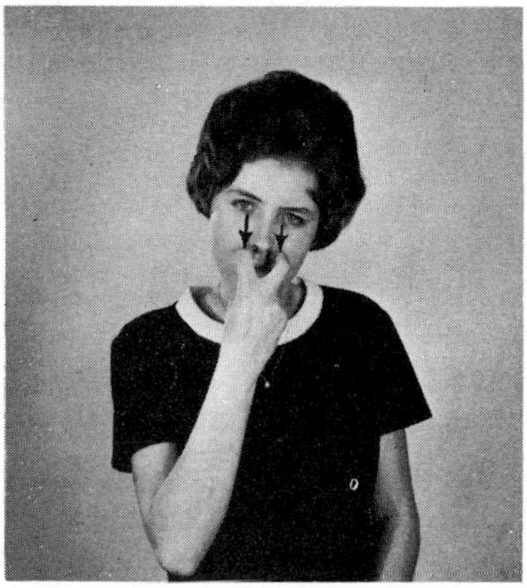 OLD

Fig. 43.2. British sign language.

taking place, however, and a number of schools are now using combined oral and manual methods.

The relative situation of deaf and hearing children at a time when formal education begins can profitably be compared. The hearing child acquires knowledge throughout his early years simply because of his ability to communicate easily with family and friends. He is also continually receiving information from other sources, from radio and television, and by hearing the conversation of others.

The situation of the preschool prelingually profoundly deaf child is vastly different. Unless special efforts have been made to communicate with him non-verbally by sign language he will not only be unable to hear and speak and have little verbal language but he will also be lacking in much basic knowledge. Gregory (1976) in a study of 122 deaf and partially hearing children under the age of five years whose parents had not been instructed in sign language found that 57 per cent relied exclusively on gesture, showing and pointing when communicating with their mothers. Lack of communication between mother and child in their early years must have important implications for the child's future development. It is vitally important, therefore, that prelingually profoundly deaf children should be given the benefit of combined oral and manual methods of communication from an early age and equally important that their parents should receive the necessary guidance and the opportunity to acquire facility in manual methods also.

Unless deaf children are exposed to sign language, their teachers will not be able to communicate easily with them and the teachers' task will be an extremely difficult one. They will have to teach the use of verbal language from the beginning, and somehow impart all that basic knowledge which hearing children so easily acquire. These are daunting obstacles and many intelligent deaf children never do gain a good command of verbal language and do not learn to speak intelligibly. Many acquire lipreading skills, but they are only able to lipread when all the conditions are right, i.e. when face to face, in good light, and, most important of all, when simple language is used. They are unable to follow normal conversation. Conrad (1976) in a study of some 360 children aged 15 to $16\frac{1}{2}$ years in schools for the deaf and partially hearing in England and Wales found that of those with hearing losses greater than 85 decibels, half had a reading age of less than $7\frac{1}{2}$ years, half lipread worse than the average hearing child and only 10 per cent had speech rated by their teachers as being easy to understand. It is hardly surprising that the prelingually deaf, whether or not they have been taught sign language in childhood, invariably come to use it eventually when communicating with other deaf people.

Deafness and mental retardation

The relationship between deafness and mental retardation is a complex one. Deafness can affect individuals of all degrees of intellect. However, some of the factors responsible for early childhood deafness, e.g. prematurity and meningitis, may result in concomitant brain damage, so that childhood deafness may be complicated by other disabilities including intellectual handicaps.

Prelingual profound deafness presents an enormous barrier to normal language development, but when it is complicated by even a minimal degree of intellectual retardation, then the acquisition of language becomes even more difficult. A normally hearing person with an intellectual handicap sufficient to preclude literacy may acquire sufficient verbal language to develop social competence, to hold down a routine job in open industry, and to marry and raise a family. Should the prelingually profoundly deaf child have an intellectual handicap only of a degree to preclude literacy, then he will be unable to acquire any such store of useful verbal language. In these circumstances, and when the intellectual handicap is not of severe degree, there will be a marked discrepancy between the child's innate intellectual potential and his or her verbal competence. The poor development of language may, unfortunately, be frequently believed to be due to a severe degree of mental retardation and there is, therefore, a grave danger that the potential of such a child will remain unrecognized and undeveloped.

To deny the prelingually profoundly deaf child who also has an intellectual handicap the chance to acquire communication skills through sign language is to deny him all communication. He will remain not only a non-verbal being but a non-communicating being.

CASE 1

PL was referred at the age of $14\frac{1}{2}$ years for advice as to management. He was born six weeks premature and weighed 2.2 kg. There was some neonatal distress. At six weeks he suffered from meningitis. His developmental milestones were delayed and he was always irritable and over-active. He failed to develop speech and at the age of about three years deafness was suspected. However, this was not confirmed until he was about six years of age when sensorineural deafness was diagnosed. He was tried with a binaural hearing aid and given auditory training but without benefit. PL's behaviour was such that his parents were unable to cope with him and he was admitted to a hospital for the mentally handicapped. His behaviour remained disturbed and psychotropic drugs brought about little change. The results of psychometric testing were thought to be unreliable because of his poor attention and distractability. Some twelve months prior to being seen attempts were made to teach PL to communicate by sign language and it was soon obvious that he had the ability to communicate by this method. His behaviour materially improved and he soon began to mimic other patients and help other more retarded patients with their personal care.

PL is profoundly deaf and in all probability has an intellectual handicap also. He is unlikely to acquire any verbal competence. He has been accepted for a school for the deaf where manual methods of communication are employed.

Mental retardation is the commonest cause of failure to develop speech and inability to speak, dumbness, is often equated with backwardness. There is a danger, therefore, that deaf children and adults without speech may be mistakenly regarded as mentally retarded (Denmark 1975).

CASE 2

FE, a prelingually profoundly deaf man, was first seen during a survey of deaf patients in a subnormality hospital in 1967. He was then 56 years of age. His father had died when he was a child and he appears to have been rejected by his mother for he was admitted to a Poor Law Institution at the age of 14. At the age of 16 he was admitted to a hospital for the subnormal.

FE has no speech and limited ability to lipread. He communicates by sign language and fingerspelling and within the limits of his language gives a good account of himself. He underwent psychometric testing using the Wechsler Adult Intelligence Scale and achieved an IQ of 104. In 1968 he was admitted to the Department of Psychiatry for the Deaf at Whittingham Hospital. He underwent rehabilitation and was discharged to a hostel in 1970 at the age of 59. He was found employment and is still working for the same employer.

In a clinical situation when the written word is used in attempts to overcome the communication difficulties of prelingually profoundly deaf people, the deaf person may not understand the questions and may answer incorrectly owing to his limited language. On the other hand, he may understand the questions, but his written answers may be grammatically and syntactically incorrect and even simple words may be mis-spelt. This may give the impression of limited intelligence. The diagnostic problems are well illustrated by the following case:

CASE 3

CM, a 25-year-old man had been remanded to prison having been charged with assault. He suffers from prelingual deafness, is without speech and his verbal language is limited. He had become aggressive when asked to leave the house of his girlfriend's mother who did not wish his association with her daughter to continue. In referring him the prison doctor had written . . . 'He may be schizophrenic, mentally defective, or anything'. Using manual communication methods CM was able to give a good account of himself, explaining that he resented being pushed out of his girlfriend's home without, he felt, good cause. He became very angry when he could not understand what was being said and because he could not communicate his own thoughts and feelings. When examined using manual communication methods there was no evidence of any material psychiatric abnormality and, using non-verbal psychological tests, he achieved a pro rated IQ of 116.

Every practising psychiatrist and clinical psychologist is likely to be faced with a prelingually deaf person at some time in his professional life, and it is important that they should have some knowledge of the implications of early profound deafness and especially of its retarding effects upon language development. In this context it is important to remember that psychological testing is fraught with difficulties when the subject is prelingually profoundly deaf. The communication problems create difficulties in establishing contact, in explaining the nature of the test situation, and in giving instructions. However, the greatest pitfalls are likely to occur in the use of inappropriate test material and in the interpretation of results.

CASE 4

WM a 19-year-old deaf youth, was referred with a history of irresponsible behaviour, inability to keep employment, and outbursts of aggressive behaviour. Some two years previously he had been referred to a psychiatric clinic and had undergone psychometric testing. He had achieved an IQ of 57 using the Terman Merril test and was, therefore, considered unemployable. WM was able to communicate by combined oral and manual methods and there was no evidence of any frank psychiatric abnormality. Using the performance items of the Wechsler Adult Intelligence Scale he achieved an IQ of 114, the scores on the sub-tests being uniformly above-average. He was recommended for vocational training and is now employed. The Terman Merril is a verbally loaded test and the discrepancy between the results of this test and that of the Wechsler test illustrates the inapplicability of using verbally loaded tests with prelingually deaf subjects.

CASE 5

PD was referred at the age of 29 years with behaviour problems. He suffers from prelingual profound deafness and is without speech. His language development is poor. He had been diagnosed as mentally retarded on more than one occasion and had been given intelligence quotients of 100, 60, and 125 by different psychologists.

It is important to remember also that children who suffer from partial hearing loss may also be mistakenly regarded as mentally retarded.

CASE 6

NM was eight years eight months old when his mother sought an appointment to discuss his management. She was concerned that he had been transferred from a primary school to a school for educationally subnormal children. She related that she had thought her son had a hearing deficit when he was about four years old and sought the opinion of her general practitioner. She stated that her doctor had performed only a very superficial examination, had told her he could find nothing wrong and that she was worrying unnecessarily.

NM developed speech and language and began primary school at four years ten months. However, his academic progress was poor and at the age of seven years he was transferred to a school for the educationally subnormal. Shortly after his transfer hearing impairment was suspected by the school doctor and subsequently confirmed by audiometry. Otological examination revealed bilateral serous otitis media. Grommets were inserted into both tympanic membranes and NM's hearing improved considerably. On psychometric testing NM achieved a full scale IQ of 102.

POSTLINGUAL DEAFNESS

Postlingual (adventitious) deafness may be of sudden onset or so insidious in development as to remain unnoticed both by the subject and by others for a considerable time. It can occur in childhood after language and speech have developed, in adolescence, or in adult life, and is very common in late age.

Reaction to deafness depends upon factors inherent in the type of deafness—its severity and its rate of development, but also upon the individual's personality, intelligence, interests, and his life style.

Man is a social being and the primary function of hearing is to maintain his relationship with his total environment and with his fellow men in particular. The most obvious handicap of the deafened person is that he loses the ability to hear easily the spoken word. He may be helped by a hearing aid and by lipreading. However, hearing aids are sometimes of limited or no benefit, and many deafened people find lipreading extremely difficult. Lipreading is moreover, confined to clearly visible speech directed at the deaf person and it demands intense concentration.

The deaf person misses not only conversation which is not directed at him, but misses also the snatches of conversation of others—the innuendos and asides of conversation, and also the tone of voice which carries so much meaning. The possibility of misunderstanding, coupled with feelings of frustration and isolation frequently result in anxiety and depression.

Deafness, however, cannot be discussed solely with reference to hearing the conversation of others. Through hearing we monitor our own speech and so control its volume and pitch, so that the deafened person is often anxious in this respect. In spite of speech therapy, many deafened people find that their speech deteriorates. This, and the fact that lipreading is so stressful and tiring, leads a few deaf and hard-of-hearing people who have lost their hearing before middle age to mix socially with the prelingually deaf and acquire manual communication skills. Many have contributed greatly to the quality of life of the prelingually deaf community.

Hearing is the channel through which we receive signals and warnings of events outside our field of vision and in darkness. Hearing contributes to our aesthetic experience in varying degrees, and for some the inability to hear music and the sounds of nature is an added deprivation.

Many deafened persons come to terms with their disability but adjustments are always necessary. Suspicion and hostility are not uncommon experiences in sensitive personalities, but the commonest feelings are those of frustration, insecurity, isolation and depression. Depression, especially in deafness of acute or sub-acute onset can be of morbid intensity. Of progressive deafness, Menninger (1924) wrote 'It is as if something vital to one's existence has been torn from him', while Lehmann (1954) describes sudden deafness as 'One of life's terrifying experiences'. Levine (1960) writes 'The abruptly deafened adult experiences in one highly concentrated measure all the pangs and agonies of years of progressive deafness'.

Deafness in adult life can affect the whole life-style of an individual—his employment, his position in society and his role within the family—and can result in severe psychiatric illness.

CASE 7

IR, aged 18, an apprentice electrical engineer, was involved in a road traffic accident. He sustained multiple fractures and was unconscious for ten days. On recovery he was found to have severe bilateral deafness, thought to be due to cochlear damage. He derived no benefit from a hearing aid. He was referred for psychiatric opinion some two years after the accident. His mother related that since the accident her son had become irritable and depressed. She had frequently heard him crying when alone in his bedroom. He complained that people were no longer interested in him. He appeared to be physically well apart from his deafness and a slight left facial paresis. There was some evidence of slight deterioration in his speech. He had some lipreading ability but most of what was said to him had to be repeated or rephrased. He had no physical complaints other than occasional blurring of vision in the left eye.

He complained of depression which he felt was the result of his deafness. He stated that his former friends ignored him because of his inability to understand them. He could no longer listen to the radio or television and no longer visited the cinema or theatre. He could not take part in casual conversation at home.

The communication problem had prevented him from continuing his technical training and he will have to be content with semi-skilled employment. All his complaints appeared to relate to his loss of hearing.

CASE 8

Mrs S B, aged 42, had lost her hearing over a period of some twelve months. At first she had not noticed her deafness, but this had been pointed out to her by neighbours. They had thought she had ignored their knocking at her door. Her hearing had gradually deteriorated to the extent that she had become totally deaf. She was fully investigated and was found to have bilateral profound perceptive deafness of unknown aetiology.

She complained of severe depression. When interviewed she stated that her children no longer approached her for she could not understand them. She wrote 'There are times I feel I must be going out of my mind with frustration, of not knowing what is going on around me, and I know I am making other people miserable with my constant tears. How do other deaf people cope? I can't go and have a chat like other people do, or 'phone, or anything else a hearing person does to get over these black moods.' Mrs S B and her husband eventually attended a course for deafened people where they received intensive counselling and guidance, and afterwards she wrote 'The course has done me the world of good . . . it has given me back the will to live. I was horribly depressed and the thought of spending a lifetime of deafness horrified me. Now I can see I can live a very near normal life and things are not as black as they once were.'

Audiological and otological assessment and treatment where indicated are of prime importance and many more deaf people could benefit from treatment and help. Unfortunately, deafness is a disability of which the sufferer may not complain. Many people with progressive deafness in middle life regard it as a symptom of aging. They resent this and the idea that their efficiency may suffer. Some not only hide their disability from others but fail to accept it themselves.

The deafened person must accept his disability if he is to make a satisfactory re-adjustment. Vocational rehabilitation may be necessary but counselling and guidance should always be available for the deafened individual. This help is equally important for his family. Counselling and guidance should be provided by social workers who have knowledge in depth of the psychosocial implications of deafness and of the technical aids and resources available. Flashing lights in place of door bells, and vibrating pillows in place of alarm clocks, are simple but effective devices, and clubs and other institutions for deaf people can help lessen their isolation and help the individual to accept his disability.

THE DEAF BLIND

The results of the dual handicap of deafness and blindness depend upon many factors but especially upon the age of onset. Children who are born blind, but are otherwise normal, will have no barrier to the development of language and speech. Should they become deaf in later life, they will be able to express themselves through speech and will be able to receive communication by the deaf/blind alphabet (Fig. 43.3) and through reading Braille.

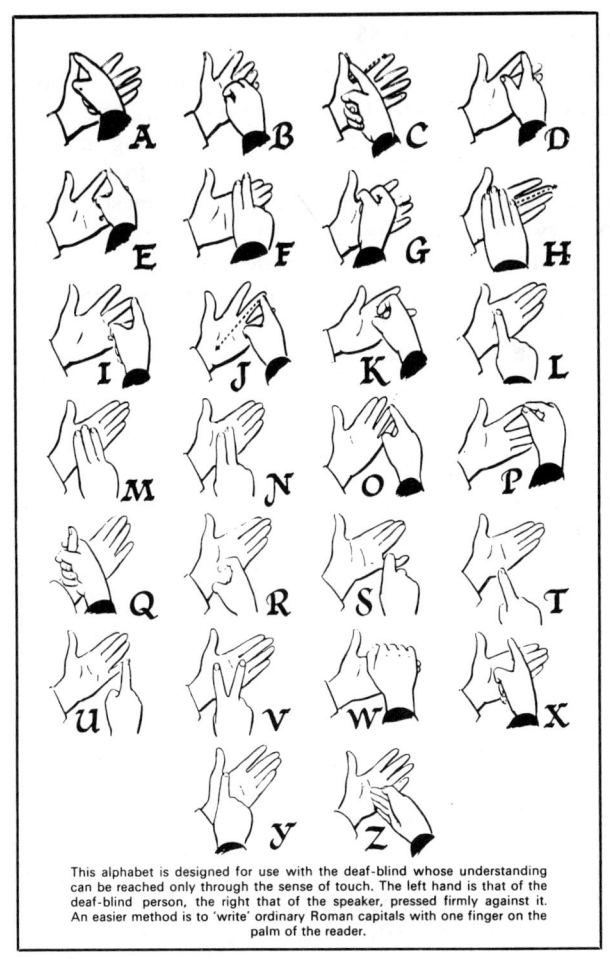

This alphabet is designed for use with the deaf-blind whose understanding can be reached only through the sense of touch. The left hand is that of the deaf-blind person, the right that of the speaker, pressed firmly against it. An easier method is to 'write' ordinary Roman capitals with one finger on the palm of the reader.

Fig. 43.3. The deaf-blind manual alphabet.

Those persons who become both deaf and blind in later life will have these abilities also. However, those who suffer from prelingual profound deafness who have poor language and speech will, if they become blind, find communication a very much more difficult problem.

There is more than a casual relationship between deafness and blindness. In 1914 Usher described a syndrome of hereditary deafness with retinitis pigmentosa. Unfortunately little is known of the natural history of this condition. Some afflicted deaf children begin to lose their sight in childhood, while others do not do so until adult life, and the rate of deterioration of vision seems to vary. However, ophthalmoscopic examination will reveal signs of the disease before visual acuity is seriously impaired and there is, therefore, a strong indication for routine ophthalmoscopic examination of all children with congenital deafness.

SOCIAL WORK AND DEAFNESS

The psychosocial implications of deafness are many and both the handicapped person and his family will need counselling and guidance. Social workers for the deaf now undertake generic training in social work and specialist training in the psycho-social aspects of deafness. They also receive training in manual methods of communication. They should be part of the multidisciplinary assessment and management teams involved with persons suffering from all degrees and types of deafness.

Deaf persons, especially those who suffer from prelingual profound deafness, are at a disadvantage in many situations because of their communication difficulties and social workers with their skills in interpretation can be of the utmost value.

PSYCHIATRIC SERVICES FOR THE DEAF

Communication between doctor and patient is of central importance in the field of psychiatry both for diagnosis and treatment. In the case of deaf patients, and especially in the case of prelingually profoundly deaf, diagnosis and treatment can be extremely difficult and time consuming. It is essential that psychiatrists and others involved in the management of deaf patients with psychiatric problems should be aware of the psychological, sociological and psychiatric aspects of deafness and, in the case of prelingually profoundly deaf patients, have facility in manual methods of communication.

In recent years there has been an increasing awareness of the need for specialized psychiatric services for the deaf, and services have been established in the United Kingdom (Denmark and Eldridge 1969; Denmark and Warren 1972), in the United States of America (Rainer and Altshuler 1963), and in Scandinavia (Remvig 1969).

Experience of workers in the field have demonstrated that specialist services can be of benefit not only to the prelingually profoundly deaf but also to the partially hearing, those who become deafened in adult life, and the deaf blind. Moreover, it seems that professionals with non-verbal communication skills (sign language) have a significant contribution to make towards the assessment of children and adults with communication disorders of all types.

ACKNOWLEDGEMENT

Figs. 43.1, 43.2, and 43.3 are reproduced with permission from *Conversation with the deaf*, published by The Royal Institute for the Deaf.

REFERENCES

CONRAD, R. (1976). Towards a definition of oral success. Paper presented at a meeting on Methods of Communication in the Education of Deaf Children, Harrogate. The Royal National Institute for the Deaf.
DENMARK, J. C. (1973). The education of deaf children. *Hearing* **28**, 284–93.
—— (1975). Early profound deafness and subnormality. M. Psy. Med. Thesis, University of Liverpool.
—— and ELDRIDGE, R. W. (1969). Psychiatric services for the deaf. *Lancet* **ii**, 259–62.
—— and WARREN, F. (1972). A psychiatric unit for the deaf. *Br. J. Psychiat.* **120**, 423–8.
GREGORY, S. (1976). *The deaf child and his family*. Allen & Unwin, London.
LEHMANN, R. R. (1954). Bilateral sudden deafness. *N.Y. St. J. Med.* **54**, 1481–5.
LEVINE, E. S. (1960). *The psychology of deafness*. Columbia University Press, New York.
MENNINGER, K. A. (1924). The mental effects of deafness. *Psychoanal. Rev.* **11**, 144–55.
RAINER, J. D. and ALTSHULER, M. D. (1966). Comprehensive Mental Health Services for the Deaf. Department of Medical Genetics, New York State Psychiatric Institute, Columbia University, New York.
REMVIG, J. (1969). Three clinical studies of deaf mutism and psychiatry. *Acta psychiat. scand.* Suppl. 210.
USHER, C. H. (1914). On the inheritance of retinitis pigmentosa. *R. Lond. ophthal. Hosp. Rep.* **19**, 130–236.

44 Tinnitus
P. D. JACKSON

DEFINITION

Although the word tinnitus is derived from the Latin *tinnire* which means to ring or to tinkle, it is used to describe the sensation of any sound which appears to be arising in the head or ears of the sufferer. Occasionally, at the onset of the tinnitus the patient may have the impression that there is an external source for the sound, but he quickly realizes this is not so. This feature distinguishes the genuine tinnitus sufferer from the so-called 'hummers'. The name has been given by Walford (1980) to a group of people, generally elderly widows over 80 years of age who complain of a low-pitched hum. This is attributed by them to machinery, electric wires, or secret defence installations, for example, and paranoid features are often present. The noise troubles the patient mostly at night time and she often complains vociferously. Even after careful measurement of ambient sound such people are not easily convinced that there is no evidence for the sound they hear. Auditory hallucinations, in which the noise takes the form of words, music or meaningful sounds are generally considered to be a manifestation of neurological or psychiatric disorder and are not generally included in the definition of tinnitus. However, Goodwin (1980) reports five of her own cases and reviews the literature of 11 other cases in which these auditory perceptions changed, generally over a period of a few weeks, to the more recognizable form of tinnitus. Hitherto 'tinnitus' has been subdivided into (i) subjective tinnitus and (ii) objective tinnitus; in the latter the sound is heard not only by the patient, but is also heard, or potentially can be heard, by another observer. Since by definition tinnitus is what is experienced by the patient, it can be argued that the term 'objective tinnitus' is inconsistent and there is no certainty an observer is hearing the same sound. Nevertheless, the term is a useful one for clinicians in their management of patients.

CLASSIFICATION OF TINNITUS

Although in recent years the subject of tinnitus has attracted much work and interest, it must be admitted that 'the cause is only rarely known and the mechanism is not known at all' (Douek 1981). The ordering of such information as is available into systems of classification may be valuable in research and in the diagnosis and management of the problem. Much of the following scheme was suggested by the working party at the CIBA Foundation Symposium on Tinnitus, No. 85, held in London in January 1981.

A. Classification from subject's description

(i) Number of sounds. A substantial minority of patients can distinguish more than one component of the tinnitus. Each separate sound or at least the most troublesome should then be further described as follows.

(ii) Loudness: e.g. faint, moderately loud, or very loud.

(iii) Pitch: e.g. low, medium, or high pitch, or without identifiable pitch.

(iv) Localization: e.g. apparently arising from the right ear, or mostly from the right ear, or from the left ear, or both ears, or centrally or elsewhere in the head.

(v) Temporal chatacteristics: continuous, or if intermittent then further information about on-duration and off-duration, and other temporal variability in quality.

(vi) Annoyance: mild, moderate, severe, or very severe.

(vii) Effect of environmental noise: against a noisy background, is the tinnitus much reduced, slightly reduced, unchanged, or worse?

B. Classification by probable site

Tinnitus may arise from one or more sites even in the same patient. If the patient has a hearing loss as well as tinnitus it is tempting to correlate the cause of the deafness with the site of the origin of the tinnitus. In many cases this will be an incorrect assumption. Sites to be considered are:

(i) Extra-auditory: e.g. vascular or from nasopharyngeal or extratympanic musculature.

(ii) Peripheral: external ear, middle ear, cochlear, or eighth cranial nerve.

(iii) Central: in the central auditory neural pathways with its various subdivisions.

(iv) Unknown.

C. Classification by measured characteristics

Although in the tinnitus patient there may be relevant associated phenomena which can be measured, the tinnitus itself, being subjective, can only be measured using subjective psycho-accoustic methods. Matching and masking techniques are the most widely used.

D. Classification by presence or absence of associated phenomena

For example:

(i) Deafness: absent, or if present its type and features.

(ii) Vestibular abnormality.

(iii) Acoustic emmission.

E. Classification by diagnosis of underlying condition

For example: Ménière's disease, noise-induced, physical trauma, 'depression', drug-induced.

F. Classification by response to treatment

For example: masking, medication, ablative surgery, or electric stimulation. An analysis of the cause of deafness in patients presenting with tinnitus is given in Table 44.1.

TABLE 44.1. *An analysis of the cause of deafness in patients presenting with tinnitus*

Cause of deafness	Jackson (1980)	Hazell (1975)
	%	%
Unknown	24	58
Acoustic trauma	17	10
CSOM	10	7
Post-stapedectomy	7	6
Viral/vascular	0	6
Ménière's	10	4
Meningitis	0	4
Congenital	3	3
H.injury	7	2
?Drug-induced	10	
Barotrauma	3	
Otosclerosis	3	
Post middle-ear surgery	3	

INCIDENCE

It is probably normal to experience transitory episodes of tinnitus occuring perhaps once a month or thereabouts. These come on suddenly and die away over a few seconds with concomittent or immediately preceding sense of dullness of hearing. Further a proportion of normal people become aware of a continuous quiet sound when in a silent sound-treated booth (Heller and Bergmann 1953). Hinchcliffe (1961) found in two samples of rural populations in the United Kindom, variously 17 to 30 per cent had experienced abnormal episodes of tinnitus and that the proportion increased with age (Fig. 44.1). An epidemiological investigation is currently being carried out by the Medical Research Council Institute of Hearing Research, Nottingham. Among results so far available the prevalence of tinnitus (which lasted more than five minutes) in four cities in Great Britain (Cardiff, Glasgow, Nottingham, and Southampton) was 14.7 to 17.7 per cent (Haggard 1980). Of those over 40 years old, 14.5 per cent reported tinnitus, whereas of those over 60 years old 22.2 per cent reported tinnitus. Severe annoyance was reported by 0.4 to 1.5 per cent, severe loss of ability to lead a normal life by 0.5 per cent, and interference with getting to sleep by 4.0 to

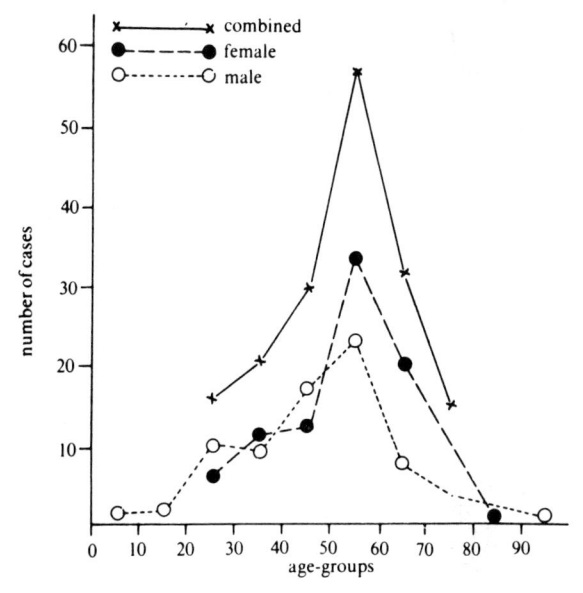

Fig, 44.1. Distribution of tinnitus cases by age at presentation. (From Hazell 1975, Courtesy of the *British Journal of Hospital Medicine*.)

6.8 per cent. An epidemiological investigation in the United States (1960–62) showed an incidence of about 2 per cent of the population (US Department of Health 1968).

MEASUREMENT OF TINNITUS

If our aim is to help people with tinnitus, there would be point in measuring the level of tinnitus before treatment and again after treatment hoping to find some improvement. But also measurement may give some indication of the underlying cause of the tinnitus and may shed further light of the working of the auditory system. A thorough assessment would include an analysis of the frequency spectrum of the noise, its loudness and its temporal characteristics. Generally attempts at measurement have so far been by using matching and masking techniques. In a qualitative way the tinnitus is matched by presenting a sound which can be varied in pitch and band-width and which can be given a variable rhythmic quality. Probably the most thorough work on the frequency content has been carried out by Hazell (1975). He has used a music synthesizer in a 'free field' and by patiently adjusting the sound to match that heard by the subject, he can reduplicate the patient's tinnitus and record this on tape. This work reveals that whereas for the majority the tinnitus consists of one component, there may be a mixture of steady and rhythmic components, the latter not necessarily in time with the pulse (Table 44.2).

The sounds are sometimes quite bizarre and it can be understood why the

TABLE 44.2. *Analysis of tinnitus using a music synthesizer (Hazell 1975)*

Number of sound components in tinnitus		% of tinnitus patients	
1		62	
2		30	
3		5	
4		2	
5		1	
Steady	83%	Rhythmic	17%
Narrow-band sound	52%	Wide-band sound	14%

patient often describes the noise in words with emotional overtones such as screeching, hissing, or shrieking. Hazell's work has been of importance in demonstrating to doctors and the lay-public the suffering the patient undergoes. Possibly tinnitus causes more handicap than the deafness itself, and one understands how from time to time patients are driven to suicide. This technique of matching takes too much time to be of value in the general management of patients. But it does reveal the shortcomings of matching techniques in which a pure-tone audiometer is used, even if this incorporates a facility for producing narrow-band and wide-band noise. More generally, workers have presented the noise to the contralateral ear (where the tinnitus is unilateral) provided this ear is not deaf. Reed (1960) used an audiometer, presenting pure tones and sounds of various band-widths. The width of the central frequency was then adjusted by trial and error to match the patient's subjective assessment of his tinnitus. The loudness of the tinnitus can then be assessed (Fowler 1944) presenting the selected matched sound to the contralateral ear to determine its threshold for that sound and then increasing the intensity until the patient perceives it as equal to the intensity of the tinnitus in the offending ear, the difference being accorded as the loudness of the patient's tinnitus. This is then repeated until reproducable results are obtained.

AUDIOMETRIC ASSESSMENT

For practical, logistic reasons this is at present the most widely used method of assessment.

Matching

A recommended matching procedure is to be published in CIBA Symposium 85. In general a pure-tone audiogram is determined for the contralateral ear. (If the tinnitus cannot be described as mostly in one ear rather than the other, the patient is asked to consider one ear as the reference when making judgements. Similarly, if there are several components to the tinnitus he is asked to consider only the loudest when making his assessment.) Vernon (1981) recommends that at this stage the patient is asked to match the loudness of his tinnitus against a 1-KHz tone, but this is by no means a universal routine. The patient is then presented with a pure tone, narrow-band, or wide-band noise and asked which most clearly represents his tinnitus sound. Unless he chooses wide-band sound the pitch is then adjusted to obtain the best match. It is probably advisable at this stage to test for 'octave confusion' presenting tones an octave above and an octave below the tone the patient has initially chosen. In a similar way, the intensity of the sound is adjusted to obtain loudness match at the chosen frequency. The sensation level is the difference between the level in decibels of the sound chosen as the match and the threshold of this sound. Reed notes that this procedure requires great patience on the parts of the technician and patient, particularly for the elderly and there must be considerable doubt as to the validity of such measurements.

Masking

Another measurement which may assess a character of the tinnitus is to determine the loudness of a sound which obliterates the tinnitus. Masking is carried out by presenting a sound whose intensity can be varied and the patient is then asked to select the quietest level which obliterates his own tinnitus. Generally, masking is carried out ipsilaterally, but it may be carried out bilaterally. The presented sound may be pure-tone and using this technique Feldman (1971) described five types (Fig. 44.2). Feldman asked is there a specific pattern related to the kind of tinnitus and does the pattern reveal anything of the underlying pathological process? Using contralateral masking he finds that at times the intensity to abolish tinnitus is greater and at times less than the ipsilateral tinnitus intensity and he concludes that the pattern of hair cells or nerve fibres whose spontaneous activity is responsible for tinnitus is not identical with the pattern activated by an external sound evoking the same subjective sensation. He asks further with regard to the conflicting findings with contralateral masking whether some central neural mechanism of contralateral inhibition is responsible. However, in general this technique of white noise masking is widely used (Morrison 1975). Both for matching and masking it may be helpful to use an intermittent pulsed tone so that the patient can be less confused between the tinnitus and the input sound. This technique makes it possible to carry out ipsilateral masking. These methods have to be appropriately modified where there is a severe unilateral hearing loss, when, for example only contralateral masking may be possible, and are obviously unsuitable in the totally deaf. It may be impossible to mask out tinnitus using generally available instruments if the hearing loss is severe. And matching is impossible in those who seem to experience tinnitus of a pitch above their audible range. Accepting these limitations these techniques of matching and masking are the best currently available and the importance of the method of adjustments is becoming increasingly recognized.

980 *Tinnitus*

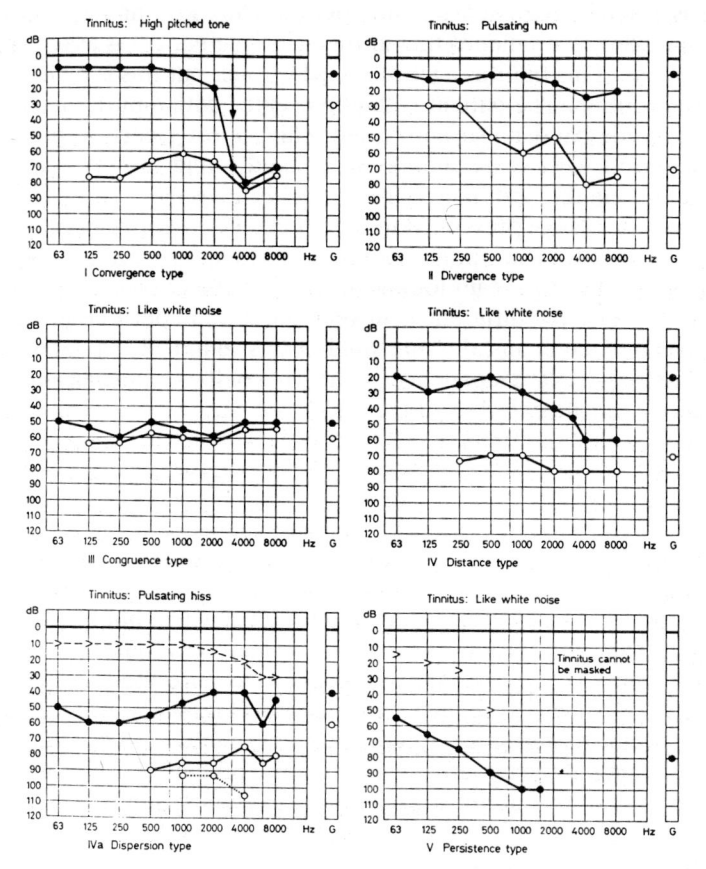

Fig. 44.2. Pure-tone masking of tinnitus. Black filled circles indicate the pure-tone threshold. Open circles indicate the level of pure-tone required to mask the tinnitus. (From Feldman, courtesy of *Audiology*.)

CRITICISM OF MATCHING TECHNIQUES

When one tries to repeat a match the subject in the majority of cases does not choose the same frequency or the same loudness each time. Because the tinnitus is very unlikely to be identical with the sound that the audiometer can produce the subject has to be instructed to find the best match. The subject may well say 'that's a perfect match' and then after further careful deliberation again determine what he calls a 'very good' or 'perfect' match when the dial readings are quite different. But if this, to the patient, represents the same sound then pitch discrimination may be at fault. Only in a minority will the figures be nearly the same on repeated testing. This means that limited reliance can be put on figures for frequency and intensity which are obtained by only one attempt at matching. By using the method of adjustments the patient can himself vary the output of the instrument (Voroba 1979) which has the advantage of better motivating the patient and keeping his attention. The patient can then produce a number of matches in a few minutes which are then available for statistical analysis. However, this has other drawbacks. Where the patient has in the contralateral ear a hearing loss which affects some frequencies of sound more than others then simply moving the output frequency control will affect the subjective impression of loudness. He may thus accept as a 'best match' a sound which is not as close to his tinnitus as the audiometer could produce. One way of overcoming this is, having determined the pure-tone audiogram, incorporate this with the audiometer in such a way that the intensity scale now represents sensation level. This technique is being used currently at the MRC Institute of Hearing Research (Tyler 1981). But there is still the problem of recruitment. A sound with a 2-dB sensation level where there is a drop in the audiogram, at say 4 KHz, may have the same subjective loudness as one with 30 dB at a lower frequency where the hearing is more normal. Because of this problem, Hazell recommends using the absolute level of loudness rather than the sensation level as the more useful figure. On the other hand Tyler (1981) emphasizing the psycho-accoustic nature of the problem, measures the loudness in sones. Some of these facilities can only be of application in research and not in the day-to-day clinical situation because of the time involved.

An alternative or supplementary technique is to have the patient record his own assessment of the tinnitus, say three times a day. In some ways this may be more useful in the management of the patient (Fig. 44.3). The degree of

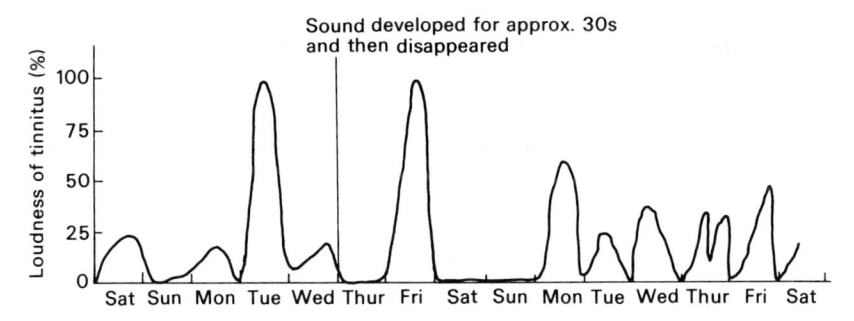

Fig. 44.3. Patient's self-recorded assessment of the loudness of his tinnitus. Note that this patient, unlike the majority, is least troubled at night and at weekends. His symptom is worst during his most active period of the day.

disability produced by tinnitus is manifest in the behaviour of the patient and this may be affected differently by an identical level of tinnitus depending on the personality of the sufferer and his mood at the time. Should the criterion for successful management be reduction in the tinnitus level or simply an improvement in the patient's acceptance of it?

OBJECTIVE TINNITUS

In a small proportion, the noise heard by the patient can also be heard (or potentially heard) by another person, typically, for example, by the spouse when both are lying in bed. The causes of such objective tinnitus can usefully be divided mainly into muscular or vascular. Involuntary rhythmic contractions (myoclonus) of the palatal, tensor tympani, or stapedial muscles give rise to a regular 'clicking' type of tinnitus, the rhythm of which bears no relation to the pulse. Although the onset of this symptom is generally in the young and middle aged (Bjork 1954) it may well persist to affect the elderly. Haemic causes giving a pulsatile tinnitus in rhythm with the heart beat may be due to vascular malformations (Arenberg and McGeary 1971), arteriovenous aneurysms, and glomus tumours. In a series of 15 patients with pulse synchronous tinnitus, three patients had no detectable murmur and no abnormal findings on angiography whereas the remaining twelve had both a murmur and a demonstrable vascular abnormality (Harris, Brishar, and Cronqvist 1979). A haemic cause for objective tinnitus is found in Paget's disease (Gibson 1973); this has been helped by carotid ligation. Turbulent blood flow over atherosclerotic plaques might also be expected to produce a pulsatile tinnitus. The presence of cervical arterial bruits increases with age and a prospective study (Heyman et al. 1980) has shown that such bruits are associated with a significantly higher risk of stroke and death from ischaemic heart disease in men (but not women). The inference is that this finding is an indication of the general state of the arterial system. The incidence of these cervical bruits was 8 per cent in the age group 75 years and over. Many of these patients may not complain of tinnitus but nevertheless the symptom of a pulsatile tinnitus affected and often relieved temporarily by firm pressure in the neck on the carotid artery below the angle of the jaw or by posture is common in the group of late middle aged or elderly patients and is presumably due to similar changes. At times one can hear in some patients a pulsatile sound by using a sensitive microphone in the patient's ear and it is possible to confirm that this objective sound is obliterated at the same time the subject says that he has obliterated the sound by gentle pressure on the neck. House (1981) says that in such cases ipsilateral ligature of the internal jugular vein abolishes the noise and may be well worth carrying out. In the examination, the mastoid, neck, skull, and eye should be auscultated. The electronic stethoscope, though not widely used, has been shown to have a place in the examination of young people with pulsatile tinnitus (Goldie 1960) and may prove worthwhile in the elderly. Tewfik (1974) used electronic recording equipment and found that where objective tinnitus was associated with hypertension then adequate treatment of the hypertension abolished both the sound as recorded in his instrument and the patient's tinnitus. In this connection, however, a case of tinnitus apparently caused by the antihypertensive drug, propranolol, has been reported (Mostyn 1969).

Although the contrary view is sometimes stated, in general the cause of objective tinnitus, particulary of vascular origin, if often not easy to find nor to treat. In the absence of other alarming symptons, angiography can seldom be recommended because of its risks and surgery for localized atheromatous plaques in the carotid arteries has not been shown to have a worthwhile result in terms of survival (Heyman *et al.* 1980). Angiography itself has apparently caused tinnitus. Embolism by gelatin sponge after selective angiography has been reported as giving a temporary cure for pulsatile tinnitus (Harris *et al.* 1979). A glomus jugulare or a glomus tympanicum may present with pulsatile tinnitus, a conductive hearing loss, and a red mass seen in the external canal or seen through an intact tympanic membrane. Myoclonus of the middle-ear muscles may be demonstrated by impedance audiometry even though movement of the tympanic membrane may not be visible on otoscopy (Coles, Snashall, and Stephens 1975). The tinnitus of stapedial myoclonus may be helped, but not always permanently, by stapedius tendon section. Carbamezapine is also said to have been helpful in the treatment of palatal myoclonus (Rahko 1979) and a case of synkinesis between the facial nerve and the stapes tendon presenting with tinnitus which was abolished by surgical division of the fibrous attachment has been described.

Kemp and Chum (1980) have found that the healthy ear can generate a sound, the evoked mechanical cochlear response (EMCR) or echo, which can be detected by a microphone in the external acoustic meatus a few milliseconds after the input of sound into the ipsilateral ear. Subsequently, Wilson (1980) and Kemp, using the same recording equipment, have found a number of normal subjects without tinnitus but with a continuous sound coming out of the ear. However, tinnitus, when present, does not necessarily have the same frequency characteristics as that of the tonal emission. Only certain defined areas of the basilar membrane are apparently responsible for the emissions which have been studied. Of the tinnitus sufferers with a sensory hearing loss the regions of the basilar membrane corresponding to the hearing loss are not the same regions as are the source of the emission. The acoustic power available to drive the stereo cilia is not enough to initiate a nerve impulse. Kemp postulates a positive feedback mechanism, dependent on energy from biological mechanisms which results in resonance of a component of the spiral organ (and may thus be partly responsible for cochlear tuning). Kemp points out that if there has been damage of the spiral organ from drugs or from noise, the phenomenon of EMCR does not occur. Clearly this spontaneous emission of sound from the cochlea is not what clinicians would call tinnitus though it may possibly be relevant to the tinnitus found immediately after noise exposure. Its significance in the subject of tinnitus needs much further study. Glanville, Coles and Sullivan (1971) reported the finding of continuous tones being emitted by a father and two of his children. It seems these sounds were not heard by the subjects themselves.

SUBJECTIVE TINNITUS

Research into tinnitus is difficult because of the subjective nature of the symptoms: it is frustrating because the disability fluctuates and is dependent on the mood and personality of the victim. And although tinnitus may rarely drive a person to suicide, it does not of itself cause death and hence the study of post-mortem material is limited. It would be helpful if there were an animal model, but animals, if they do suffer from tinnitus, do not complain of it as far as we know. A possible approach would be to give an animal drugs known to produce tinnitus in man and to study any changes in histology and neurophysiology. Similary surgical assaults could perhaps be made and the effects studied. Thus Evans (1981) established an animal model by giving salicylates in doses producing blood concentrations which would evoke tinnitus in man. He asks whether tinnitus is a manifestation of (i) an increased, or (ii) a decreased level of spontaneous neural activity (the spontaneous neural activity in the absence of external sound being interpreted as silence). Using a cat poisoned with salicylate (which produced a reversible dose-related tinnitus in man) he recorded electrical activity from the cochlear nerve fibres and found there was a marked change in auditory threshold. This indicated a peripheral action for salicylates. With regard to spontaneous activity recorded from the cochlear nerve he found that, with salicylate poisoning there was an increased discharge rate.

A closer analysis, however, revealed two populations of nerve fibres, one group (a) with a low rate of spontaneous activity, and a second group (b) with a higher rate of spontaneous activity. With salicylates, the spontaneous activity in group (a) fibres decreased while that in group (b) increased.

Tonndorf (1979) pointed out that tinnitus is a feature of noise-induced hearing loss and of antibiotic ototoxicity. He experimentally produced noise-induced hearing loss in the guinea pig and found some of the stereocilia on the hair cells had blebs on the summit of the hairs. He considers these are dying hair cells and postulates that this change leads to an increase in background 'noise' level of spontaneous emission interpreted as tinnitus. His concept is set out in Table 44.3.

He also suggests, from comparative animal work and histopathological changes, the correlation shown in Table 44.4.

Brown (1981) has made two lists of drugs which produce tinnitus, one in which the drugs also cause a hearing loss, either temporary or permanent (this includes aminoglycosides) and a second in which there is no associated hearing loss. Using both electric response audiometry and scanning electron microscopy, he found in the rat that aminoglycosides potentiated the damage caused by acoustic trauma whereas sodium salicylate did not. On the other hand, chloramphenicol (not recognized as an ototoxic drug) also potentiated the damage caused by noise. Could it be that this potentiation occurs when either agent separately produces an area of temporary or subliminal damage and this is only revealed when there is a further insult to the same region? Although there was no direct assessment of tinnitus in the

TABLE 44.3.

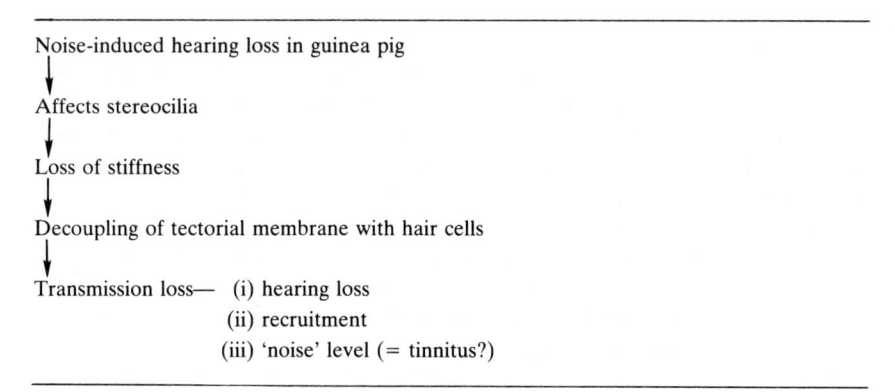

Noise-induced hearing loss in guinea pig
↓
Affects stereocilia
↓
Loss of stiffness
↓
Decoupling of tectorial membrane with hair cells
↓
Transmission loss— (i) hearing loss
(ii) recruitment
(iii) 'noise' level (= tinnitus?)

TABLE 44.4.

Aetiology	Site of cochlear lesion	Type of tinnitus
Acoustic trauma	Upper basal turn	Narrow-band 4 kHz
'Fluctuating hearing loss' (e.g. hydrops)	Apical turn	'Low-pass' roaring
Advanced antibiotic ototoxic changes	Widespread, starting in basal turn	Broad-band, high-frequency

experimental animals, the work is likely to be of relevance to tinnitus in man both with regard to prevention and to the understanding of underlying mechanisms. Tinnitus is a manifestatation of disorder in the auditory system and it is widely held that it is a feature of patients with hearing loss. Although Fowler quotes 85 per cent of patients with otological disease as having tinnitus, nevertheless of patients attending a tinnitus clinic, 20 to 30 per cent are found to have normal hearing, and conversely, many patients with a 'dead ear' do not complain of tinnitus. Among those most to be pitied must surely be people who have little or no hearing together with continuous tinnitus.

The distribution of the causes of deafness, where it occurs, in patients with tinnitus taken from the figures of two tinnitus clinics in London is approximately as given in Table 44.1.

Tinnitus is one symptom of vestibulo cochlear schwannoma and is the sole presenting symptom in 11 per cent of such cases in a large series reported by House and Brackman (1981). Probably sensorineural hearing loss from any of the many known causes may be associated with tinnitus. It is certainly a feature in adults with profound congenital hearing loss. Graham (1981) studied children in a Partially Hearing Unit and in a school for the deaf. About half the children (age 12 to 18 years) experienced tinnitus but it was more common in the group with less hearing loss. Indeed, where tinnitus was unilateral, it was in the better hearing ear in more than 80 per cent. On the other hand, of the 150 children, only two had constant tinnitus.

Tinnitus is a symptom in very many, if not all, patients with a syphilitic hearing loss. Conductive hearing loss with tinnitus occurs in chronic suppurative otitis media (CSOM) particularly after mastoidectomy, after middle-ear surgery and myringoplasty, and is a feature of otosclerosis. In many cases as we have seen, no aetiological factor is found. Very commonly the patient gives a history of experiencing tinnitus on waking up one morning and it has peristed unchanged ever since, and in the majority of cases it comes on suddenly and persists unchanged. One sees nowadays a number of patients who say that tinnitus began on descent to the ground after flying. Otitic barotrauma is not simply related in most of these as only sometimes has there been accompanying otalgia.

Exposure to a sufficiently loud sound produces deafness which may be temporary together with tinnitus which may persist for a variable period after hearing loss recovers. More prolonged exposure to hazardous noise (e.g. industrial noise) may produce a gradually increasing noise-induced hearing loss but tinnitus is only sometimes a feature, and then a late one, and the factor of aging cannot be quantified. Recently patients presenting with tinnitus for the first time were most commonly in the 50 to 60 age group. This age group included many who would have been subjected to acoustic trauma during the war years and although Hinchcliffe (1961) found no correlation between tinnitus and exposure to acoustic hazard at work the findings of the recent Nottingham survey referred to earlier are suggestive that environmental noise is a factor.

PATIENT MANAGEMENT

With regard to the history, examination, and investigation, these will be along the general lines of those for a deaf patient. Of particular relevance are enquiries about previous drug administration. From the extensive list of Brown referred to earlier, the most important include aminoglycoside antibiotics, anti-inflammatory agents, quinine, tricyclic antidepressants, and beta blockers. Auscultation, with amplification where possible, is particularly important in those with a rhythmic element to the tinnitus. Electrophysiological methods in which the electrical activity in the auditory pathway can be detected is so far without promise in measuring or assessing tinnitus as it depends on the use of a computer to 'average out' the background activity, and in so doing any activity due to or associated with continuous tinnitus would be lost. However, electrocochleography may be of value in the examination of the totally deaf ear (Graham 1979) in that the site of deafness, whether cochlear or retrocochlear, and hence the presumed site of tinnitus can be revealed.

Perhaps 80 per cent or so of patients referred to a tinnitus clinic can be helped simply by interview together with the relevant examination and investigation, followed by reassurance where this can be given. But patients all too often become depressed, suicidal, and a burden to those who care for them. This is particularly a feature of the elderly patient with tinnitus when activity and other interests are waning and time seems to hang heavily. In general once tinnitus is troublesome it can be expected to persist so that its incidence in the population increases with age. Most elderly patients with tinnitus will have had this symptom for many years and although the noise may not have become quieter, it has become for them a fact of life. The patient involved in community work for his or her peers will generally make light of the symptom.

But on the other hand people in this age group are prone to depression and the depressed patient with tinnitus is a not infrequent attender both at psychiatric and tinnitus clinics. It seems the state of mind makes the tinnitus worse, and the tinnitus in turn makes the depression worse. The patient with endogenous depression may tend to rationalize his feelings, and if tinnitus is present 'as it often is in the early involutional period the patient becomes preoccupied with it to the exclusion of all else . . . telling himself (or more generally herself) that "these noises are spoiling my life and driving me mad"' (Kennedy 1953). Although it is demanding to see such patients, particularly where the physician may feel himself unable to help, nevertheless it is probably beneficial to the patient to have follow up appointments at suitably long intervals. Some of these patients may already be on tranquillizers, and if one simply takes them off diazepam for example, one is rewarded by seeing at the next visit a much brighter happy patient, even though the tinnitus is still present. Others may be on an inappropriate hypertensive, reserpine for example, which may cause or exacerbate the depressive mood.

For those who have a hearing loss but retain useful hearing, a hearing aid may not only give improved communication, but also amplification of the ambient sound such as effectively to mask the tinnitus. Unfortunately some will find that the amplification distorts speech sound and makes communication more difficult but before this is abandoned consideration should be given to the use of bilateral hearing aids if the hearing loss affects both ears.

Provided he is not profoundly deaf, a sound of sufficient loudness can often make the patient oblivious of his tinnitus and many prefer hearing this external noise to his own noises. It is now possible to provide a masking device like a hearing aid, which produces a masking noise. On the simpler machines which produce 'white noise' the volume control can be adjusted by the patient. Other devices have additionally a frequency adjustment and some have a hearing aid as well as a masking instrument. Vernon has the most experience in this field. He stresses the importance of matching the masker to the patient's tinnitus, and of carefully assessing the patient's tinnitus. In addition to the procedures already given he looks for residual inhibition. The patient may find maskers in both ears a significant improvement on the unilateral masker and find that conversation is still possible. The percentage of the patients who can be helped in this way varies in different series (Schleuring, Johnson, and Vernon 1980; Rosen and Price 1980; Rose 1980). If, as commonly occurs, the patient finds the tinnitus most obtrusive when trying to sleep, it may be possible to try a masker which fits under the pillow, but just as cheap and at least as effective is a bedside radio which will switch itself off after the patient has gone to sleep. A masker is of limited help to the profoundly deaf as the masking tone will not be heard loudly enough to obliterate the tinnitus (Fig. 44.4).

There is on the other hand a sizeable group very differently affected in which the tinnitus is more troublesome when there is background noise or when trying to concentrate or engaged in activity.

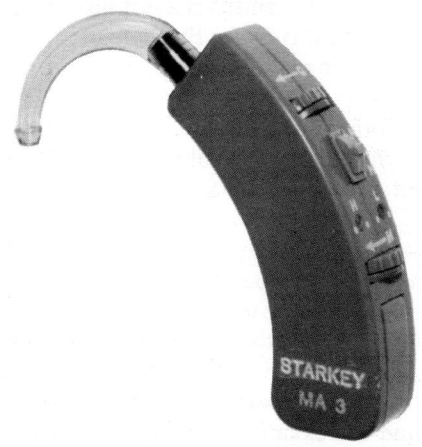

Fig. 44.4 An ear-level hearing aid incorporating a masking device with frequency control.

SURGERY

For those with a conductive hearing loss plus tinnitus it is tempting to consider reconstructive surgery in the hope that by improving the hearing there would be an increased awareness of ambient sound which would have a masking effect. All too frequently, however, this type of surgery, be it myringoplasty or ossicular reconstruction, while it may improve the hearing does not improve the tinnitus and may make it worse. Tinnitus with otosclerosis is not necessarily improved by stapedectomy and in the group of ostosclerotics whose chief presenting complaint is tinnitus (rather than hearing impairment) perhaps 50 per cent or more are made worse by stapedectomy; those who have undergone a 'failed stapedectomy' are among the sufferers from the worst tinnitus. If the patient has a profoundly deaf ear which is the source of tinnitus, then destruction of the ipsilateral vestibulocochlear nerve may be considered. Ideally the patient should be shown to have poor speech discrimination even with amplification, and good hearing on the opposite side. However here again the results are disappointing, the tinnitus being improved in 25 to 50 per cent of patients in various series (Morrison 1975). This must be because the tinnitus is arising centrally.

Even if the cause of the associated hearing loss is peripheral (e.g. from a perilymph fistula or after stapedectomy) there is no certainty that the tinnitus, by the time the patient is seen, is arising peripherally. It may be possible in the future to determine what is the site of origin of the tinnitus and so lead to a better pre-operative selection.

It has been recently shown to be possible to abolish tinnitus by electrical stimulation. Portmann, Cazals, Negrevergne, and Aran (1979) have applied an electrode variously to the round windows and to the promontories of patients with tinnitus and delivered positive and negative currents at various frequencies. With the postive electrode in position, they found the patient would declare supression of the tinnitus using current strength generally between 50 to 300 µA at frequencies between 200 to 3200 Hz. One could envisage the development of a simple device which may be of benefit particularly to those with a dead ear or perhaps with a mastoid cavity. This may pose another good reason for not embarking too readily on nerve section as treatment for tinnitus because clearly after this has been carried out the peripheral electrical suppression technique can no longer be offered.

DRUGS

Gejrot (1976) reported that, when using intravenous lignocaine (lignocaine = lidocaine) for the treatment of acute attacks of Ménière's disease, there was suppression of both the vertigo and the tinnitus. Melding, Goodey, and Thorne (1978) confirmed this observation and also found that the tinnitus which accompanied middle ear disease was not affected by lignocaine. They felt at that time that the value of lignocaine may be in determing the source of the noise but they and others (Emmett and Shea 1980) considered that in those patients in whom lignocaine abolishes the tinnitus, the tinnitus is arising centrally. However, in those patients selected for cochlear nerve section as treatment for their tinnitus, there has been correlation in a small series between the abolition of the tinnitus by lignocaine and its abolition by the section; furthermore those who fail preoperatively to respond to lignocaine do not have tinnitus abolished by subsequent nerve section, though there has been in a small series one exception to this observation (Jackson 1980). Although an early view was that a response or non-response to lignocaine may be useful in classifying tinnitus (Melding et al. 1978), it gives ground for optimism that a similar effective drug could be found which would have a prolonged bio-availability when given by mouth. A number of such drugs allied to lignocaine having a similar cardiac antidysrhythmic action is at present undergoing evaluation and preliminary reports are encouraging (Emmet and Shea 1980) (Fig 44.5). Naftidrofuryl is also a powerful local anaesthetic and apparently inhibits the destruction of ATP. Gibson, Moffat, and Ramsden (1977) found that this drug altered the electrocochleogram in Ménière's disease. Patients have occasionally reported that their tinnitus does seem to be helped by this drug. Also one sees patients from time to time who claim that their tinnitus has been relieved by

LIGNOCAINE

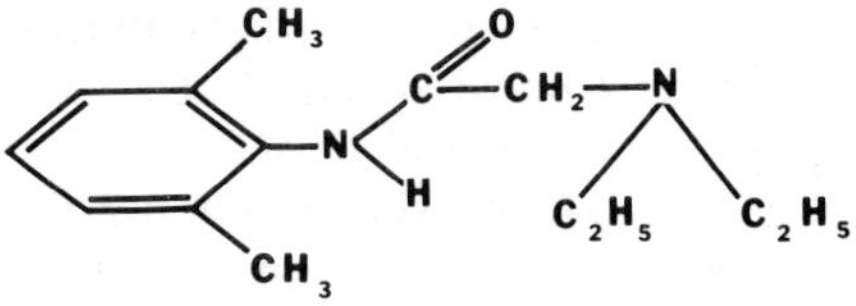

TOCAINIDE

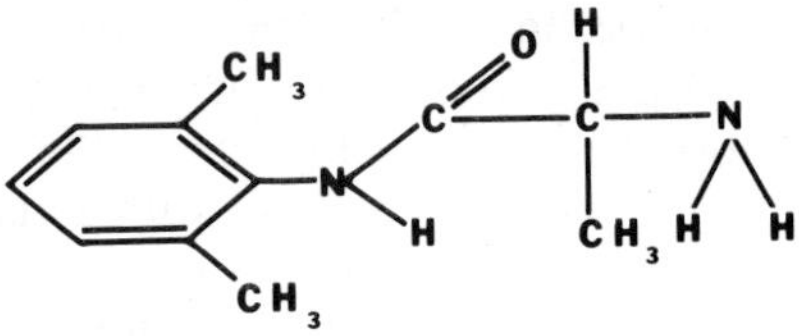

LORCAINIDE

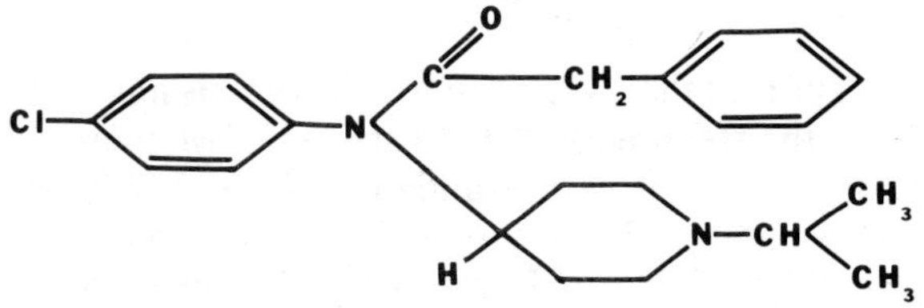

MEXILETENE

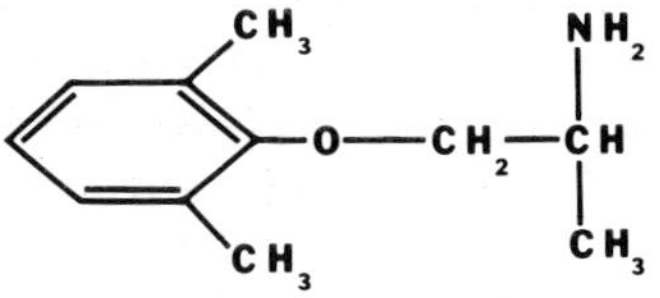

Fig. 44.5. Structural formula of lidocaine and related drugs with cardiac antidysrhythmic action undergoing trials for the treatment of tinnitus.
(Note: lignocaine = lidocaine.)

betahistine and by prochloperazine. Donaldson (1979) has found that amylobarbitone has relieved tinnitus. Patients with tinnitus do not respond to placebo given in the form of either saline injection or inactive oral preparations (Jackson 1980). Because lignocaine proved effective in abolishing the epileptic attacks of the experimental animal (Bernhard and Bohm 1954), anti-epileptic drugs have been used in tinnitus. In this connection perhaps most work has been done with carbamezapine and in spite of some encouraging initial reports, it has now been largely abandoned in the treatment of subjective tinnitus because of its side effects (Shea and Harrell 1979). A psychotherapeutic drug to improve the mood of the depressed patient with tinnitus is often helpful (Williamson 1980) but such long-term drug therapy can be criticized as threatening the wholeness of the personality, and a drug which would specifically take away the tinnitus would be generally preferable. Diabetes and dyslipoproteinaemia, if discovered in the course of investigations for tinnitus, may themselves require medical treatment. The hearing impairment associated with dyslipoproteinaemia may at times be reversed by dieting together with an improvement in the serum lipoprotein levels; it is reasonable to hope that the tinnitus too would be improved.

On the basis that in the elderly the cochlear damage and hence the tinnitus might be due to impaired circualtion, drugs aimed at improving the circulation have been used, e.g. naftidrofuryl, as mentioned earlier, cyclandelate, and nicotinic acid.

BIOFEEDBACK

Some sucess is claimed in American reports for biofeedback (House 1978; Grossman 1979). This technique has not been widely used in the United Kingdom so far. The principle is to induce the patient to relax by picking up action potentials in, for example, the frontalis muscle and making this electrical activity visible or audible to the patient. House (1978) reports that 47 per cent of patients undergoing this form of therapy were improved though it is admitted that it could well be the patient's attitude to his tinnitus is improved rather than there being any change in the sensation level.

MISCELLANEOUS

Portmann has found experimentally that a direct current applied to an electrode on the round window can suppress tinnitus without at the same time affecting the hearing. The suppression was initially found to be lasting only so long as the current flowed. The technique seems to be well tolerated. Perhaps further work along these lines may well result in the development of a technique useful particularly for the patient with inactive otitis media.

One sees from time to time patients who claim that acupuncture and faith healing have been helpful.

CONCLUSION

Many patients experiencing tinnitus for the first time are particularly anxious lest they may have a cerebral tumour or that it may be a feature of impending deafness. If after investigations it is possible to reassure the patients about their fears then this in itself is therapeutic and the patient may well find the symptom more acceptable. Likewise for the severely depressed patient psychotherapy and encouragement to become involved in active pursuits will improve the quality of life, reducing the effect of the tinnitus.

The recently formed British Tinnitus Association gives the opportunity for patients to meet fellow sufferers (who are likely to be sympathetic) and for keeping them informed of progress in the field and of facilities as they become available. The American Tinnitus Association performs a similar service. These have given hope to many patients who have endured their symptons for years.

Thus there is no simple panacea for tinnitus and in general at the present time when the doctor is expected to 'cure' the patient he himself feels inadequate and helpless: he dreads seeing the tinnitus patient and is glad when he is gone. One hopes that the present activities aimed at the study of tinnitus, both causation and management, will help to improve this frustrating situation.

REFERENCES

ARENBERG, I. K. and MCCREARY, H. S. (1971). Objective tinnitus aurium and dural arterio-venous malformation of the posterior fossa. *Ann. Otol. Rhinol. Lar.* **80**, 112–20.

BERNHARD, C. G. and BOHM, E. (1954). Epilepsy abolished by lidocaine. *Acta physiol. scand.* **31** Suppl. 114, 5.

BJORK, H. (1954). Objective tinnitus due to clonus of the soft palate. *Acta oto-lar.* Suppl. 16, 39–45.

BROWN, D. (1981). CIBA Foundation Symposium No. 85. London.

COLES, R.R. A., SNASHALL, S.E., and STEPHENS, S.D.G. (1975). Some varieties of objective tinnitus. *Br. J. Audiol.* **9**, 1–6.

DONALDSON, I. (1979). Tinnitus: a theorectical view and a therapeutic study using amylobarbitone. *J. Lar. Otol.* **92**, 123–30.

DOUEK, E. (1981). Classification of tinnitus. CIBA Foundation Symposium No. 85. London.

EMMETT, J. R. and SHEA, J. J. (1980). Treatment of tinnitus with tocainide hydrochloride. *Otolar. Head Neck Surg.* **88**, 442–6.

EVANS, E. F. (1981). CIBA Foundation Symposium No. 85. London.

FELDMAN, H. (1971). Homolateral and contralateral masking of tinnitus by noise bands and pure tones. *Audiology* **10**, 138–44.

FOWLER, E. P. (1944). Head noises in normal and in discordered ears: significance measurement differentiation and treatment. *Archs Otolar.* **39**, 498–503.

GEJROT, T. (1976). Ménière's, tinnitus and lidocaine. *Acta oto-lar.* **82**, 301.

GIBSON, R. (1973). Tinnitus in Paget's disease with external carotid ligation. *J. Lar. Otol.* **87**, 299–301.

GIBSON, W. P. R., MOFFAT, D., and RAMSDEN, M. (1977). The immediate effects of naftidrofuryl on the human electrocochleogram in Ménière's disorder. *J. Lar. Otol.* **91**, 679–96.

GLANVILLE, J.D., COLES, R.R.A., and SULLIVAN, B. M. (1971). A family with high-tone obective tinnitus. *J. Lar. Otol.* **85**, 1–10.

GOLDIE, L. (1960). Phonocraniography. The recording of cephalic bruits. Third International Conference on Medical Electronics. Motor and Nervous Systems II.

GOODWIN, P. E. (1980). Tinnitus and auditory imagery. *Am. J. Otol.* **2**, 5–9.

GRAHAM, J. (1979). The role of evoked response audiometry in evaluation of the tinnitus patient. Paper read at 1st International Tinnitus Seminar, New York City, June 1979.

—— (1981). CIBA Foundation Symposium No. 85. London.
GROSSMAN, M. (1979). Treatment of subjective tinnitus with biofeedback. *Ear, Nose Throat J.* **55**, 22–8.
HAGGARD, M. (1980). Epidemiology of tinnitus. Paper read at meeting of British Society of Audiology, Nottingham, June 1980.
HARRIS, S., BRISHAR, J., and CRONQVIST, S. (1979). Pulsatile tinnitus and therapeutic embolism. *Acta oto-lar.* **88**, 220–6.
HAZELL, J. W. P. (1975). Determination of tinnitus quality. Presented to British Society of Audiology, 12 December 1975.
HELLER, M. F. and BERGMAN, M. (1953). Tinnitus aurium in normally hearing persons. *Ann. Otolar.* **62**, 73–82.
HEYMAN, A. et al. (1980). Risk of stroke in asymptomatic persons with cervical bruits. *New Engl. J. Med.* **302**, 838–41.
HINCHCLIFFE, R. (1961). Prevalence of the commoner ear nose and throat conditions in the adult rural population of Great Britain. *Br. J. Prev. Soc. Med.* 15, 128–140.
HOUSE, J. and BRACKMAN, D. (1981). CIBA Foundation Symposium No. 85.
HOUSE, P. (1978). Treatment of severe tinnitus with biofeedback training. *Laryngoscope, St. Louis* **88**, 406–12.
HURST, J. W., HOPKINS., L. C., and SMITH, R. B. (1980). Noises in the neck. *New Engl. J. Med.* **302**, 862–3.
JACKSON, P. D. (1980). Tinnitus: An enigma with variations. Paper read at the Royal College of Surgeons of England, February 1979.
KEMP, D. T. and CHUM, R. (1980). Properties of the generator of stimulated acoustic emissions. *Hear. Res.* **2**, 213–32.
KENNEDY, A. (1953). Cochlear, neural and subjective factors in tinnitus. *Proc. R. Soc. Med.* **825**, 829–32.
KIMURA, Y. (1976). Tinnitus without hearing loss. *Otolaryngology, Tokyo* **45**, 819.
LEVEQUE, H., BIALOSTOZKY, F., BLANCHARD, C. L., and SUTER, C. M. (1979). Tympanometry and evaluation of vascular lesions of the middle ear and tinnitus of vascular origin. *Laryngoscope, St. Louis* **89**, 1197–218.
MELDING, P. S. and GOODEY, R. J. (1979). The treatment of tinnitus with oral anticonvulsants. *J. Lar. Otol.* **93**, 11–22.
—— ——, and THORNE, P. R. (1978). The use of intravenous lignocaine in the diagnosis and treatment of tinnitus. *J. Lar. Otol.* **92**, 115–21.
MORRISON, A. (1975). *Management of sensorineural deafness*, Chapter 5. Butterworth, London.
MOSTYN, R. H. L. (1969). Tinnitus and Propranolol. *Br. med. J.* i, 766.
PORTMANN, M., CAZALS, Y., NEGREVERGNE, M., and ARAN, J. M. (1979). Temporary tinnitus suppression in man through electrical stimulation of the cochlea. *Acta oto-lar.* **87**, 294–9.
PULEC, J. L., HODELL, S. E., and ANTHONY, P. F. (1979). Tinnitus—diagnosis and treatment. *Ann. Otol. Rhinol. Lar.* 87, 821–33.
RAHKO, T. and Hakkinen, V. (1979). Carbamezapine in the treatment of objective myoclonus tinnitus. *J. Lar. Otol.* 93, 123–7.
REED, G. F. (1960). An audiometric study of 200 cases of subjective tinnitus. *Archs Otolar.* **71**, 84–94.
ROESEN, R. J. and PRICE, D. R. (1980). Clinical experience with tinnitus maskers. *Ear Hear.* **1**, 63–8.
ROSE, E. D. (1980). Tinnitus maskers: a follow up. *Ear Hear.* **1**, 69–70.
SCHLEURING, A. J., JOHNSON, R. A., and VERNON, J. (1980). Evaluation of a tinnitus masking program. *Ear Hear.* **1**, 71–4.

SHEA, J. J. and HARRELL, M. (1979). Management of tinnitus aurium with lidocaine and carbamezapine. *Laryngoscope, St. Louis* **88**, 1477–84.
TEWFIK, S. (1974). Phonocephalography—an objective diagnosis of tinnitus. *J. Lar. Otol.* **88**, 869–75.
TONNDORF, J. (1979). Tinnitus and physiological correlates of the cochleovestibular system. Paper read at 1st International Tinnitus Seminar, New York City, June 1979.
TYLER, R. S. (1981). CIBA Foundation Symposium No. 85. London.
US DEPARTMENT OF HEALTH (1968). Hearing status and ear examination—findings among adults in United States (1960–1962: *Vital and health statistics*, Vol. 11, No. 32). US Department of Health, Education and Welfare, Public Health Service.
VERNON, J. (1977). Attempts to relieve tinnitus. *J. Am. audiol. Soc.* **2**, 124–31.
—— (1981) CIBA Foundation Symposium No. 85. London.
—— JOHNSON, R., SCHLEUNING, A., and MITCHELL, C. (1980). Masking and tinnitus. *Audiol. hear. Educ.* Summer, 5–9.
VOROBA, B. (1979). Tinnitus research frontiers. *Hear. Instrum.* **30**, 31–3.
WALFORD, R. (1980). Acoustical techniques for diagnosing low frequency tinnitus in noise complainants know as hummers. Proc. Inst. of Acoustic, Spring Meeting.
WILLIAMSON, J. (1980). Aspects of depression. *Geriat. Med.* **9**, 15–19.
WILSON, J. F. (1980). Evidence for a cochlear origin for acoustic re-emission threshold, fine structure and tonal tinnitus. *Hear. Res.* **2**, 233–52.

Index

abnormal auditory adaptation (AAA) 380, 381, 384, 423–6
achondroplasia 602
acoustic impedance bridges and meters (also oto-admittance meters, ME analysers, tympanometers) 228–40
   calibration 238–40
   electroacoustic 227 ff.
   electromechanical 228–9
acoustic impedance, compliance, admittance 145 ff., 228, 232–4, 376, 377
acoustic measurements 141–4, 831–5, 847, 848
acoustic neuroma 41, 377, 378, 398, 415–40, 507–9, 761, 776, 796–8, 985
   flow chart for investigation 421
   various surgical approaches 508–9
acoustic stapedial reflex 229, 230, 234, 235, 238, 372, 373, 380, 710–13, 718, 719, 915, 916, 921, 922
   adaptation 380, 426, 427, 717
   artefacts 239, 711
   differential diagnosis: cochlear/retrocochlear 715–18
   sensation level (SL) 716–18
aditus 18, 46
adults with acquired total deafness 518
aminoglycosides and ototoxicity (streptomycin, kanamycin, gentamycin, amikacin, tobramycin) 573–92
   concentration in perilymph 587
   in pregnancy 584–5
amplifiers 193
anaesthetics and sedatives for general anaesthesia 809–15
   atropine 810, 811
   cetacaine® 813
   chlorpromazine 814
   diazepam 813
   enflurane 815
   halothane 766, 811, 813
   ketamine 766, 809–11, 813
   nitrous oxide 809, 811, 813
   pentobarbital 814
   promethazine HCl 814
   quintalbarbitone 814
   thiopentone 814
   trimeprazine 813
annulus tympanicus, see tympanic ring
anterior horn cells 38

anterior inferior cerebellar artery 43, 67, 73, 436, 512
antibiotics, see drugs
aqueduct of the cochlea 40, 69, 587
aqueduct of the vestibule 30, 32
arachnoid cyst 437
assisted resonance 138
ataxic neuropathy 629
athetoid cerebral palsy 632, 633
atresia of auricular structures 694–6
attic 11, 46
audiological medicine 937, 939, 957
   science of 938
audiometers 161
   Békésy 366, 368, 917, 918
   calibration of 168–75
   computer-based 179, 180
   peep-show 180
   pure-tone 161–5
   routine checking of 180–4
   sound field 178, 179
   speech 175–8
audiometric room 138–41
auditory nerve action potential (AP or CAP) 75, 98, 196, 428, 429, 543, 574, 755, 766, 781, 798
auditory ossicles 11–13, 17, 105, 106, 152, 154, 156, 493–501, 694, 702
   abnormalities 694, 696, 697
   blood supply 22
   lever ratio 106, 152, 153, 493–5, 816–19, 821, 822
   resonance of 494, 495
auditory pathway 36
   placode 50
   vesicle 50, 64
auditory threshold 121
   variability of 369
auditory tube, see Eustachian tube
auricle (pinna) 3–6, 41, 104, 246, 694–6, 702
   extrinsic muscles 4, 5
autograft 497
averaging (computer), time domain 188–91
   sampling rate 190, 191
axodendritic synapse 56, 543

basilar artery 43, 73
basilar membrane 35, 41, 50, 51, 53, 56, 59, 67, 69, 70, 73, 82, 108, 109, 113, 983

Békésy audiometers, audiometry 366, 368, 917, 918
  Jerger's classification 371
biofeedback for tinnitus 991
bony cochlea 17, 30, 104
  dysplasias affecting IAM 512
  labyrinth 17, 28, 29, 40, 41, 108
  promontory 112
  spiral lamina 30, 41, 53, 76, 89
brainstem
  conduction time 801
  disorders of, affecting hearing 383–5
  electric (or evoked) responses (BSER) 575, 655, 656, 719, 755, 757, 758, 761, 765–7, 798–801, 923–5
  in acoustic neuroma 429
  in relation to cochlear implantation 558, 559
branchial arches 12
British sign language 665
Bruyn's cerebellar nystagmus 432

canal of Hugier 16
canal for tensor tympani 25
canalis reuniens 31
carotid canal 20, 25
cartilage grafts 497
cerebello-pontine angle 41
cerebral cortex, hemispheres 36, 45
cerumen 441–2, 948
cholesteatoma 268–71, 437, 482, 709, 714, 715, 824
  of cerebello-pontine angle 509
cholesterol granuloma 266–8
cialit 493, 496, 497
Claudius' cells 34
clinical, non-audiometric, test of hearing 320–64
cochlea 34, 50, 51, 60, 61, 63, 68, 70, 72, 79, 113, 152, 154, 156, 245, 258, 296, 394, 541–72, 816–26, 970
cochlear artery 68
cochlear deformity or dysplasia 817–20
cochlear duct 34, 35, 40, 50, 52, 66, 70
cochlear ganglion cells (Types 1–3) 85–9
cochlear implantation 511, 512, 541–72
cochlear microphonic (CM) 73, 111–13, 115, 196, 428, 429, 492, 756, 781–98
  separation from AP 784, 785
cochlear nerve, see under nerves
cochlear nerve ending 61, 63
cochlear nerve fibre tuning curves 546–9
cochlear nucleus (dorsal, ventral) 36
coding in cochlear nerve fibres 566
collagen in myringoplasty 490–3
  T-antigen 490
colliculus facialis 44
computerized tomography (CAT or CT scan) 436, 438

concha 3
cone cells in retina 38
cone of light 15
congenital hearing defects
  autosomal dominant 310–13
  autosomal recessive 303–10
  hypothyroidism 624
coning 435
contingent negative variation (CNV) 373, 759, 760
contrast cisternography 796, 824
cortical ERA (or V-potential) 755, 758, 759, 761, 767, 801–8
  d.c. perstimulatory potentials 755, 759
  disorders affecting hearing 385, 386
  medicolegal use 801
  for NOHL 806, 923–8
counselling for adult deaf 530, 531
cribriform plate (of IAM) 30, 36, 41
critical band, ratio 125
crossed acoustic reflex (CAR), see post-auricular myogenic response
crus commune 29
cryptophthalmos syndrome 307
CSF fistula 820
cued speech 665, 673
cuticular plate 60

Deiter's cells, see phalangeal cells
delayed auditory feedback (DAF) 920, 921
delayed speech feedback (DSFB) 920, 921
development
  of external ear 246
  of inner ear 249
  of middle ear 246
diabetes mellitus 295
dilator tubae muscle 27
diotic and dichotic hearing 127
diplacusis 124
diplöe, diploic spaces 24
distraction tests for infants 648–52
Doerfler–Stewart test 402, 921
drugs and other preparations
  acetylcysteine 457
  adrenaline (epinephrine) 700
  amikacin 573, 580, 589
  aminosalicylic acid 462
  amoxycillin 448, 451
  ampicillin 452, 455, 461
  amylobarbitone (amobarbital) 470, 990
  azathioprine 464
  azidocillin 447, 455
  betahistine 460, 990
  brompheniramine 455
  bupivacaine 469
  calcitonin 458
  carbamazepine 470, 983, 990
  carbamine (urea) 455
  cephalothin 585

chlorambucil 465
chloramphenicol 984
clioquinol 446
co-trimoxazole 451, 452, 455
cyclandelate 467, 991
dextran 40, 458
diazepam 471, 772, 789, 796, 987
dihydrostreptomycin 585
ephedrine 455, 699
erythromycin 448
ethacrynic acid 582, 584
furosemide (frusemide) 583, 584
gentamycin 573, 580, 582, 589
glycerol 511
heparin 466
hydrochlorothiazide 459
isoniazid 463
kanamycin 573, 580, 585, 588, 589
lidocaine (lignocaine) 470, 989, 990
lorcainide 990
metronidazole 444
mexilitine 470, 990
naftidrofuryl 469, 989, 991
neomycin 573, 577, 582
nicotinamide 465
nicotinic acid 465, 991
nitrazepam 471
norephedrine 455
penicillamine 458
phenoxyethanol 445
phenoxymethylpenicillin 448
phenylephrine 455
phenytoin 470
piracetam 467
practolol 946
prednisolone 462, 464
prednisone 461, 465
prochlorperazine 990
propanodol 982
retinol (vitamin A) 456
silver protein 699
sodium fluoride 458
sodium salicylate 984
streptomycin 573, 577, 585, 949
sulfadiazine 450
sulfadimidine 450
sulfafurazole 455
sulfalene (sulfametopyrazine) 454
sulfamerazine 450
sulfamethoxypyridazine 453, 454
temazepam 471
thalidomide 946
tobramycin 573, 581, 582, 587, 588
tocainide 470, 989, 990
triiodobenzoic acid derivatives 466
trimethoprim 451, 452
trisulfapyridine 448
vincamine 466
ACTH and steroids 468

alcohol (ethanol) 772
antilymphocyte serum 463
bismuth iodoform paraffin paste (BIPP) 698, 703
ferritin 67
iodophendylate (Myodil) 796, 824
metrizamide 824
phenol 954
ductus endolymphaticus 31, 32, 40
ductus reuniens 51
dura 41
dynamic range of cochlear nerve fibres 548, 549
dysacusis 472
dyslipoproteinaemia 991
dysostosis mandibulofacialis, see Treacher-Collins' syndrome

ear canal, see external auditory meatus
ectasia of basilar artery 437
educational management of hearing-impaired children 663–77
efferent (olivocochlear) fibres and endings 61, 64
electric (evoked) response audiometry (ERA)
  in the diagnosis of acoustic neuroma 428, 429, 457, 761
  in the diagnosis of NIHL (noise induced hearing loss) 923–8
  NIHL claims evaluation (Canada) 980
  technique of 751–8
electrical impedance 145–9
electrical stimulation of the cochlea 39, 98, 541–72
electrical suppression of tinnitus 989
electrocochleography (ECochG) 98, 953, 954, 986, 989
  in diagnosis of acoustic neuroma 430–4, 508, 761
  for adults 761, 923
  for children 655–6, 764–7
  after glycerol dehydration 511
  in ototoxicity 574–6
  in RW membrane rupture 507
electrodes for stimulation of cochlear nerve 553–7, 559–68
embryology of the ear 50, 51
endolymph 35, 40, 41, 52, 57, 59, 64, 67, 70, 108, 110
endolymphatic duct, see ductus endolymphaticus
endolymphatic hydrops 225
endolymphatic potential 65, 108, 111, 755, 757
endolymphatic sac 32, 52, 510, 511
environmental aids (for the deaf) 534–7
Eustachian (Eustacean) tube 10, 13, 20, 25, 46, 482–5, 694, 697, 723–51

Eustachian tube—*contd*
  blood supply 27
  closing forces 727–9
  functions of 726
  growth changes 27
  methods indicating opening in
    subject with intact drum 730–8
    subject with perforated drum 739–40
  muscular opening 727
  nerve supply 27
  pressure opening 727
  tubal orifice 27, 104
evoked mechanical cochlear response 983
evoked potential 186–99
external auditory meatus 3, 6, 8–10, 24, 46, 104, 152, 153, 157, 246, 486, 517, 518, 947, 948, 983

facial canal 19, 20, 45, 46
facial ganglion, *see* geniculate ganglion
facial nerve, *see* nerves
facial palsy or paresis 947, 970
facial recess 19
fenestra cochleae, *see* oval window
fenestra vestibuli, *see* round window
feigned hearing loss 323–5
  Callahan's test 325
  Erhard's test 323
  Hummel's test 325
  Lombard's test 324, 918
ferritin 67
filtering, anti-aliasing 191
filters, filtering 187, 193
fissura antefenestram 29
fissures of Santorini 8
footplate of stapes 17, 22, 23, 29, 109, 499–501
foramen of Hüschke 8
foramen ovale 21, 26
foramen spinosum 21, 26
formants 124
fossa incudis 19
fourth ventricle 34, 44
fractures of temporal bone 253–8
frequency coding disorders
  binaural diplacusis 348–50
  echoic diplacusis 350
  isocusis 350
  monaural diplacusis 347, 348
  paracusis duplicata 347
  paracusis sclerotica 346, 347
functional volume of middle ear and mastoid cells 485

gelatine film (Gelfilm) 498
gelatine sponge (Gelfoam, Sterispon) 498
general educational management of hearing impaired children 663–77
giant nerve fibres in organ of Corti 89

'glue ear' 699–701
Golgi apparatus 20, 45
Gradenigo's index vocalis for detecting recruitment 325

hair cells 34, 40, 57, 60–4, 73, 77, 78, 82, 89, 91, 109, 111, 112, 115, 245, 258
handicap measures for the hearing impaired adult 520–2
Hearing Aid Council 954, 955, 957
hearing aids 117, 200–26, 393, 397, 954, 955, 961, 963, 966, 969, 987
  automatic gain control 213
  choice of, for children 679–84
    narrow band FF noise tests and 681–4
  CROS and BICROS aids 215, 216
  earmoulds 217–19
  educational 219–21
  with induction loop 221–7
  non-electronic 226
  performance 207–11, 407
  with radio-microphone system 224–6
  in rehabilitation of the adult 525–30, 892, 893, 900
  types 200
hearing loss due to trauma 256–9, 887, 898
helicotrema 31
helix 4
Hensen's cells 59
hiatus canalis facialis 20, 21, 45
holographic studies of tympanic membrane 448
homograft ossicles 495, 497, 499
horse radish peroxidase 59, 66, 77
Hughes' audiometer 366
Hughson–Westlake technique of threshold determination 368
hyperprolinaemia 622, 623, 646
hypothalamus 45

impedance of the ear 105, 106
impedance matching by the ear 106
infection
  of external ear (also malignant external otitis) 259–60
  of middle ear 260
    (acute) 260, 261
    (chronic) 261–71
    (secretory) 271–3
inferior colliculus 36
inferior petrosal sinus 43
inner ear 3, 28, 46, 108
  hair cells 36, 38
integration of hearing impaired children 669–74
intensity coding abnormalities (recruitment or regression) 351–3
  Chandler's test 351
  Corradi's test 353, 354

Lever pocket-watch tests 355
monochord tests 354
reflex tests 356
uncomfortable loudness level (ULL) 353–4
Weber's test for recruitment 353
whistle tests 354, 355
intensity discrimination tests 382
interaction of inner and outer hair cell 96–8
interaural attenuation 126
internal auditory artery 22, 43, 67, 73
internal auditory (acoustic) meatus 31, 32, 41, 85, 95, 767, 817–26
blood-vessels of 43
internal carotid artery 20, 26
internal jugular vein, j. bulb 20
Inverse Square Law 135

jugular fossa 20

kanamycin 551, 573, 580, 585, 588, 589
ketamine anaesthesia 776, 809–11, 813
kinocilia 35
knuckle pad, leuconychia deafness syndrome 599

labyrinthine artery, *see* internal auditory artery
lagena 34
lateral lemniscus 36, 39, 46
lateral line organ 61
lateral pterygoid muscle 26
lateral semicircular canal 18
lenticular process of incus 22
leontiasis ossea 601
Lewis report 663
'light' cells 66
limbus 66, 69
lip reading, *see* speech reading
loop diuretics (ethacrinic acid, furosemide or frusemide) 537, 582–4
and aminoglycosides (synergistic action) 583
loudness 123
loudness discomfort level (LDL) 422

Macewan's triangle, *see* suprameatal triangle
malformation of middle ear 246, 247; *see also* 573–92
malformation of inner ear 249, 282
manual methods of communication 524, 962, 963, 965
British Sign Language 964
deaf–blind manual alphabet 971
manual alphabet 963
masking 124–7, 369, 374–6
of cochlear nerve response 549, 550
level difference (MLD) 128, 129
of tinnitus 979–81

mastoid air cells 10, 20, 21, 24
pneumatization of 24, 25
mastoid antrum 9, 20, 21, 24, 46
nerve supply 24
mastoid process 24
Meckel's cartilage 246
medial geniculate body 36, 39
medulla 34, 36, 39, 42
membrana tectoria 35, 50, 60, 64, 66, 110
membranous labyrinth 28, 31, 40, 50–2, 67, 70
semicircular canals 31
Mendelian principles of inheritance 302, 303
Ménière's disease 255, 296, 297, 370, 378, 392, 394, 398, 409, 417, 437, 459, 460, 761, 798, 975, 989
surgical management 509–11
meningioma 280, 437, 767
meningitis 646
mid-brain 36
middle ear (tympanic cavity) 3, 10, 11, 18, 25, 27, 46, 104, 246
blood supply 21
cranial fossa 20
latency (evoked) responses 755, 757–9
meningeal artery 20, 21, 22
muscles 107
nerve supply 20, 21
transformer action 152–4
migration of epithelium 10
modiolus 30, 36, 52, 53, 72, 108
mucopolysaccharidosis 608–10
mucosal folds of middle ear 20
multiple sclerosis 437, 778, 779, 800
muscular dystrophy 617
myelin sheath 41, 76, 544
myopathy and lactic acidosis 617
myringoplasty 487–93

nasopharynx 25–7
National Health Service (NHS) 936–9, 942
narrowing of internal auditory meatus 512
neomycin 99, 573, 577, 582
neoplasms
cerebello-pontine angle (except Schwannoma) 288
chordoma of clivus 509
external ear 273–8
haemangioma of internal auditory meatus 509
inner ear 284–8
primary cholesteatoma 822
Schwannoma, *see* acoustic neuroma
leukaemia and lymphoma (incl. Waldenstrom's macroglobulinaemia) 289, 290, 465, 466
meningioma of cerebello-pontine angle, or IAM 509
metastatic tumour of the ear 288, 289, 509

middle ear 280–4
  glomus tumour 822, 983
  meningioma 280
  paraganglioma 281, 282
  rhabdomyosarcoma 283, 284
  squamous carcinoma 282, 283
  neuroma of nerves V, VI, VII, IX, X, XI 509
  pontine glioma 509
  temporal bone 278–80
    histiocytosis-X 279, 280
nerves
  V 9, 17, 21, 25, 28, 42, 417, 418, 437, 509
  VI 44, 418, 509
  VII 4, 41, 44, 45, 46, 260, 417, 419, 420, 437, 507, 509, 512, 694, 696, 711, 712, 719, 821, 822, 947, 951, 983
  VIII cochlear (auditory) nerve 4, 36, 40, 42, 72, 76, 84, 89, 98, 99, 111, 215, 260, 284–8, 398, 507–10, 512, 541–72, 711, 712, 715, 716, 717, 822, 949, 975, 988, 989
    vestibular nerve 42, 73, 76, 417, 507, 510
  IX 260, 420, 437, 509, 789
    tympanic branch 17, 18, 20, 21
  X 260, 420, 437, 509
    auricular branch 9, 17, 46, 417
    recurrent laryngeal branch 952
  XI 420, 509
  XII 260, 420
  other neural structures
    anastomosis of Oort 72, 73
    cervical sympathetic trunk 72
    lesser superficial petral nerve 20
    pharyngeal branch of sphenopalatine ganglion 28
    stellate ganglion 73
    sympathetic plexus on internal carotid artery 20
  nerve fibres within the organ of Corti
    basilar fibres 79, 80, 85, 86
    inner radial fibres 79, 85, 86
    inner spiral fibres 78
    outer spiral fibres 79, 80, 85, 86
neurofibromatosis 437, 766
NIHL (noise induced hearing loss) 848, 936, 942, 945, 947, 953, 984, 986
  assessment of handicap and compensation (UK) 855–8
  compensation under Statute Law in the UK 853–5
  DHSS Handicap Assessment Scheme 858
  non-organic hearing loss in context of NIHL 586
NIHL assessment method in Australia 904–8, 986
  compensation and Common Law settlements 900

  financial aspects of NIHL 902, 903
  hearing aids 900
  lump sum payments, various Australian States 899, 900
  National Acoustic Laboratories procedure for evaluating percentage hearing loss 902–8
  non-compensable component 902, 903
  presbyacusis correction 902
  traumatic hearing loss 898
NIHL assessment methods in Canadian Provinces 882–6
  AAOO (and derivatives) in Canada 884, 885
  cash settlements in lieu of pensions 887
  hearing conservation, audiometric screening 894
  number of claims and awards 1961–67 889
  Provincial claim evaluation arrangements 890–2
  Rehabilitation, hearing aids 892, 893
  tinnitus, tinnitus maskers 888
  traumatic hearing loss 887
  Workers Compensation Boards in Canada 880, 881, 883
NIHL assessment formulae for the USA
  AAOO – AMA formula 870–2
  1947 AMA method 869, 870
  Californian variation of AAOO formula 872
  Fletcher 8-point formula 869
  summary of various aspects of compensation laws for all States of the USA 876–78
noise hazards in industry 829–45
  Code of Practice 843
  ear muffs, ear plugs 836–8
  Health and Safety at Work Act 842
  hearing protection 836–8
  industrial audiometry 838–41
  measuring instruments (sound level meters, integrating meters, dosimeters) 831–5, 848
  noise control 835
  Noise Immission Level (NIL) 848
  noise measurements 831–5
non-organic hearing loss (NOHL)
  in adults 370–3, 794, 796, 800, 856, 891, 910–31
    Békésy audiometry in 917, 918
    delayed speech feedback (DSFB) 920, 921
    detection 912, 913
    differential diagnosis 916
    Doerfler–Stewart test 921
    electric response audiometry (cortical ERA, ECochG, BSER) 923–8
    Harris's test 917
    incidence 911, 912

Lombard test 918
psychogalvanic skin response (PGSR) 923
speech audiometry 914, 915
Stenger test 919, 920, 926
stapedial reflex thresholds 915, 916, 921, 922
routine hearing tests in 913, 914
in children 685–93, 767
  apparent simulation 692
  delayed speech feedback test (DSFB) 691
  electrophysiological test for 688–90
  recruitment in 687, 690, 691
  stapedial reflex 687
  type of NOHL 685
  unilateral 687–8
notch of Rivinus 13, 15
nystagmus 418, 431–4, 574, 575, 581

objective tinnitus 982, 983
occipital bone 24
olivary nucleus, olive 39, 41, 78
olivocochlear efferent fibres 39
onychydystrophy 598
organ of Corti 35, 39, 40, 50–2, 56, 59, 67, 69, 70, 73, 74, 76, 79, 85, 90, 93, 98, 245, 850
ossicular chain, see auditory ossicles
  discontinuity 714
osteitis deformans (Paget's disease) 294, 601
osteogenesis imperfecta 294, 600
osteopetrosis 294
osteoporosis with syndactyly 601
otic ganglion 21
otitis externa 442–7
otitis media 447–57
otosclerosis 290–4, 313, 314, 392, 499–501, 457, 458, 713, 714, 825, 826, 986, 988
  cochlear 458
ototoxicity, ototoxic drugs 297–300, 573–92, 948, 984
oval window 11–13, 17, 45, 104

Paget–Gorman sign system 665, 666, 673
palatal muscles 26, 27
papilloedema 418
para-aminobenzoic acid 452
parietal bone 24
parotid gland 9, 21
pars flaccida 15
pars tensa 15
partial ossicular replacement (PORP) 498
perilymph 11, 17, 35, 40, 41, 52, 56, 57, 59, 67, 70, 108, 109, 225, 500, 501
  fistula 499, 506
petrotympanic fissure 17, 20, 21
petrous part of temporal bone 19, 29
phalangeal (Deiter) cells 56–9, 80

pharyngobasilar fascia (phar. aponeurosis) 27
pharynx 27
pili torti 598
pinna, see auricle
pinnaplasty 486
Plastipore 495, 498
Plowden Report 663
polytomography under anaesthesia 694
pons 34, 36, 41
porus (acousticus) of the IAM 41, 43
post-auricular myogenic response 769–80
  bilateral nature of 773, 774
  in children 774–6
  effect of muscle tone 722
  in neurological diagnosis 776–9
  in multiple sclerosis 778, 779
postcentral gyrus 45
posterior auricular artery 21, 22
posterior cranial fossa 24, 41
post-stimulus time (PST) histogram 546–9
precentral gyrus 44
prelingually deaf adult 517
presbyacusis 295, 296
processus cochleariformus 20
promontory electrodes for electrical stimulation of cochlea 568
Proplast 495, 498
psychological assessment of hearing-impaired children
  Benton visual retention test 677
  Frostig test 377
  Hiskey Nebraska Scale 677
  Leiter International Performance Scale 677
  Merrill–Palmer Scale 677
  Snijder–Oomen Scale 677
  Terman–Merrill Test 968
  Wechsler Performance Scale 677, 967, 968
psychophysical tuning curves 55
pterygoid plexus 17, 21
pterygoid region 16
pure-tone audiometry (infants and children) 653–5

radiography
  in diagnosis of acoustic neuroma 434–6
  in paedoaudiology 656
radiology of the ear 816–26
  acoustic neuroma, diagnosis of 822–4
  inner ear dysplasia, diagnosis of 819, 820
  Myelodil cisternography 824
  Stenver's projection 816
  submento-vertical projection 817
  tilted lateral projection 816
  tomography, hypocycloidal 766, 794, 795, 816, 818–21, 824–6
  Towne's projection 816

Rainville test 375
ratio of innervation IHC/OHC '79, 80
receiver operating characteristic (ROC) curve 122
recruitment of cochlear nerve fibres 548
recruitment of loudness 123, 394
recruitment tests 378–80
Reference Equivalent Threshold Sound Pressure Level (RETSPL) 166, 167, 170, 171, 173
rehabilitation (auditory) 516–40
Reichert's cartilage 246
Reissner's (vestibular) membrane 34, 52, 67, 108
res ipsa loquitur 947, 950
residual hearing in education 666–9
resistance changes in organ of Corti 111
reticular lamina 56, 57
retrograde degeneration of cochlear nerve fibres 90–3
rod cells (retina) 39
rods of Corti 35, 41
room acoustics 136–41
Rosenthal's canal (spiral canal) 36, 39, 72
round window 17, 29, 104, 112
  membrane, see secondary tympanic membrane
  membrane rupture 507
rubella deafness 633–6, 645
Runge test 346

saccule 30, 31, 50–2
saccus endolymphaticus 32, 52, 510, 511
safety of intracochlear electrodes 567, 568
salpingopharyngeus muscle 27
sarcoidosis 462, 463
satellite cell 97, 98
scala media 34
scala tympani 18, 30, 34, 35, 40, 41
scala vestibuli 30, 34, 40
Scarpa's (vestibular) ganglion 32
Schwann cells 82
Schwann sheath 41
screening tests of hearing 641–4
secondary auditory area (of cortex) 36
  tympanic membrane 17, 18
semicircular canals 29, 50
Sensorineural Acuity Level (SAL) 375, 376
sensory radicular neuropathy 629
shearing forces in organ of Corti 109, 110
Shrapnell's membrane, see pars flaccida
sigmoid sinus 24, 43
signal detection theory 121, 122
signal-to-noise (S/N) ratio 186, 187, 189
sinus of Morgagni 21
sinus tympani 19
social and employment aspects of auditory rehabilitation 537, 538
sodium–potassium ratio 40

soft palate 26
sound localization 127, 128
spaces of Nuel 40, 51, 57, 59
specific acoustic impedance 136
speech audiometry 391–414
  in central deafness 400–2
  in detection of non organic hearing loss 402, 403
  material for 369, 382
  phonetically balanced (PB) words 393
  sentence intelligibility 392
  speech detection threshold (SDT) 393, 394, 404, 409, 411
  speech reception threshold (SRT) 382, 393, 408–11
  speech redundancy 369, 394, 407, 411, 413
speech production in the adult deaf 524
speech reading 532, 533, 962, 963, 965, 966, 969, 970
  with electronic supplement 534
  with manual supplement 523–4
sphenoid bone 26
spine of Henle 24
spiral canal (Rosenthal's) 36
spiral ganglion 36, 38, 39, 69, 72, 85, 89
spiral ligament 53, 56, 64, 68, 69, 73
spiral prominence 68
split hand and foot syndrome 603
stapedectomy 499–501, 506, 947, 951, 988, 989
  acoustic impedance after 500, 501
  perilymph fistula after 500, 501, 506, 989
  result of surgery 501
stapedial artery 13
stapedial prostheses 499–501
static compliance of the middle ear 708, 709
Stenger test 371, 402, 919, 920, 926
stereocilia (or cilia) 35, 60, 62, 109, 111, 983
stria vascularis 34, 40, 50, 51, 52, 64, 65, 68, 69, 70, 73
styloid process 47
stylomastoid foramen 8, 19, 46
subarachnoid space 40, 41
subarcuate fossa 24
summating potential (SP) 75, 111, 112, 113, 115, 196, 755, 756, 781–98
  separation from AP 786–8
superior colliculus 36
superior constrictor muscle 27
superior salivatory nucleus 44
superior temporal gyrus 36
supramastoid crest 24, 61
suprameatal triangle 4, 9, 24
syndromes associated with hearing loss
  cryptophthalmos syndrome 307
  knuckle pad, leuconychia and deafness syndrome 599

myopathy and lactic acidosis syndrome 617
osteogenesis imperfecta 294, 600
osteopetrosis 294
osteoporosis with syndactyly 601
split hand and foot syndrome 603
syndromes (eponymous) with hearing loss (see 596–7 for classification)
  Alberg–Schönberg disease 601, 602
  Alport's syndrome 313, 620–2
  Apert's syndrome 602–7
  Cockayne's syndrome 618
  Cogan's syndrome 463, 619, 620
  Crouzon's syndrome 248, 603
  Down's syndrome 594, 628, 630, 631
  Fanconi's syndrome 632
  Franceschetti, see Treacher–Collins
  Friedrich's ataxia 629
  Goldenhar's syndrome 818
  Hallerman–Streif syndrome 623
  Hallgren's syndrome 618
  Hirschsprung's disease 4, 628, 629
  Hunter/Hurler syndrome (gargoylism) 248, 608, 609, 647
  Jaksch–Wartenhorst syndrome 463, 464
  Jervell and Lange-Neilson 252, 304, 306, 307, 309, 631, 632
  Kearn's syndrome 616
  Klippel–Feil syndrome 248, 249, 614, 615, 647, 818
  Kniest disease 602
  Laurence–Moon–Biedl syndrome 603
  Leber's disease 619
  Leigh's syndrome 779
  Marfan's syndrome 600
  Marotaux–Lamy syndrome 609
  Mobius' syndrome 616
  Mundini defect 306, 820
  Ollier's disease 603
  osteogenesis imperfecta (van der Hoeve's syndrome) 294, 600
  Paget's disease of bone 252, 601, 825
  Pendred's syndrome 252, 304, 306, 307, 309, 623–5
  Pierre–Robin syndrome 613, 614
  Refsum's syndrome 618, 619
  Siebermann and Bing syndrome 305
  Treacher–Collins' syndrome 248, 312, 610–13, 614, 623, 647, 821
  Turner's syndrome 630
  Unverich's syndrome 623
  Usher's syndrome 304, 307, 617, 618, 972
  Von Recklinghausen's disease 776
  Vogt–Kayanagi–Harada syndrome 463
  Waardenberg syndrome 252, 311, 312, 626–8, 647
syphilis of the ear 439, 460–2

T-antigens 496
taste disorders, electrogustometry 419
T-cells 497
tectorial membrane, see membrana tectoria
tectospinal tract 38
Teflon 498
tegmen tympani 24
temporal bone 46, 245, 816–26
temporal lobe 20, 400, 401
test environment for paedoaudiology 641
thalamus 45
tight (occluding) junctions
  in relation to hair cells 35, 56
  stria vascularis 65, 66
  Reissner's membrane 34, 67, 70
tinnitus 417, 468–72, 507, 512, 888, 947, 948, 974–94
  maskers 888, 987, 988
total ossicular replacement (TORP) 498
transtympanic electrocochleography 197
trapezoid body, nucleus 36
trauma
  external ear 252
  inner ear 253–8
  middle ear 253
Trautmann's triangle 24
travelling (Békésy) wave on basilar membrane 113–15
tuning curves of cochlear nerve fibres 252, 547
tuning forks 135, 484
  physical considerations 327–9
tuning fork tests 326–48
  Bing 337–9
  Callahan's 333
  Chimani–Moos' 333, 334
  Escat's 344, 345
  Frederici's 342
  Gellé's 345, 346
  Lewis' 342
  Pomeroy's 377
  Rinne (or Polansky–Rinne) 339–42
  Schwabach 334–6
  Stenger's 332, 333
  Teal's 330–2
  Weber's (Schmaltz–Weber) 342–4
  Woolaston's 334
tunnel or Corti (cells, rods) 35, 40, 51, 56–8, 79, 109
tympanic branch of maxillary artery 22
tympanic cavity, see middle ear
tympanic membrane 3, 8, 11, 13, 15, 18, 27, 39, 106, 152, 155, 156, 487–93, 697–700, 702, 703, 715, 948, 949, 968, 983
  blood supply 16
  mechanics of 487–90
  nerve supply 16
tympanic part of temporal bone 9
tympanic ring (annulus) 8, 15
tympanic sulcus 8

tympanogram, types A, B, C 709, 710
tympanometry 709, 710

umbo 15
utricle 30, 31
utricular duct 52

vancomycin 573
variability in hearing testing 118, 119
vertebral artery 73
vertebro-basilar insufficiency 467
vestibular (Scarpa's) ganglion 32

vestibular membrane, see Reissner's membrane
vestibular nuclei 34
vestibule 29, 52, 60, 61
vestibulo-cochlear nerve, see nerves
viral hearing loss 646, 647
visual evoked response (VER) 779
voice tests of hearing 321–6
vokoder 568
volley theory 114

Warnock Report 663, 675